SETHI'S
HPTLC

High Performance Thin Layer Chromatography

Quantitative Analysis of Pharmaceutical Formulations

SETHI'S
HPTLC

High Performance
Thin Layer Chromatography

Quantitative Analysis of Pharmaceutical Formulations

Volume 3

Dr. P.D. Sethi
M.Pharm., Ph.D.

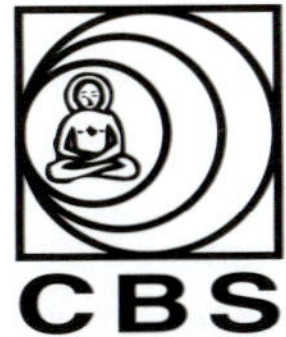

CBS PUBLISHERS & DISTRIBUTORS PVT. LTD.
New Delhi • Bengaluru • Pune • Kochi • Chennai

ISBN : 978-81-239-2279-9

First Edition : 2013

Published by:
Satish K. Jain and produced by Vinod K. Jain for CBS Publishers & Distributors Pvt. Ltd.,
4819/XI Prahlad Street, 24 Ansari Road, Daryaganj, New Delhi - 110002 (India)
E-mail: cbspubs@airtelmail.com, delhi@cbspd.com • www.cbspd.com

Branches:

- ***Bengaluru:*** 2975, 17th Cross, K.R. Road,
  Bansankari 2nd Stage, Bengaluru - 560070
  Ph.: +91-80-26771678/79
  E-mail: cbsbng@gmail.com, bangalore@cbspd.com
- ***Pune:*** Bhuruk Prestige, Sr. No. 52/12/2+1+3/2,
  Narhe, Haveli (Near Katraj-Dehu Road By-pass), Pune - 411051
  Ph.: +91-20-64704058/59, 32342277 • E-mail: pune@cbspd.com
- ***Kochi:*** 36/14, Kalluvilakam, Lissie Hospital Road, Kochi - 682018, Kerala
  Ph.: +91-484-4059061-65 • Fax: +91-484-4059065
  E-mail: cochin@cbspd.com
- ***Chennai:*** 20, West Park Road, Shenoy Nagar, Chennai - 600030
  Ph.: +91-44-26260666, 26208620 E-mail: chennai@cbspd.com

Printed at :
Aegean Offset Printers, Greater Noida (UP)

To

The woman, USHA,
my wife, my friend
who stood by me all the time.

Life is all about aspiration, struggle, failures, triumph and achievement.

Dedicated to fellow analysts exploring wider application of TLC/HPTLC, a versatile analytical technique.

Please remember, how good analyst you may be but one can't do inspired analysis without aesthetic qualities, the gift possessed by relatively very few like skill of a musician or a painter but one can emulate their mentors, teachers/gurus.

"Guru/teacher/mentor is like a live-map; if you can read the map, you know the right path to go, without map it may take life-time to find the right path."

Preface

Quality level of any analytical work depends on appropriate analytical method, performance of analytical instruments, certified standard substances, reagents, suitable sample preparation and analysts having adequate scientific knowledge of the analytical chemistry and practical experience. The analytical data so generated for any decision-making process must be technically sound, defensive and with very low level of uncertainty. Please remember, analytical data may be dealt with computers and human intellect but intuition is exclusively human.

High performance thin layer chromatography (HPTLC) works on the same principles as other chromatographic techniques such as HPLC/GC with added advantages of fastness, high sample throughput analysis, less labour intensive sample cleanup procedures, and simultaneous parallel analysis of several samples under identical conditions avoiding system suitability test (SST), disposable stationary phase, and static detection. Now HPTLC system is fully automated thus enhancing the system reproducibility allowing reliable, accurate and precise analytical results. These advantages have made HPTLC a comprehensive analytical technique for application in different fields (pharma and herbal analysis, food, cosmetology, environmental analysis, clinical laboratories, forensic and biochemistry) providing same level of quality results as that of HPLC/GC. However, there are many challenges which the analyst shall often face while working with this technique successfully as HPTLC being an open system method, is highly affected by experimental and environmental conditions which need to be controlled and regulated for reproducible results in each chromatoplate. It need to be borne in mind that consistency of performance of each application shall squarely depend on controlling various influencing factors. This compilation is an attempt to demonstrate how HPTLC fits in a well-managed analytical laboratory as an independent analytical technique on its own merit.

There is no contemporary monograph on application of HPTLC in analysis of multi-component pharmaceutical formulations except the one authored by me in 1996. The old monograph was primarily based on experimental work carried out at CDL (now CDTL), Mumbai (Bombay) and the work was based on single point validation. Since 15 years, HPTLC is the most prevalent analytical technique in pharmaceutical analysis, it was considered appropriate to fill this gap by updating the available information to help the young and novice analysts to advance their analytical knowledge. The entire text has been written in very clear, concise and simple language avoiding scientific jargon to improve the readability and understandability for bench analysts those not possessing very advanced academic qualifications. The present text in 3 volumes series contains detailed procedures for more than 500 multi-component formulations. Each formulation contains detailed analytical procedure as protocol along with typical densitogram of the sample/standard or both, and also overlaid UV-spectra of analytes to help analysts select suitable wavelength for densitometric scanning. Efforts have been made to provide all possible details under protocols to enable the analysts to repeat the method without recourse to original literature.

In addition to comprehensive introduction and a special chapter on validation of HPTLC method, the analytical methods for different formulations have been arranged in broader pharmacological activities i.e. cardiovascular system, musculoskeletal disorders, antibiotics, central nervous system, respiratory system, alimentary system, preparations for external use, and miscellaneous formulations such as vitamins and enzymes, antidiabetic drugs, cholesterol lowering drugs, etc. The methods described may not be the only one available, better alternative may well exist in literature or one may develop in the laboratory.

Most of the methods embodied in this compilation are based on work carried out in academic institutions and are claimed to have been validated as per international guidelines by the reporting authors, however, one may experience untoward surprises as institutions rarely include vigorous validation programme. It is, therefore, suggested that the method may be optimized in the given laboratory conditions before adopting for final use. For several formulations, methods by both NP-HPTLC and RP-HPTLC have been described. Such RP-HPTLC methods can help analysts to transfer such methods to RP-HPLC with reasonable success. Please remember skill obtained during actual method development can never be obtained through written description of a method. Learn from your experience and find your own solution. Analytical methods with higher accuracy and precision are difficult to perform. It may be mentioned that for majority of methods included in this monograph authors have used pre-coated plates manufactured by Merck probably due to cost and easy availability. However, pre-coated plates from other manufacturers (Whatman, Analtech, Altech, etc.) can be used but it must be kept in mind that plates from different manufacturers are likely to vary in certain specifications such as particle size, pore distribution, amount and type of binder used, etc. which are important for reproducibility of analytical results and need to be considered while revalidating or optimizing a given method. **A word of caution:** Frequent change of brand of pre-coated plates is not advisable.

From my personal experience, I can claim with belief that when other available analytical methods do not elicit the desired analytical information due to complexity of samples, HPTLC may provide the answer. Think logically, it may be a great surprise for you to observe how well this technique provides the desired answer for a separation and quantitation problem. Chromatographers are advised to read carefully **practical tips** before starting experimental work, these will help you to be a better chromatographer.

It should not be forgotten that certain minimum amount of basic knowledge and experience is needed for effective application of this technique. Attempt has been made to provide brief, comprehensive introduction to familiarize the analysts with important steps of this technique. How far I have succeeded in this attempt is left to the analysts to judge.

New Delhi, India

P.D. Sethi, M.Pharm, Ph.D.
Pharmaceutical Analyst

After transfer of the validated method to a quality control laboratory for adopting for routine quality control work, there is still a challenge to face, as HPTLC being an open system method, is highly affected by experimental and environmental conditions, one need to check regularly the suitability of chromatographic results on each chromatoplate.

Creativity – generating an idea, and innovation – implementing the idea, both must converge to fruition (applied creativity), otherwise waste of talent.

Acknowledgement

I place on record my gratitude to analytical fraternity, students, teachers and professionals for their support and inspiration in my entire analytical career.

I am extremely obliged to all TLC/HPTLC practitioners for sharing analytical data (published and unpublished) without which this compilation would never have been possible. I am thankful to Dilip Charegaonkar, CMD, M/s Anchrom Enterprises (I) Pvt. Ltd., Mumbai, India, for extending facilities in HPTLC application laboratory for verification of several reported methods and scientific support in compilation of this monograph. Valued advice by Mr. Dilip Charegaonkar for practically-oriented presentation of the subject matter is highly appreciated.

Merck Specialities Private Limited, Mumbai, India was kind enough to provide pre-coated plates for analytical work and also permission to reproduce data and figures required. I am thankful to M/s Camag, Switzerland for permission to reproduce different figures related to their HPTLC system.

I am thankful to Prof. Nitin Dubey and his team for contributing an exhaustive chapter on validation of HPTLC method and sharing their knowledge and experience with analytical fraternity. This should help analysts in planning validation of chromatographic methods. Sharing knowledge and experience with bench-analysts for the last 35 years for ultimate successful application has been source of unmatched happiness for me. At the end, I place on record my most sincere appreciation for Mr. Dharmvir for his dedicated support not only in compilation of this monograph but also giving practical shape to many of my ideas.

New Delhi, India

P.D. Sethi, M.Pharm, Ph.D.
Pharmaceutical Analyst

"Have creative mind, evaluate critically and logically."

Contents

CHAPTER 8

Formulation No. and Name

CHAPTER 9

Formulation No. and Name

CHAPTER 10

Miscellaneous .... 1143 – 1281

Formulation No. and Name

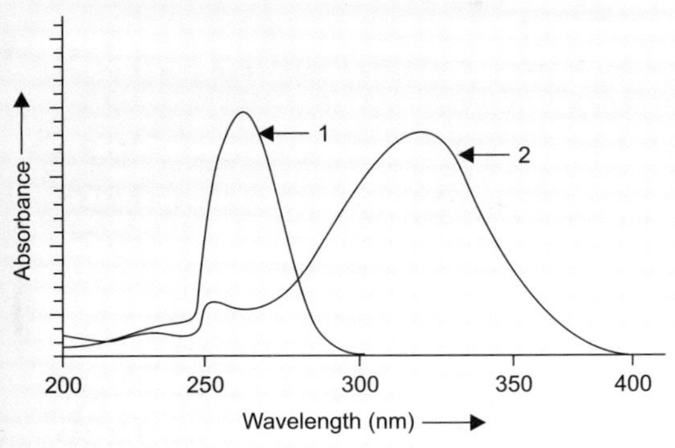

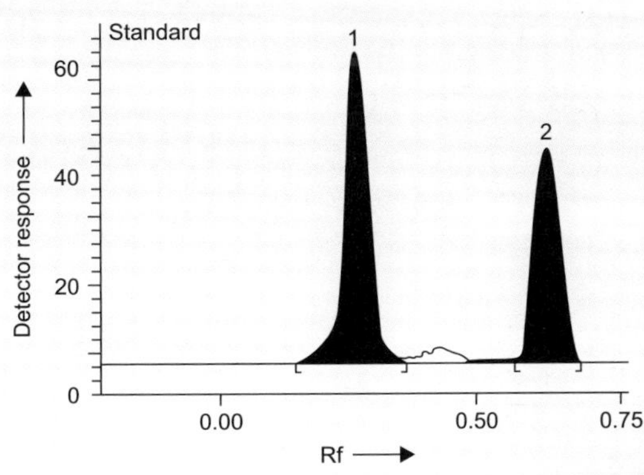

Alimentary System

- Antacids
- Ulcer-healing drugs
- Antidiarrhoeals
- Digestive enzymes

Protocols and Densitograms from 332 to 397

Every work has a starting point, method development is no exception.

HPTLC : High Performance Thin Layer Chromatography
HPTLC Densitogram

No. 332

Paracetamol

Domperidone

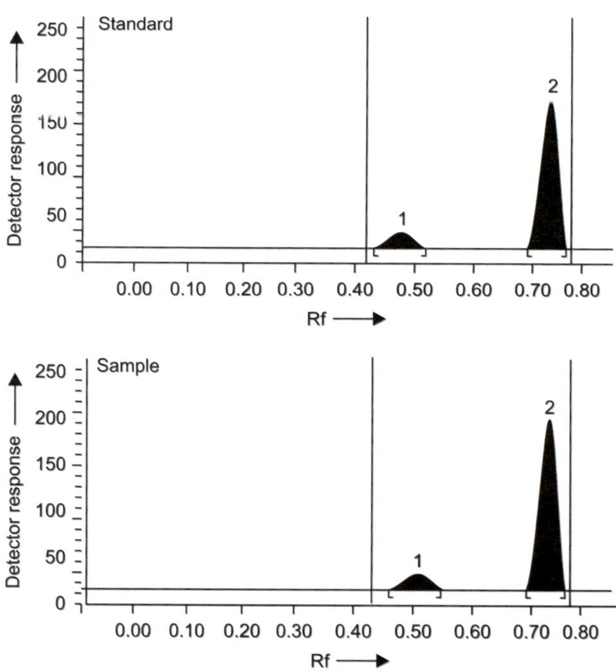

Typical densitogram of the sample and standard containing paracetamol and domperidone. For detailed experimental and chromatographic conditions, refer to Protocol No. 332. Peaks identification: 1. Domperidone; 2. Paracetamol.

PROTOCOL FOR HPTLC ANALYSIS OF PHARMACEUTICAL FORMULATION

Protocol No. 332

Formulation: Paracetamol, Domperidone

Classification: Alimentary System **Dosage form:** Tablets

Standard preparation: Dissolve pure compound in solvent to get 20 μg/ml of domperidone and 1000 μg/ml of paracetamol. Further dilutions made to get 8 μg/ml of domperidone and 400 μg/ml of paracetamol and used for analysis.

Solvent: Acetone–methanol (1 : 1 v/v).

Sample preparation: Powdered sample equivalent to 5 mg of domperidone suspended in solvent, sonicated, diluted to volume as under standard solution. Filter and dilute the filtrate to get 8 μg/ml (domperidone) and 400 μg/ml (paracetamol) and use for assay.

Chromatographic equipments:

Sample applicator: Camag Linomat–V

Development chamber: Camag twin-trough glass chamber, 20 × 20 cm

Densitometric scanner: Camag TLC Scanner–III

Chromatographic conditions:

1. Stationary phase: Silica gel $60F_{254}$ pre-coated TLC plates, 10 × 10 cm (250 μm) – Merck
2. Mobile phase (MP): Acetone–toluene–methanol (4 : 4 : 2 v/v)
3. Standard/Sample application:
   Band length: 6 mm Volume applied: 2–10 μl Spacing: 10 mm
4. Chamber saturation: 30 min (MP)
5. RH (%): 55 ± 5
6. Temperature °C: 22 ± 2
7. Separation technique: Ascending
8. Quantity of mobile phase: 20 ml
9. Migration distance: 80 mm
10. Migration time: 15 min

Densitometric evaluation:

Wavelength: UV–248 nm (paracetamol) and 285 nm (domperidone)

Scanning mode: Reflectance/Absorbance

HRF: Domperidone—52; Paracetamol—74

Linearity (ng/band): Paracetamol—800–2400; Domperidone—16–48

Recovery (%): 99.71–100.14 for both the compounds

References: Alok Yadav, Raman M. Singh, Satish C. Mathur, Pawan K. Saini and G.N. Singh, *J. Planar Chromatogr.*, **22(6)**, 421–426, 2009.

Comments: The method validated for accuracy, precision, linearity, LOD, LOQ, specificity, robustness and ruggedness.

HPTLC : High Performance Thin Layer Chromatography
HPTLC Densitogram

No. 333

Paracetamol

Domperidone

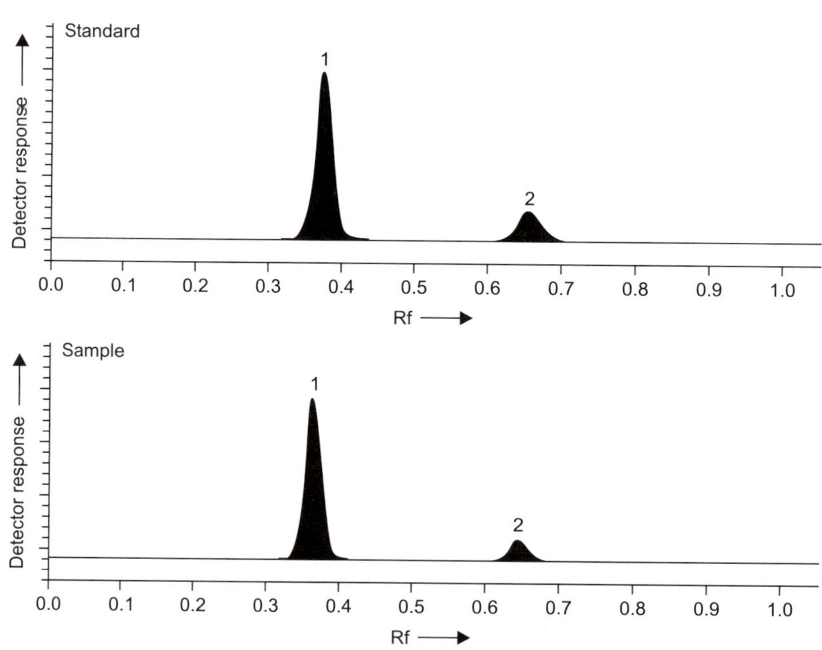

Typical densitogram of the sample and standard containing paracetamol and domperidone. For detailed experimental and chromatographic conditions, refer to Protocol No. 333. Peaks identification: 1. Paracetamol; 2. Domperidone.

PROTOCOL FOR HPTLC ANALYSIS OF PHARMACEUTICAL FORMULATION

Protocol No. 333

Formulation: **Paracetamol, Domperidone**
Classification: Alimentary System **Dosage form:** Tablets
Standard preparation: Dissolve pure compound in solvent to get 20 µg/ml of domperidone and 1000 µg/ml of paracetamol. Further dilutions made to get 8 µg/ml of domperidone and 400 µg/ml of paracetamol and used for analysis. Solvent: Acetone–methanol (1 : 1 v/v).
Sample preparation: Powdered sample equivalent to 5 mg of domperidone suspended in solvent, sonicated, diluted to volume as under standard solution. Filter and dilute the filtrate to get 8 µg/ml (domperidone) and 400 µg/ml (paracetamol) and use for assay.
Chromatographic equipments:
Sample applicator: Camag Linomat–V
Development chamber: Camag twin-trough glass chamber, 10 × 10 cm
Densitometric scanner: Camag TLC Scanner–III
Chromatographic conditions:

1. Stationary phase: Silica gel $60F_{254}$ pre-coated TLC plates, 10 × 10 cm (250 µm) – Merck
2. Mobile phase (MP): Methanol–water (7 : 3 v/v)
3. Standard/Sample application:
   Band length: 5 mm Volume applied: 1–10 µl Spacing: 10 mm
4. Chamber saturation: 30 min (MP)
5. RH (%): 55 ± 5
6. Temperature °C: 22 ± 2
7. Separation technique: Ascending
8. Quantity of mobile phase: 10 ml
9. Migration distance: 80 mm
10. Migration time: 25 min

Densitometric evaluation:
Wavelength: UV–285 nm and UV–248 nm
Scanning mode: Reflectance/Absorbance
HRF: Paracetamol—38; Domperidone—67
Linearity (ng/band): Paracetamol—800–2400; Domperidone—16–48
Recovery (%): 99.85–101.5 for both the compounds
References: —
Comments:

- The method was optimized and analytical work carried out at **Anchrom's HPTLC Application Laboratory**, Mumbai, India.
- Several market samples of similar composition were analysed by the proposed method to give reproducible results.
- See reversal of Rf values as compared to the method reported by other authors.

HPTLC : High Performance Thin Layer Chromatography
HPTLC Densitogram

No. 334

Paracetamol

Metoclopramide

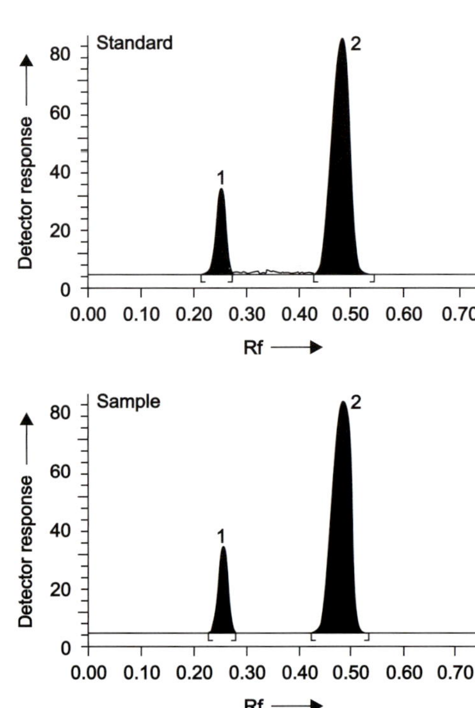

Typical densitogram of the sample and standard containing paracetamol and metoclopramide hydrochloride. For detailed experimental and chromatographic conditions, refer to Protocol No. 334. Peaks identification: 1. Metoclopramide HCl; 2. Paracetamol.

PROTOCOL FOR HPTLC ANALYSIS OF PHARMACEUTICAL FORMULATION

Protocol No. 334

Formulation: Paracetamol, Metoclopramide hydrochloride

Classification: Alimentary System **Dosage form:** Tablets

Standard preparation: (1) Prepare 500 μg/ml solution of metoclopramide HCl in methanol. (2) Weigh 50 mg of paracetamol, add 1 ml of solution (1) and dilute 10 ml with methanol. Apply 5 μl for analysis.

Sample preparation: Weigh accurately powdered sample equivalent to 50 mg of paracetamol, suspend in methanol, sonicate for 5 min and dilute to 10 ml with methanol. Apply 5 μl for assay.

Chromatographic equipments:

Sample applicator: Camag Linomat–IV

Development chamber: Camag twin-trough glass chamber, 10 × 10 cm

Densitometric scanner: Camag TLC Scanner–II

Chromatographic conditions:

1. Stationary phase: Silica gel $60F_{254}$ pre-coated HPTLC plates, 10 × 10 cm (200 μm) – Merck
2. Mobile phase (MP): Ethyl acetate–acetone–25% ammonia (6 : 4 : 0.1 v/v)
3. Standard/Sample application:
   Band length: 5 mm Volume applied: 5 μl Spacing: 10 mm
4. Chamber saturation: 10 min (MP)
5. RH (%): 55 ± 5
6. Temperature °C: 22 ± 2
7. Separation technique: Ascending
8. Quantity of mobile phase: 10 ml
9. Migration distance: 50 mm
10. Migration time: 15 min

Densitometric evaluation:

Wavelength: UV–205 nm or 300 nm Scanning mode: Reflectance/Absorbance

HRF: Metoclopramide HCl—26; Paracetamol—48

Linearity (ng/band): Metoclopramide HCl—50–500; Paracetamol—1000–5000

Recovery (%): 100.80–101.0 for both the compounds

References: P.P. Shrike, M.K. Patel, V.A. Tamhane, V.B. Tirodkar, *Eastern Pharmacist*, **37**, 155–156, 1994.

Comments: The method validated for accuracy, precision and linearity.

HPTLC : High Performance Thin Layer Chromatography
HPTLC Densitogram

No. 335

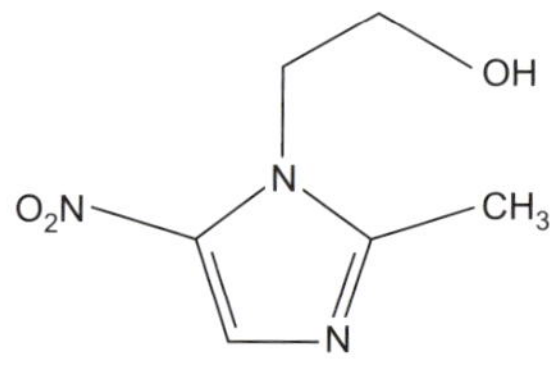

Metronidazole

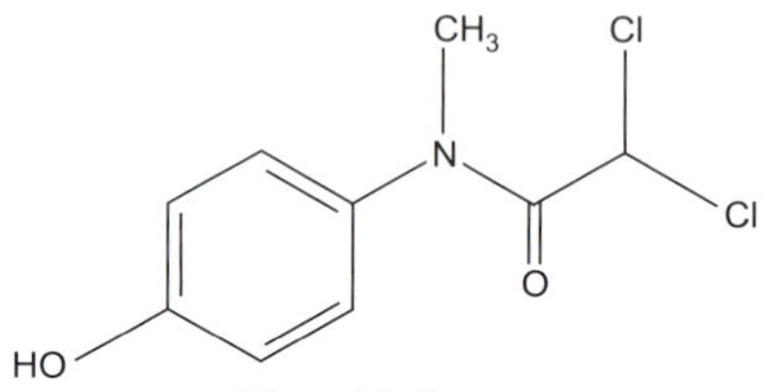

Diloxanide furoate

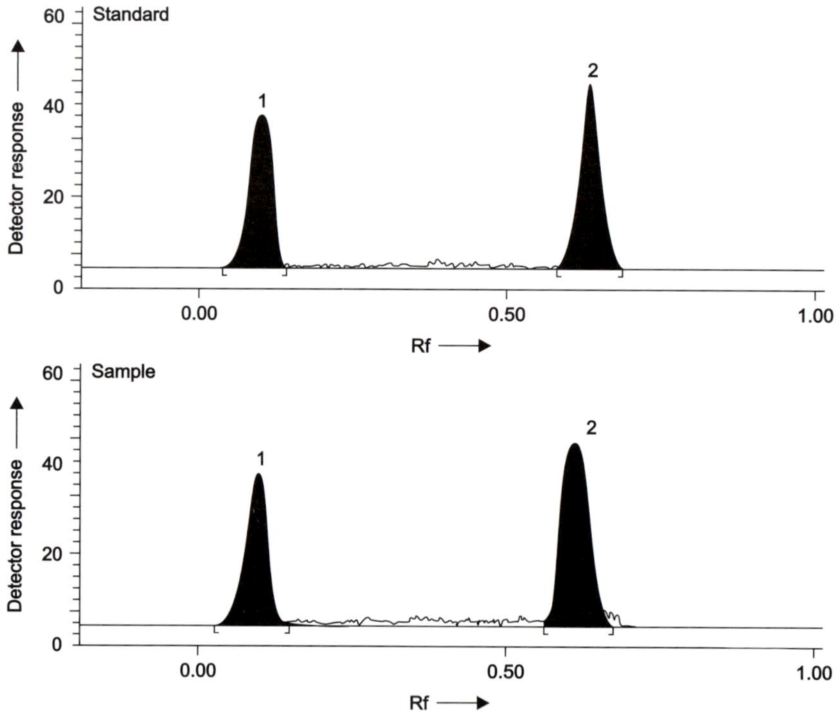

Standard

Sample

Typical densitogram of the sample and standard containing metronidazole and diloxanide furoate. For detailed experimental and chromatographic conditions, refer to Protocol No. 335. Peaks identification: 1. Metronidazole; 2. Diloxanide furoate.

PROTOCOL FOR HPTLC ANALYSIS OF PHARMACEUTICAL FORMULATION

Protocol No. 335

Formulation: Metronidazole, Diloxanide furoate

Classification: Alimentary System **Dosage form:** Tablets, Suspension

Standard preparation: Dissolve 10 mg of metronidazole and 12.5 mg of diloxanide furoate in methanol to produce 10 ml. Further dilute 0.2 ml to 10 ml with methanol and apply 10 μl for analysis.

Sample preparation: Powdered sample equivalent to 10 mg of metronidazole suspended in methanol, shake, dilute to 10 ml, filter and dilute 0.2 ml of the filtrate to 10 ml with methanol and use for estimation.

Chromatographic equipments:

Sample applicator: Camag Linomat–IV

Development chamber: Camag twin-trough glass chamber, 10 × 10 cm

Densitometric scanner: Camag TLC Scanner–II

Chromatographic conditions:

1. Stationary phase: Silica gel $60F_{254}$ pre-coated HPTLC plates, 10 × 10 cm (200 μm) – Merck
2. Mobile phase (MP): (i) Toluene–acetone–25% ammonia (8 : 2 : 0.5 v/v); (ii) Toluene–acetone–methanol (6 : 3.5 : 1 v/v); (iii) chloroform–methanol (5 : 5 v/v)
3. Standard/Sample application:
   Band length: 7 mm Volume applied: 10 μl Spacing: 10 mm
4. Chamber saturation: 10 min (MP)
5. RH (%): 55 ± 5
6. Temperature °C: 22 ± 2
7. Separation technique: Ascending
8. Quantity of mobile phase: 10 ml
9. Migration distance: 50 mm
10. Migration time: 15 min

Densitometric evaluation:

Wavelength: UV–280 nm Scanning mode: Reflectance/Absorbance

HRF: Metronidazole—10; Diloxanide furoate—60

Linearity (ng/band): Metronidazole—100–400; Diloxanide furoate—100–500

Recovery (%): 98.70–100.40 for both the compounds

References: —

Comments:

- The method was optimized and analytical work carried out at **Anchrom's HPTLC Application Laboratory**, Mumbai, India.
- Several market samples of similar composition were analysed by the proposed method with reproducible results.

HPTLC : High Performance Thin Layer Chromatography
HPTLC Densitogram

No. 336

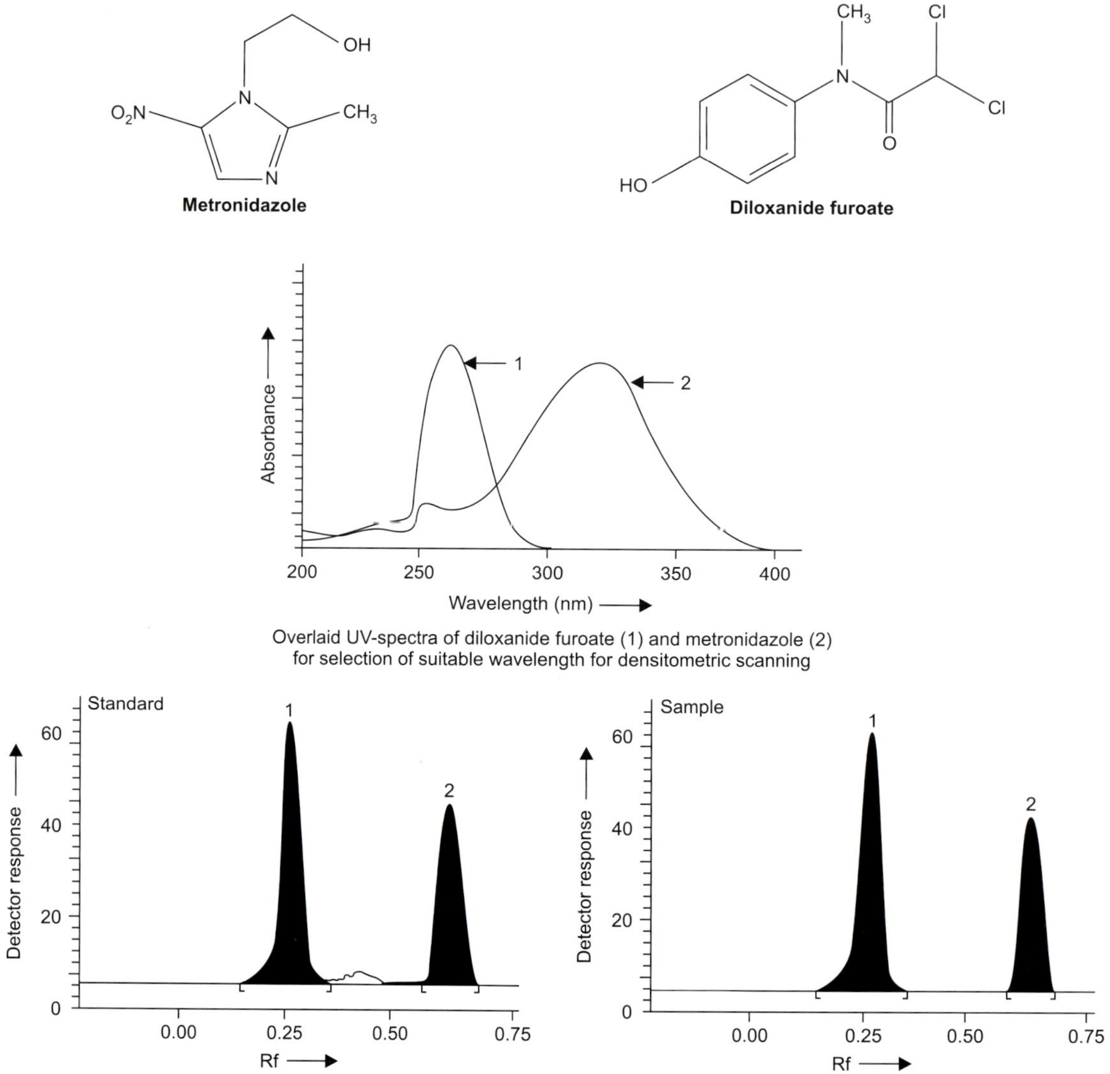

Overlaid UV-spectra of diloxanide furoate (1) and metronidazole (2) for selection of suitable wavelength for densitometric scanning

Typical densitogram of the sample and standard containing metronidazole and diloxanide furoate. For detailed experimental and chromatographic conditions, refer to Protocol No. 336. Peaks identification: 1. Diloxanide furoate; 2. Metronidazole.

PROTOCOL FOR HPTLC ANALYSIS OF PHARMACEUTICAL FORMULATION

Protocol No. 336

Formulation: Metronidazole, Diloxanide furoate

Classification: Alimentary System **Dosage form:** Tablets, Suspension

Standard preparation: Dissolve 10 mg of metronidazole and 12.5 mg of diloxanide furoate in methanol to produce 10 ml. Further dilute 0.2 ml to 10 ml with methanol and apply 10 µl for analysis.

Sample preparation: Powdered sample equivalent to 12.5 mg of diloxanide furoate suspended in methanol, shake, dilute to 10 ml, filter and 0.2 ml of the filtrate diluted to 10 ml and used for estimation.

Chromatographic equipments:

Sample applicator: Camag Linomat–IV

Development chamber: Camag twin-trough glass chamber, 10 × 10 cm

Densitometric scanner: Camag TLC Scanner–II

Chromatographic conditions:

1. Stationary phase: Silica gel 60 RP-18F_{254s} pre-coated HPTLC plates, 5 × 10 cm (200 µm) – Merck
2. Mobile phase (MP): 0.5 M sodium chloride–methanol–acetonitrile–glacial acetic acid (5 : 2 : 3 : 0.1 v/v)
3. Standard/Sample application:
   Band length: 7 mm Volume applied: 10 µl Spacing: 10 mm
4. Chamber saturation: 30 min (MP)
5. RH (%): 55 ± 5
6. Temperature °C: 22 ± 2
7. Separation technique: Ascending
8. Quantity of mobile phase: 10 ml
9. Migration distance: 50 mm
10. Migration time: 25 min

Densitometric evaluation:

Wavelength: UV–280 nm Scanning mode: Reflectance/Absorbance

HRF: Diloxanide furoate—25; Metronidazole—65

Linearity (ng/band): Metronidazole—200–400; Diloxanide furoate—200–500

Recovery (%): 99.50–100.10 for both the compounds

References: —

Comments:

- The method was optimized and analytical work carried out at **Anchrom's HPTLC Application Laboratory**, Mumbai, India.
- Several market samples of similar composition were analysed by the proposed method with reproducible results.
- RP–HPTLC resulted in reversal of retention order when compared to NP–HPTLC.

HPTLC : High Performance Thin Layer Chromatography
HPTLC Densitogram

No. 337

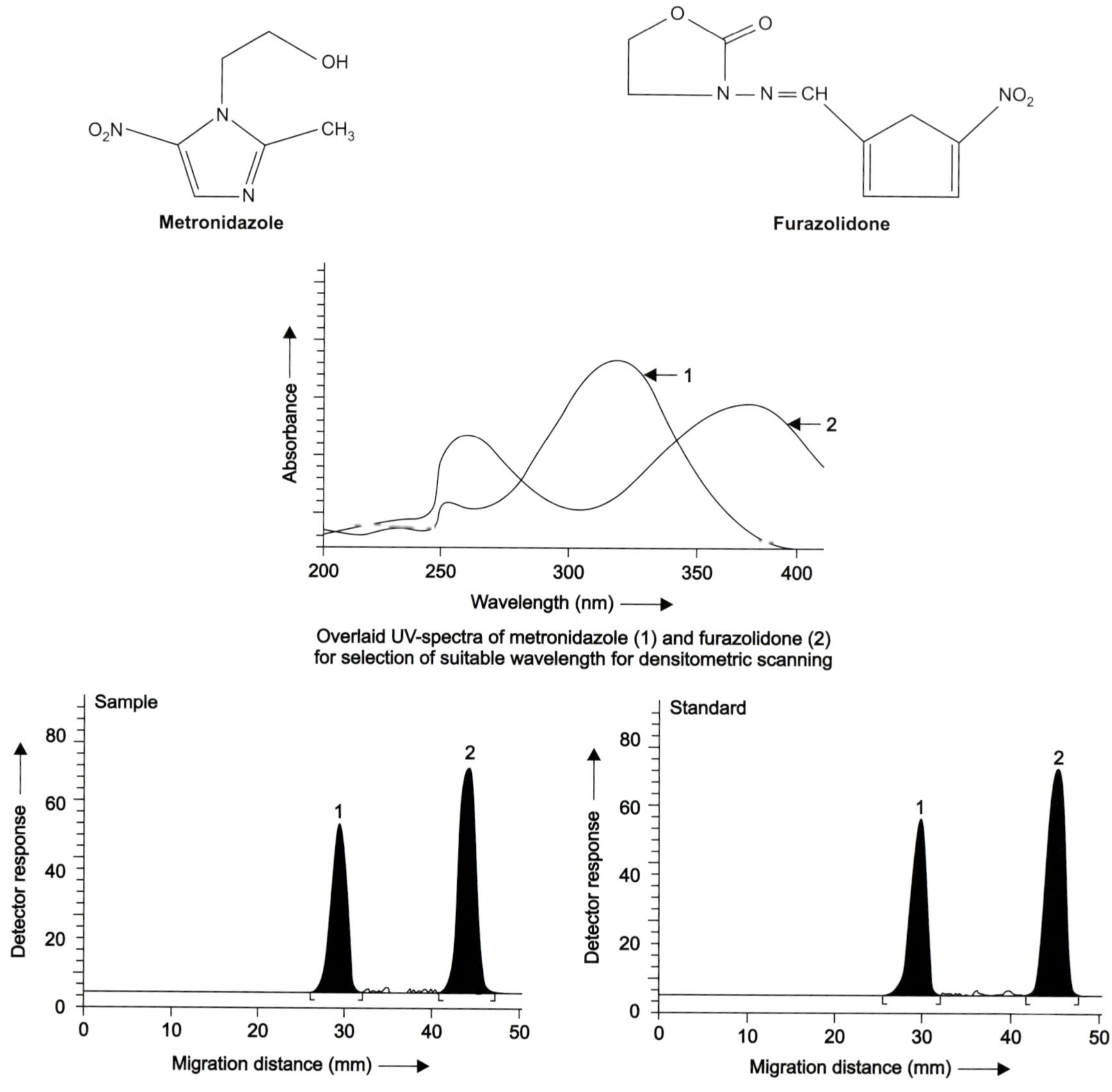

Overlaid UV-spectra of metronidazole (1) and furazolidone (2) for selection of suitable wavelength for densitometric scanning

Typical densitogram of the sample and standard containing metronidazole and furazolidone. For detailed experimental and chromatographic conditions, refer to Protocol No. 337. Peaks identification: 1. Metronidazole; 2. Furazolidone.

PROTOCOL FOR HPTLC ANALYSIS OF PHARMACEUTICAL FORMULATION

Protocol No. 337

Formulation: Metronidazole, Furazolidone

Classification: Alimentary System **Dosage form:** Tablets, Suspension

Standard preparation: Prepare 1 mg/ml solution of both the compounds in DMF with the help of sonication. Further dilutions made with methanol for analysis.

Sample preparation: Powdered sample equivalent to 50 mg of furazolidone suspended in DMF, sonicated, diluted to 50 ml with DMF, filtered and filtrate suitably diluted with methanol for assay.

Chromatographic equipments:

Sample applicator: Camag Linomat–IV

Development chamber: Camag twin-trough glass chamber, 10 × 10 cm

Densitometric scanner: Camag TLC Scanner–II

Chromatographic conditions:

1. Stationary phase: Silica gel $60F_{254}$ pre-coated HPTLC plates, 5 × 10 cm (200 μm) – Merck
2. Mobile phase (MP): Chloroform–acetone–methanol (10 : 1.6 : 0.4 v/v)
3. Standard/Sample application:
   Band length: 5 mm Volume applied: 8 μl Spacing: 5 mm
4. Chamber saturation: 10 min (MP)
5. RH (%): 55 ± 5
6. Temperature °C: 22 ± 2
7. Separation technique: Ascending
8. Quantity of mobile phase: 12 ml
9. Migration distance: 50 mm
10. Migration time: 15 min

Densitometric evaluation:

Wavelength: UV–254nm or 280 nm Scanning mode: Reflectance/Absorbance

HRF: Metronidazole—36; Furazolidone—67

Linearity (ng/band): Metronidazole—100–400; Furazolidone—50–500

Recovery (%): 99.86–100.32 for both the compounds

References: P.P. Shirke, M.K. Patel and V.B. Tirodkar, *Ind. J. Pharm Sci.*, 108–109, 1994.

Comments: The method validated for accuracy, precision, linearity, LOD and LOQ.

HPTLC : High Performance Thin Layer Chromatography
HPTLC Densitogram

No. 338

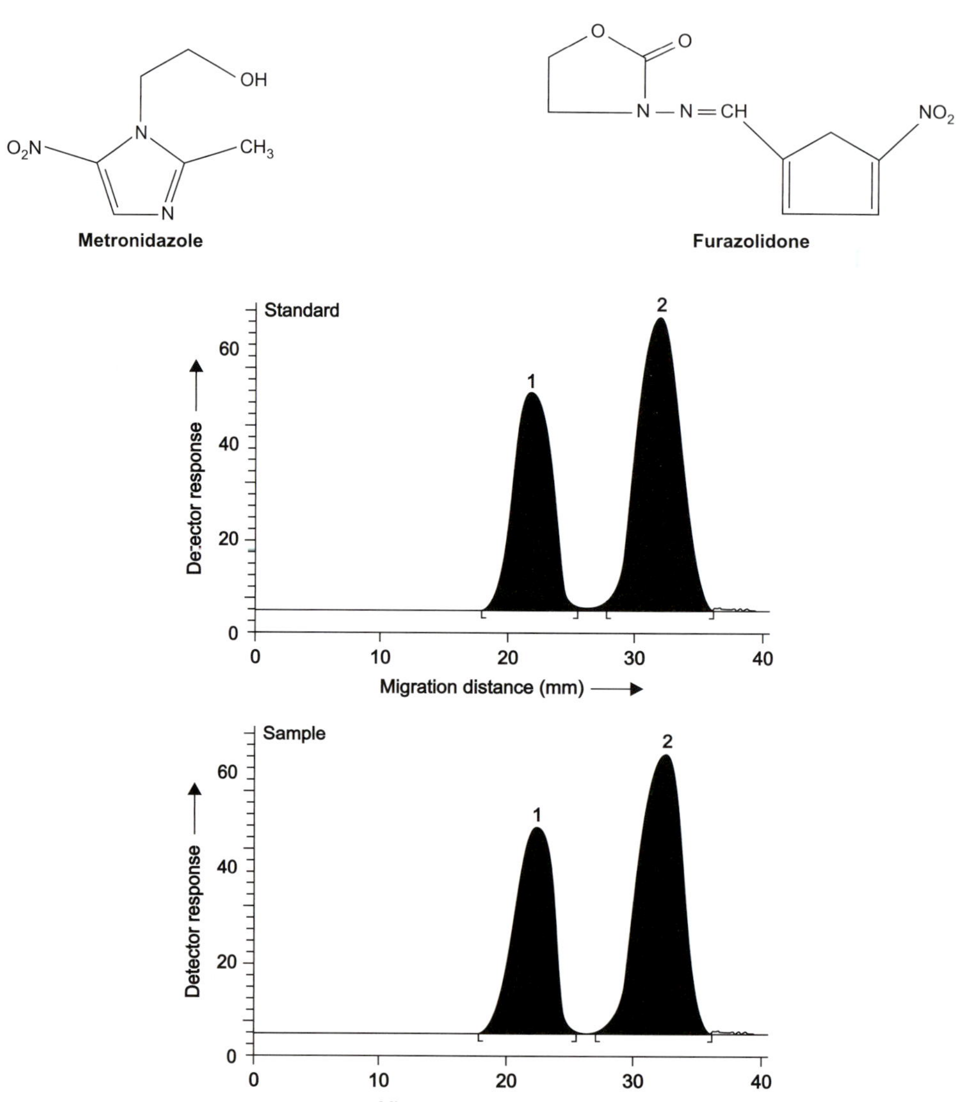

Typical densitogram of the sample and standard containing metronidazole and furazolidone. For detailed experimental and chromatographic conditions, refer to Protocol No. 338. Peaks identification: 1. Metronidazole; 2. Furazolidone.

PROTOCOL FOR HPTLC ANALYSIS OF PHARMACEUTICAL FORMULATION

Protocol No. 338

Formulation: Metronidazole, Furazolidone

Classification: Alimentary System **Dosage form:** Tablets, Suspension

Standard preparation: Prepare 1 mg/ml solution of each compound in DMF with the aid of sonication. Further suitable dilutions made with methanol for analysis.

Sample preparation: Powdered sample equivalent to 10 mg of furazolidone suspended in DMF, sonicated, diluted to 10 ml, filtered and 0.1 ml of the filtrate diluted to 10 ml with methanol and used for assay.

Chromatographic equipments:

Sample applicator: Camag Linomat–IV

Development chamber: Camag twin-trough glass chamber, 10 × 10 cm

Densitometric scanner: Camag TLC Scanner–II

Chromatographic conditions:

1. Stationary phase: Silica gel 60 RP-18F_{254s} pre-coated HPTLC plates, 5 × 7.5 cm (200 μm) – Merck
2. Mobile phase (MP): 0.5 M sodium chloride–methanol–glacial acetic acid (12 : 8 : 0.01 v/v)
3. Standard/Sample application:
   Band length: 5 mm Volume applied: 8 μl Spacing: 5 mm
4. Chamber saturation: 20 min (MP)
5. RH (%): 55 ± 5
6. Temperature °C: 22 ± 2
7. Separation technique: Ascending
8. Quantity of mobile phase: 20 ml
9. Migration distance: 50 mm
10. Migration time: 25 min

Densitometric evaluation:

Wavelength: UV–254nm or 280 nm Scanning mode: Reflectance/Absorbance

HRF: Metronidazole—40; Furazolidone—54

Linearity (ng/band): Metronidazole—100–400; Furazolidone—50–500

Recovery (%): 99.85–101.50 for both the compounds

References: —

Comments:

- The method was optimized and analytical work carried out at **Anchrom's HPTLC Application Laboratory**, Mumbai, India.
- Several market samples of similar composition were analysed by the proposed method with reproducible results.

HPTLC : High Performance Thin Layer Chromatography
HPTLC Densitogram

No. 339

Metronidazole **Furazolidone**

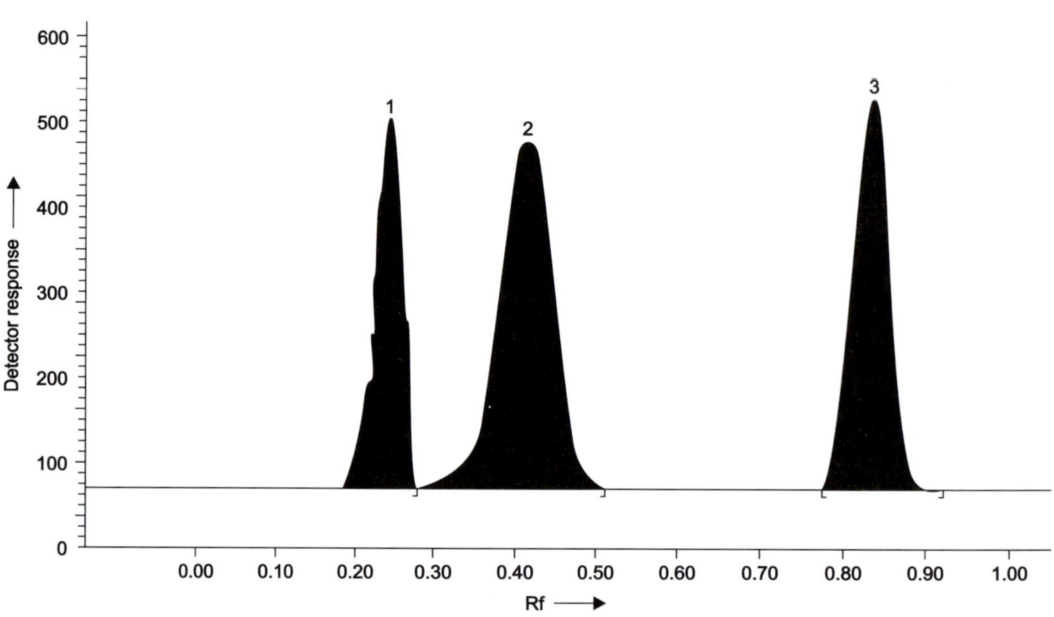

Typical densitogram of the standard containing metronidazole and furazolidone. For detailed experimental and chromatographic conditions, refer to Protocol No. 339. Peaks identification: 1. Metronidazole; 2. Furazolidone; 3. Diloxanide furoate (IS).

PROTOCOL FOR HPTLC ANALYSIS OF PHARMACEUTICAL FORMULATION

Protocol No. 339

Formulation: Metronidazole, Furazolidone

Classification: Alimentary System **Dosage form:** Tablets, Suspension

Standard preparation: Dissolve 10 mg of furazolidone, 30 mg of metronidazole and 20 mg of diloxanide furoate (IS), all in 10 ml of chloroform. Further dilute 1.25 ml to 25 ml with chloroform and carry out the analysis by spotting 10 μl of the resulting solution.

Sample preparation: Weigh powdered sample equivalent to 100 mg of furazolidone or 300 mg of metronidazole, suspend in 80 ml of chloroform, shake, dilute to 100 ml, filter and dilute 1.25 ml of the filtrate to 25 ml with chloroform after adding 2 ml of IS solution (2 mg/ml) and use for assay.

Chromatographic equipments:

Sample applicator: Camag Linomat–IV

Development chamber: Camag twin-trough glass chamber, 10 × 10 cm

Densitometric scanner: Camag TLC Scanner–II

Chromatographic conditions:

1. Stationary phase: Silica gel $60F_{254}$ pre-coated HPTLC plates, 10 × 10 cm (200 μm) – Merck
2. Mobile phase (MP): Toluene–acetone–methanol (6 : 3.5 : 1 v/v)
3. Standard/Sample application:
   Band length: 10 mm Volume applied: 10 μl Spacing: 10 mm
4. Chamber saturation: 20 min (MP)
5. RH (%): 55 ± 5
6. Temperature °C: 22 ± 2
7. Separation technique: Ascending
8. Quantity of mobile phase: 10 ml
9. Migration distance: 75 mm
10. Migration time: 20 min

Densitometric evaluation:

Wavelength: UV–254nm Scanning mode: Reflectance/Absorbance

HRF: Metronidazole—22; Furazolidone—40; Diloxanide furoate (IS)—84

Linearity (ng/band): Metronidazole—150–750; Furazolidone—50–250

Recovery (%): 99.35–99.15 for both the compounds

References: S.S. Zarapkar, A.A. Dhanvale, V.J. Doshi, U.B. Salunkhe and S.V. Sawant, *Indian Drugs*, **31(1)**, 368–471, 1994.

Comments: The method validated for accuracy, precision, linearity, LOD, LOQ, specificity, robustness and ruggedness.

HPTLC : High Performance Thin Layer Chromatography
HPTLC Densitogram

No. 340

Metronidazole **Tinidazole**

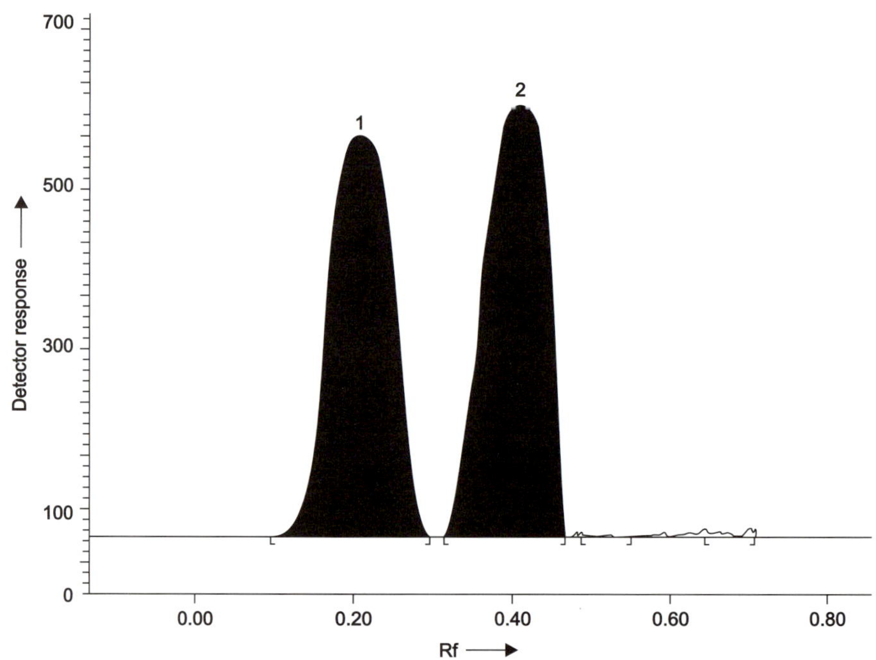

Typical densitogram of the sample containing metronidazole and tinidazole. For detailed experimental and chromatographic conditions, refer to Protocol No. 340. Peaks identification: 1. Metronidazole; 2. Tinidazole.

PROTOCOL FOR HPTLC ANALYSIS OF PHARMACEUTICAL FORMULATION

Protocol No. 340

Formulation: Metronidazole, Tinidazole

Classification: Alimentary System **Dosage form:** Infusion

Standard preparation: Prepare 1.5 mg/ml solution of each compound in methanol and use for analysis.

Sample preparation: An appropriate quantity of the sample diluted with methanol to get 1.5 mg/ml of each compound and used for analysis.

Chromatographic equipments:

Sample applicator: Camag Linomat–IV

Development chamber: Camag twin-trough glass chamber, 10 × 10 cm

Densitometric scanner: Camag TLC Scanner–II

Chromatographic conditions:

1. Stationary phase: Silica gel $60F_{254}$ pre-coated HPTLC plates, 10 × 10 cm (200 μm) – Merck, pre-washed with methanol, dried prior to use
2. Mobile phase (MP): Dichloromethane–acetone–diethylether (5 : 5 : 2.5 v/v)
3. Standard/Sample application:
   Band length: 2 mm Volume applied: 200 nl Spacing: 5 mm
4. Chamber saturation: 10 min (MP)
5. RH (%): 55 ± 5
6. Temperature °C: 22 ± 2
7. Separation technique: Ascending
8. Quantity of mobile phase: 12.5 ml
9. Migration distance: 40 mm
10. Migration time: 15 min

Densitometric evaluation:

Wavelength: UV–311 nm Scanning mode: Reflectance/Absorbance

HRF: Metronidazole—20; Tinidazole—40

Linearity: 60–360 ng for both the compounds

Recovery (%): 99.8–101.9 for both the compounds

References: Hennele Salomies, *J. Planar Chromatogr.*, **5**, 291–293, 1992.

Comments: The method validated for accuracy, precision, linearity, LOD, LOQ, specificity, robustness and ruggedness.

HPTLC : High Performance Thin Layer Chromatography
HPTLC Densitogram

No. 341

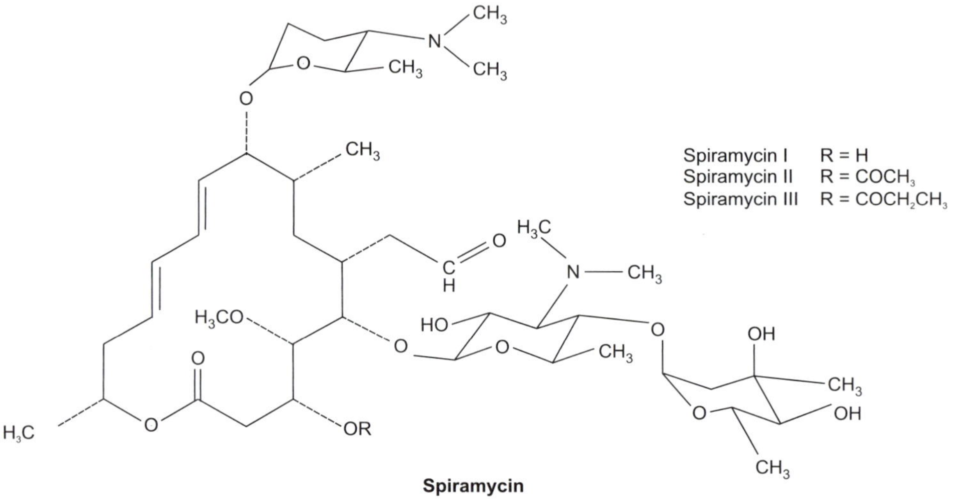

Spiramycin I R = H
Spiramycin II R = $COCH_3$
Spiramycin III R = $COCH_2CH_3$

Spiramycin

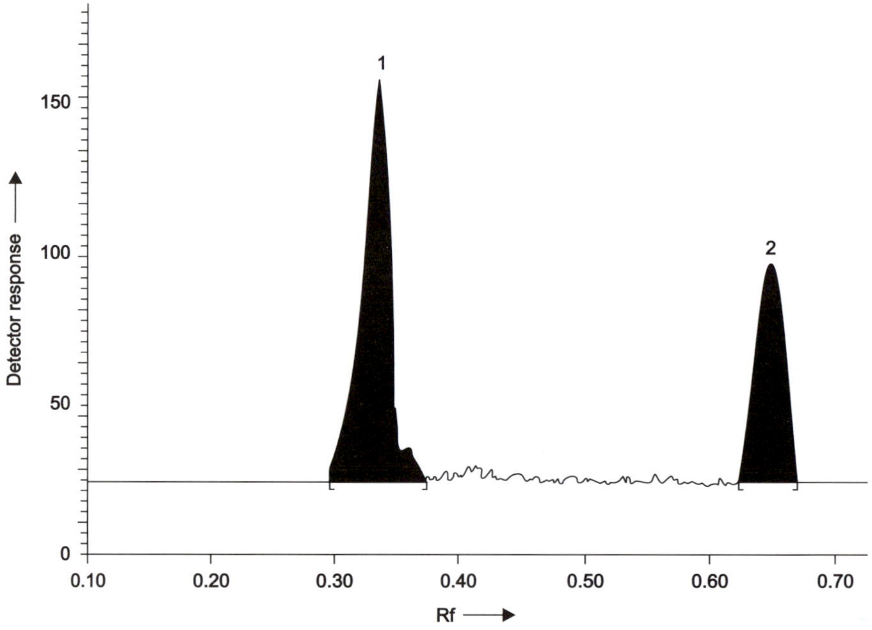

Typical densitogram of the standard containing metronidazole and spiramyxin. For detailed experimental and chromatographic conditions, refer to Protocol No. 341. Peaks identification: 1. Metronidazole; 2. Spiramycin.

PROTOCOL FOR HPTLC ANALYSIS OF PHARMACEUTICAL FORMULATION

Protocol No. 341

Formulation: Metronidazole, Spiramycin
Classification: Alimentary System **Dosage form:** Infusion
Standard preparation: Prepare 1 mg/ml solution of each compound in methanol. Further serial dilutions made with methanol to get 100–200 μg/ml (metronidazole) and 80–200 μg/ml (spiramycin). Apply 10 μl of each solution for linearity profile.
Sample preparation: Powdered sample equivalent to 50 mg of metronidazole and 68 mg of spiramycin suspended in 40 ml of methanol, sonicated for 30 min, diluted to 50 ml and filtered. Further suitably diluted with methanol to get 100 μg/ml of metronidazole and 136 μg/ml of spiramycin. Apply 10 μl for assay.
Chromatographic equipments:
Sample applicator: Camag Linomat–IV sample applicator
Development chamber: Camag twin-trough glass chamber, 20 × 10 cm
Densitometric scanner: Camag TLC Scanner–III
Chromatographic conditions:

1. Stationary phase: Silica gel $60F_{254}$ pre-coated TLC plates, 20 × 10 cm (250 μm) – Merck (MP), pre-washed with methanol, activated (100°C) for 5 min prior to use
2. Mobile phase (MP): Methanol–chloroform (9 : 1 v/v)
3. Standard/Sample application:
   Band length: 8 mm Volume applied: 10 μl Spacing: 10 mm
4. Chamber saturation: 30 min (MP)
5. RH (%): — 6. Temperature °C: 25 ± 2
7. Separation technique: Ascending
8. Quantity of mobile phase: 20 ml
9. Migration distance: 90 mm
10. Migration time: 40 min

Densitometric evaluation:
Wavelength: UV–240 nm Scanning mode: Reflectance/Absorbance
HRF: Metronidazole—35; Spiramycin—65
Linearity (μg/ml): Metronidazole—100–200; Spiramycin—80–200
Recovery (%): 99.07–99.32 for both the compounds
References: Hadir M. Maher and Rasha M. Youssef, *Chromatographia*, **69(3/4)**, 345–350, 2009.
Comments:

- The method validated for accuracy, precision, linearity, LOD, LOQ, specificity and robustness.
- The method compared with RP–HPLC. Spiramycin appeared as one spot by NP-HPTLC; whereas in RP-HPLC peaks corresponding to SPY-I and SPY-II were obtained.

HPTLC : High Performance Thin Layer Chromatography
HPTLC Densitogram

No. 342

Metronidazole

Tetracycline

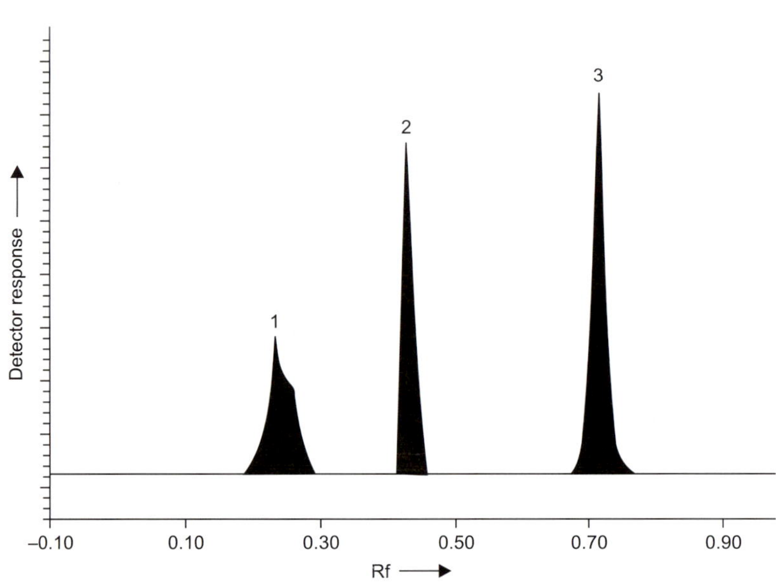

Typical densitogram of the standard containing metronidazole and tetracycline hydrochloride. For detailed experimental and chromatographic conditions, refer to Protocol No. 342. Peaks identification: 1. Ofloxacin (IS); 2. Metronidazole; 3. Tetracycline HCl.

PROTOCOL FOR HPTLC ANALYSIS OF PHARMACEUTICAL FORMULATION

Protocol No. 342

Formulation: Metronidazole, Tetracycline hydrochloride

Classification: Alimentary System **Dosage form:** Capsules

Standard preparation: Prepare 1 mg/ml solution of each compound in methanol. Further serial dilutions are made with methanol, each solution containing 1000 μg/ml of ofloxacin as IS. Carry out linearity studies.

Sample preparation: Powdered sample equivalent to 400 mg of metronidazole suspended in minimum amount of methanol, add 1 ml of (IS) solution, dilute to 10 ml with methanol, sonicate and filter. The filtrate suitable diluted with methanol for chromatographic evaluation.

Chromatographic equipments:

Sample applicator: Camag Linomat–V

Development chamber: Camag twin-trough glass chamber, 10 × 10 cm

Densitometric scanner: Camag TLC Scanner–III

Chromatographic conditions:

1. Stationary phase: Silica gel 60F_{254} pre-coated TLC plates, 10 × 10 cm (250 μm), pre-washed with methanol and activated at 110°C for 5 min prior to use
2. Mobile phase (MP): Benzene–ethyl acetate–toluene–methanol–glacial acetic acid (9.5 : 2 : 5 : 1.5 : 0.5 v/v)
3. Standard/Sample application:
   Band length: 6 mm Volume applied: 10 μl Spacing: 10 mm
4. Chamber saturation: 30 min (MP)
5. RH (%): 60 ± 5
6. Temperature °C: 25 ± 2
7. Separation technique: Ascending
8. Quantity of mobile phase: 18 ml
9. Migration distance: 80 mm
10. Migration time: 20 min

Densitometric evaluation:

Wavelength: UV–283 nm Scanning mode: Reflectance/Absorbance

HRF: Ofloxacin (IS)—25; Metronidazole—43; Tetracycline HCl—74

Linearity (μg/band): Metronidazole—0.5–2.5; Tetracycline HCl—0.75–3.75

Recovery (%): 99.95–100.10 for both the compounds

References: S. Shamma and M.C. Shamma, *Int. J. Pharm. Tech. Res.*, **3(2)**, 1169–1173, 2011.

Comments: The method validated for accuracy, precision, linearity, LOD, LOQ, specificity, robustness and ruggedness.

HPTLC : High Performance Thin Layer Chromatography
HPTLC Densitogram

No. 343

Tinidazole

Diloxanide furoate

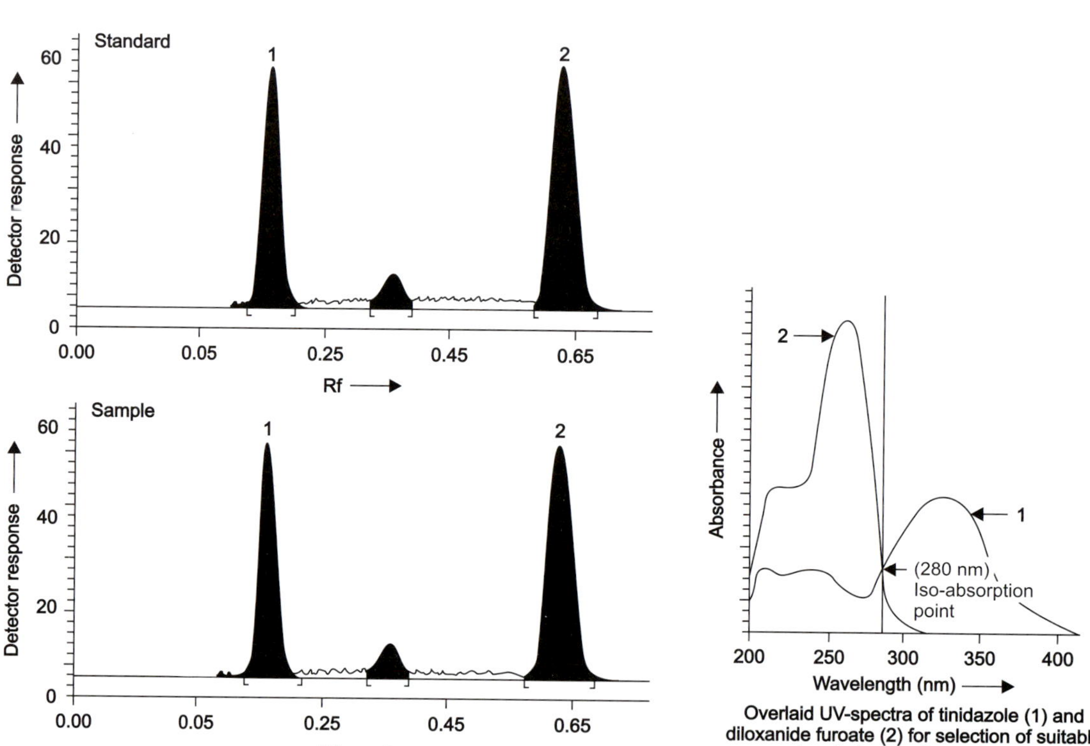

Overlaid UV-spectra of tinidazole (1) and diloxanide furoate (2) for selection of suitable wavelength for densitometric scanning

Typical densitogram of the sample and the standard containing tinidazole and diloxanide furoate. For detailed experimental and chromatographic conditions, refer to Protocol No. 343. Peaks identification: 1. Tinidazole; 2. Diloxanide furoate.

PROTOCOL FOR HPTLC ANALYSIS OF PHARMACEUTICAL FORMULATION

Protocol No. 343

Formulation: Tinidazole, Diloxanide furoate

Classification: Alimentary System **Dosage form:** Tablets

Standard preparation: Dissolve 30 mg of tinidazole in 5–6 ml of methanol, add 25 mg of diloxanide furoate, dilute to 10 ml with methanol and use for analysis.

Sample preparation: To powdered sample equivalent to 300 mg of tinidazole add 60–70 ml of methanol, sonicate and dilute to 100 ml. Filter and dilute 0.2 ml of the filtrate to 10 ml with methanol and use for application.

Chromatographic equipments:

Sample applicator: Camag Linomat–IV

Development chamber: Camag twin-trough glass chamber, 10 × 10 cm

Densitometric scanner: Camag TLC Scanner–II

Chromatographic conditions:

1. Stationary phase: Silica gel $60F_{254}$ pre-coated HPTLC plates, 10 × 10 cm (200 μm) – Merck
2. Mobile phase (MP): Toluene–acetone–25% ammonia (8 : 2 : 0.5 v/v)
3. Standard/Sample application:
   Band length: 5 mm Volume applied: 5 μl Spacing: 5 mm
4. Chamber saturation: 10 min (MP)
5. RH (%): 55 ± 5
6. Temperature °C: 22 ± 2
7. Separation technique: Ascending
8. Quantity of mobile phase: 10 ml
9. Migration distance: 50 mm
10. Migration time: 20 min

Densitometric evaluation:

Wavelength: UV–280 nm Scanning mode: Reflectance/Absorbance

HRF: Tinidazole—12; Diloxanide furoate—65

Linearity (ng/band): Tinidazole—60–360; Diloxanide furoate—100–500

Recovery (%): 98.5–99.2 for both the compounds

References: —

Comments:

- The method was optimized and analytical work carried out at **Anchrom's HPTLC Application Laboratory**, Mumbai, India.
- Several market samples of similar composition were analysed by the proposed method with reproducible results.

HPTLC : High Performance Thin Layer Chromatography
HPTLC Densitogram

No. 344

Tinidazole

Diloxanide furoate

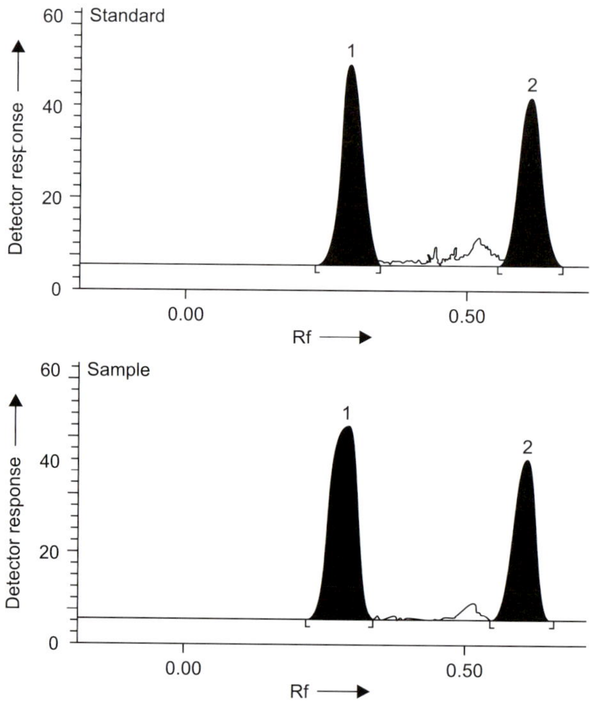

Typical densitogram of the sample and the standard containing tinidazole and diloxanide furoate. For detailed experimental and chromatographic conditions, refer to Protocol No. 344. Peaks identification: 1. Diloxanide furoate; 2. Tinidazole.

PROTOCOL FOR HPTLC ANALYSIS OF PHARMACEUTICAL FORMULATION

Protocol No. 344

Formulation: Tinidazole, Diloxanide furoate

Classification: Alimentary System **Dosage form:** Tablets

Standard preparation: Dissolve 30 mg of tinidazole in 5–6 ml of methanol, add 25 mg of diloxanide furoate, dilute to 10 ml with methanol and use for analysis.

Sample preparation: To powdered sample equivalent to 300 mg of tinidazole add 60–70 ml of methanol, sonicate and dilute to 100 ml. Filter and dilute 0.2 ml of the filtrate to 10 ml with methanol and use for chromatographic application.

Chromatographic equipments:

Sample applicator: Camag Linomat–IV

Development chamber: Camag twin-trough glass chamber, 10 × 10 cm

Densitometric scanner: Camag TLC Scanner–II

Chromatographic conditions:

1. Stationary phase: Silica gel 60 RP-18F_{254s} pre-coated HPTLC plates, 5 × 7.5 cm (200 μm) – Merck
2. Mobile phase (MP): 0.5 sodium chloride–methanol–acetonitrile–glacial acetic acid (5 : 2 : 3 : 0.1 v/v)
3. Standard/Sample application:
   Band length: 5 mm Volume applied: 5 μl Spacing: 5 mm
4. Chamber saturation: 30 min (MP)
5. RH (%): 55 ± 5
6. Temperature °C: 22 ± 2
7. Separation technique: Ascending
8. Quantity of mobile phase: 10 ml
9. Migration distance: 50 mm
10. Migration time: 25 min

Densitometric evaluation:

Wavelength: UV–280 nm Scanning mode: Reflectance/Absorbance

HRF: Diloxanide furoate—30; Tinidazole—60

Linearity (ng/band): Tinidazole—60–360; Diloxanide furoate—100–500

Recovery (%): 99.37–100.95 for both the compounds

References: —

Comments:

- The method was optimized and analytical work carried out at **Anchrom's HPTLC Application Laboratory**, Mumbai, India.
- Several market samples of similar composition were analysed by the proposed method with reproducible results.
- RP chromatography resulted in reversal of retention order as compared to NP-chromatography.

HPTLC : High Performance Thin Layer Chromatography
HPTLC Densitogram

No. 345

Tinidazole

Furazolidone

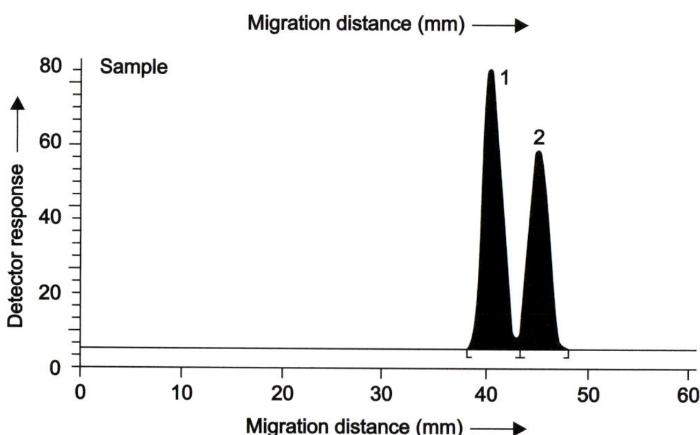

Typical densitogram of the sample and the standard containing tinidazole and furazolidone. For detailed experimental and chromatographic conditions, refer to Protocol No. 345. Peaks identification: 1. Furazolidone; 2. Tinidazole.

PROTOCOL FOR HPTLC ANALYSIS OF PHARMACEUTICAL FORMULATION

Protocol No. 345

Formulation: Tinidazole, Furazolidone

Classification: Alimentary System **Dosage form:** Tablets, Suspension

Standard preparation: Prepare 1 mg/ml solution of each compound in DMF. Mix 0.2 ml of solution of furazolidone and 0.6 ml of solution of tinidazole and dilute to 10 ml with methanol and use for analysis.

Sample preparation: The sample equivalent to 100 mg of furazolidone suspended in 50–60 ml of DMF, sonicate, dilute to 100 ml with DMF. Filter and dilute 0.2 ml of filtrate to 10 ml with methanol and use for assay.

Chromatographic equipments:

Sample applicator: Camag Linomat–IV

Development chamber: Camag twin-trough glass chamber, 10 × 10 cm

Densitometric scanner: Camag TLC Scanner–II

Chromatographic conditions:

1. Stationary phase: Silica gel $60F_{254}$ pre-coated HPTLC plates, 5 × 10 cm (200 μm) – Merck
2. Mobile phase (MP): Chloroform–methanol–25% ammonia (9 : 1 : 0.1 v/v) or chloroform–acetone–methanol–25% ammonia (10 : 1.5 : 0.5 : 0.1 v/v)
3. Standard/Sample application:
   Band length: 5 mm Volume applied: 6 μl Spacing: 5 mm
4. Chamber saturation: 15 min (MP)
5. RH (%): 55 ± 5
6. Temperature °C: 22 ± 2
7. Separation technique: Ascending
8. Quantity of mobile phase: 12 ml
9. Migration distance: 50 mm
10. Migration time: 22 min

Densitometric evaluation:

Wavelength: UV–280 nm Scanning mode: Reflectance/Absorbance

HRF: Furazolidone—58; Tinidazole—70

Linearity (ng/band): Tinidazole—60–360; Furazolidone—50–500

Recovery (%): 99.95–104.50 for both the compounds

References: B.S. Desai, U.M. Shine and N.M. Tendulkar, Abstract No. E–07; 46th IPC, 1994.

Comments: The method validated for accuracy, precision, linearity, LOD, LOQ, specificity, robustness and ruggedness.

HPTLC : High Performance Thin Layer Chromatography
HPTLC Densitogram

No. 346

HN N N CH_3 F O COOH

Norfloxacin

OH N O_2N CH_3 N

Metronidazole

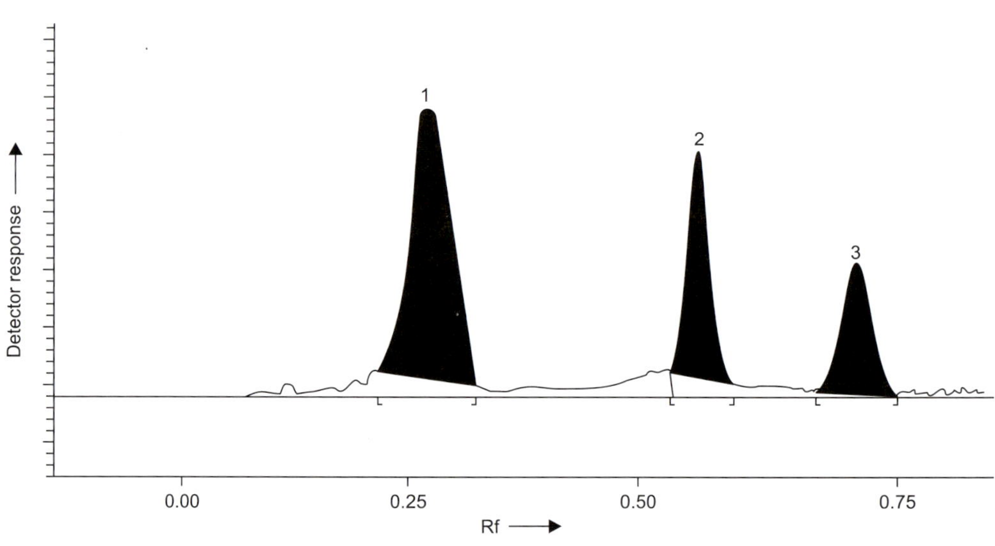

Typical densitogram of the sample containing norfloxacin and metronidazole. For detailed experimental and chromatographic conditions, refer to Protocol No. 346. Peaks identification: 1. Norfloxacin; 2. Metronidazole; 3. Tinidazole (IS).

PROTOCOL FOR HPTLC ANALYSIS OF PHARMACEUTICAL FORMULATION

Protocol No. 346

Formulation: **Norfloxacin, Metronidazole**

Classification: Alimentary System **Dosage form:** Tablets

Standard preparation: Prepare standard solution of both the compounds in the solvent to get 500 μg/ml of norfloxacin and 400 μg/ml of metronidazole. Further dilutions made to get different concentrations for linearity range. Each solution contains 37.5 μg/ml of tinidazole as (IS). Apply 10 μl of each solution for analysis.

Sample preparation: Powdered sample equivalent to 500 mg of metronidazole or 400 mg of norfloxacin suspended in solvent, sonicated, diluted to 100 ml, filtered. Dilute 0.25 ml of the filtrate to 25 ml with solvent after adding 3.75 ml of (IS) solution (4000 μg/ml in solvent).

Solvent: Mixture of dichloromethane–methanol (1 : 1 v/v).

Chromatographic equipments:

Sample applicator: Camag Linomat–IV

Development chamber: Camag twin-trough glass chamber, 10 × 10 cm

Densitometric scanner: Camag TLC Scanner–II

Chromatographic conditions:

1. Stationary phase: Silica gel $60F_{254}$ pre-coated HPTLC plates, 10 × 10 cm (200 μm) – Merck
2. Mobile phase (MP): Chloroform–methanol–diethylamine–water (9 : 2 : 0.4 : 0.2 v/v)
3. Standard/Sample application:
   Band length: 10 mm Volume applied: 10 μl Spacing: 10 mm
4. Chamber saturation: 25 min (MP)
5. RH (%): 55 ± 5.6
6. Temperature °C: 22 ± 2
7. Separation technique: Ascending
8. Quantity of mobile phase: 11 ml
9. Migration distance: 70 mm
10. Migration time: 30 min

Densitometric evaluation:

Wavelength: UV–254 nm Scanning mode: Reflectance/Absorbance

HRF: Norfloxacin—27; Metronidazole—55; Tinidazole (IS)—74

Linearity (μg/ml): Norfloxacin—10–50; Metronidazole—12.5–62.5

Recovery (%): 98.0–101.0 for both the compounds

References: S.S. Zarapkar and N.S. Kanyawar, *Indian Drugs*, **36(5)**, 293–295, 1999.

Comments: The method validated for accuracy, precision, linearity, LOD, LOQ, specificity, robustness and ruggedness.

HPTLC : High Performance Thin Layer Chromatography
HPTLC Densitogram

No. 347

Norfloxacin

Tinidazole

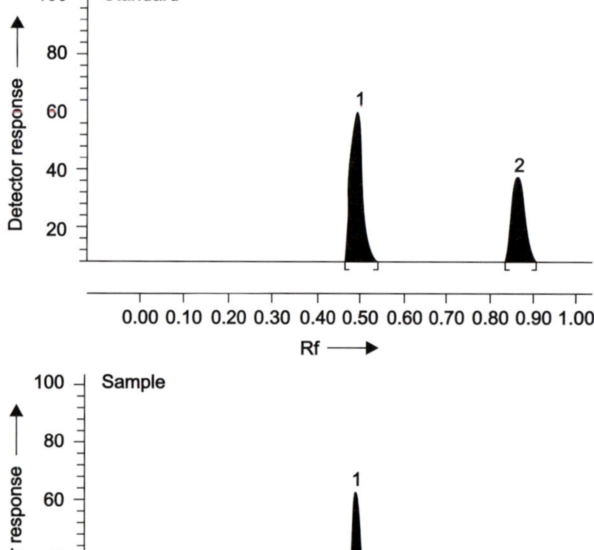

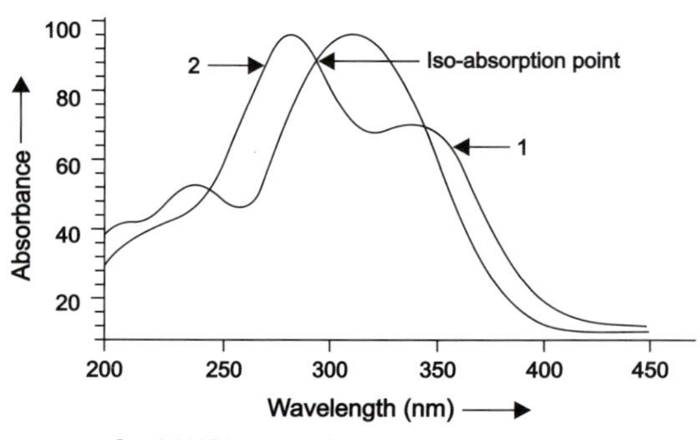

Overlaid UV-spectra of tinidazole (1) and norfloxacin (2) for selection of suitable wavelength for densitometric scanning

Typical densitogram of the sample and the standard containing tinidazole and norfloxacin. For detailed experimental and chromatographic conditions, refer to Protocol No. 347. Peaks identification: 1. Norfloxacin; 2. Tinidazole.

PROTOCOL FOR HPTLC ANALYSIS OF PHARMACEUTICAL FORMULATION

Protocol No. 347

Formulation: Norfloxacin, Tinidazole

Classification: Alimentary System **Dosage form:** Tablets

Standard preparation: Prepare 1 mg/ml solution of each compound in methanol. Further dilutions made with methanol to get 5 μg/ml solution of each and apply 5 μl for chromatographic analysis.

Sample preparation: An appropriate quantity of powdered sample extracted with solvent mixture of dichloromethane–methanol (1 : 1 v/v) to get 500 μg/ml of tinidazole. Further dilutions made with methanol for assay. Apply 5 μl for assay.

Chromatographic equipments:

Sample applicator: Camag Linomat–IV
Development chamber: Camag twin-trough glass chamber, 10 × 10 cm
Densitometric scanner: Camag TLC Scanner–III

Chromatographic conditions:

1. Stationary phase: Silica gel $60F_{254}$ pre-coated HPTLC plates, 10 × 10 cm (200 μm) – Merck
2. Mobile phase (MP): Chloroform–methanol–toluene–diethylamine–water (4 : 4 : 2 : 1.4 : 0.8 v/v)
3. Standard/Sample application:
   Band length: 5 mm Volume applied: 5 μl Spacing: 5 mm
4. Chamber saturation: 20 min (MP)
5. RH (%): 55 ± 5
6. Temperature °C: 25 ± 2
7. Separation technique: Ascending
8. Quantity of mobile phase: 12 ml
9. Migration distance: 70 mm
10. Migration time: 25 min

Densitometric evaluation:

Wavelength: UV–290 nm (iso-absorption point)
Scanning mode: Reflectance/Absorbance
HRF: Norfloxacin—48; Tinidazole—86
Linearity: 5–50 ng/band for both the compounds
Recovery (%): 101.97–102.95 for both the compounds

References: —

Comments:

- The method was optimized and analytical work carried out at **Anchrom's HPTLC Application Laboratory**, Mumbai, India.
- Several market samples of similar composition were analysed by the proposed method with reproducible results.
- The method was routinely used to study the dissolution profile of both the compounds in fixed-dose combinations.

HPTLC : High Performance Thin Layer Chromatography
HPTLC Densitogram

No. 348

HN N N CH_3 F O COOH

Norfloxacin

NO_2 O O S N CH_3 N CH_3

Tinidazole

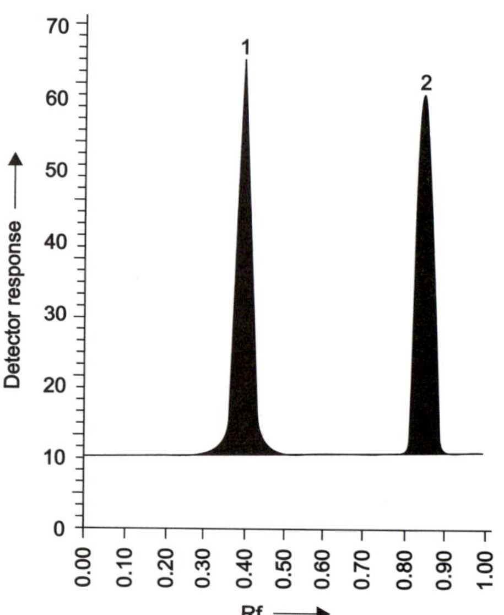

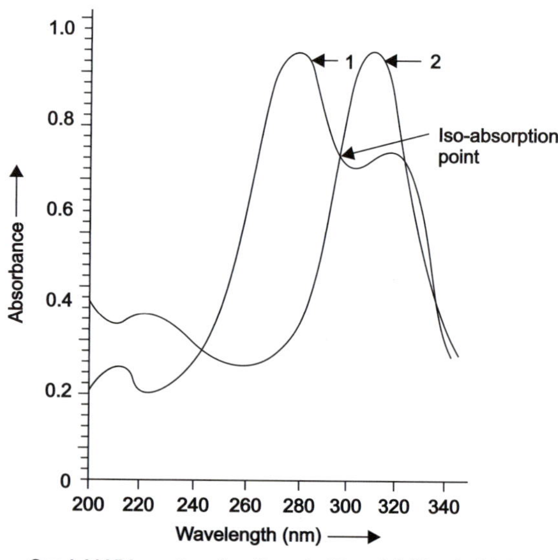

Overlaid UV-spectra of norfloxacin (1) and tinidazole (2) for selection of suitable wavelength for densitometric scanning

Typical densitogram of the sample containing norfloxacin and tinidazole. For detailed experimental and chromatographic conditions, refer to Protocol No. 348. Peaks identification: 1. Norfloxacin; 2. Tinidazole.

PROTOCOL FOR HPTLC ANALYSIS OF PHARMACEUTICAL FORMULATION

Protocol No. 348

Formulation: Norfloxacin, Tinidazole

Classification: Alimentary System **Dosage form:** Tablets

Standard preparation: Dissolve 50 mg of norfloxacin and 75 mg of tinidazole in solvent to produce 50 ml. 1 ml of resulting solution diluted to 100 ml with methanol and used for analysis.

Solvent: 10% v/v solution of glacial acetic acid in acetonitrile.

Sample preparation: Powdered sample equivalent to 50 mg of norfloxacin suspended in 40 ml of solvent, sonicated for 10 min, diluted to 50 ml, filtered through Whatman No. 42 filter paper and 1 ml of the aliquot diluted to 100 ml with methanol and used for analysis.

Chromatographic equipments:

Sample applicator: Camag Linomat–IV

Development chamber: Camag twin-trough glass chamber, 10 × 10 cm

Densitometric scanner: Camag TLC Scanner–II

Chromatographic conditions:

1. Stationary phase: Silica gel $60F_{254}$ pre-coated HPTLC plates, pre-washed with 5% ammonical methanol, air dried prior to use
2. Mobile phase (MP): n-butanol–ethylalcohol–12.5% ammonia (4 : 1 : 2.2 v/v)
3. Standard/Sample application:
   Band length: 8 mm   Volume applied: 1–10 μl   Spacing: 10 mm
4. Chamber saturation: 20 min (MP)
5. RH (%): 55 ± 5
6. Temperature °C: 22 ± 2
7. Separation technique: Ascending
8. Quantity of mobile phase: 14 ml
9. Migration distance: 70 mm
10. Migration time: 30 min

Densitometric evaluation:

Wavelength: UV–293 nm (iso-absorption point)

Scanning mode: Reflectance/Absorbance

HRF: Norfloxacin—40; Tinidazole—85

Linearity (ng/band): Norfloxacin—10–200; Tinidazole—15–300

Recovery (%): 99.94–100.13 for both the compounds

References: A.P. Argekar, S.U. Kapadia and S.V. Raj, *J. Planar Chromatogr.*, **6(3)**, 1996.

Comments: The method validated for accuracy, precision, linearity, LOD, LOQ, specificity, robustness and ruggedness.

HPTLC : High Performance Thin Layer Chromatography
HPTLC Densitogram

No. 350

Ofloxacin

Tinidazole

Overlaid UV-spectra of ofloxacin (1) and ornidazole (2) for selection of suitable wavelength for densitometric scanning

Typical densitogram of the sample containing ofloxacin and ornidazole. For detailed experimental and chromatographic conditions, refer to Protocol No. 350. Peaks identification: 1. Ofloxacin; 2. Ornidazole.

PROTOCOL FOR HPTLC ANALYSIS OF PHARMACEUTICAL FORMULATION

Protocol No. 350

Formulation: Ofloxacin, Ornidazole

Classification: Alimentary System **Dosage form:** Tablets

Standard preparation: Standard solution of both the compounds was prepared in methanol to get final concentration of 100 μg/ml (ofloxacin) and 250 μg/ml of ornidazole.

Sample preparation: Powdered sample equivalent to 10 mg of ofloxacin extracted with methanol with the aid of sonication, filtered through Whatman No. 1 filter paper and suitably diluted to get 100 μg/ml of ofloxacin and 250 μg/ml of ornidazole and used for assay.

Chromatographic equipments:

Sample applicator: Camag Linomat–V

Development chamber: Camag twin-trough glass chamber, 10 × 10 cm

Densitometric scanner: Camag TLC Scanner–III

Chromatographic conditions:

1. Stationary phase: Silica gel $60F_{254}$ pre-coated HPTLC plates, 20 × 10 cm (200 μm) – Merck, pre-washed with methanol and air-dried prior to use
2. Mobile phas (MP): n-butanol–ethanol–25% ammonia (5 : 5 : 0.4 v/v)
3. Standard/Sample application:
   Band length: 5 mm Volume applied: 1–5 μl Spacing: 5 mm
4. Chamber saturation: —
5. RH (%): 55 ± 5
6. Temperature °C: 22 ± 2
7. Separation technique: Ascending
8. Quantity of mobile phase: 10 ml
9. Migration distance: 82 mm
10. Migration time: 30 min

Densitometric evaluation:

Wavelength: UV–295 nm Scanning mode: Reflectance/Absorbance

HRF: Ofloxacin—59; Ornidazole—86

Linearity (ng/band): Ofloxacin—1–5; Ornidazole—2.5–12.5

Recovery (%): 102.27–103.04 for both the compounds

References: M. Gandhimathi, T.K. Ravi and Nilima Shukla, *Ind. J. Pharm Sci.*, **68(6)**, 838–840, 2006.

Comments: The method validated for accuracy, precision, linearity, LOD, LOQ, specificity, robustness and ruggedness.

HPTLC : High Performance Thin Layer Chromatography
HPTLC Densitogram

No. 351

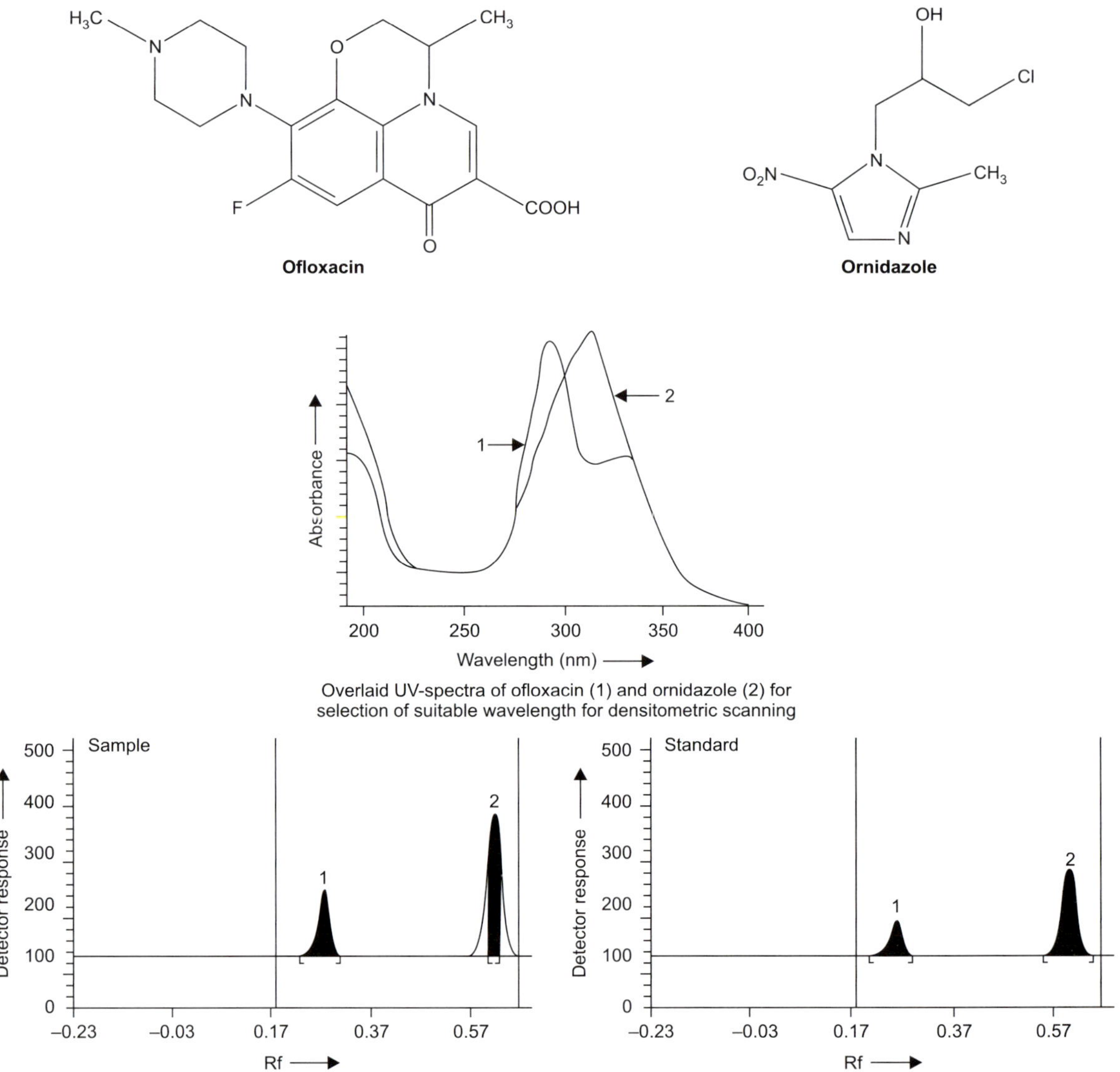

Overlaid UV-spectra of ofloxacin (1) and ornidazole (2) for selection of suitable wavelength for densitometric scanning

Typical densitogram of the sample and standard containing ofloxacin and ornidazole. For detailed experimental and chromatographic conditions, refer to Protocol No. 351. Peaks identification: 1. Ofloxacin; 2. Ornidazole.

PROTOCOL FOR HPTLC ANALYSIS OF PHARMACEUTICAL FORMULATION

Protocol No. 351

Formulation: Ofloxacin, Ornidazole

Classification: Alimentary System **Dosage form:** Tablets

Standard preparation: Prepare 100 μg/ml solution of ofloxacin and 250 μg/ml of ornidazole, both in methanol. Further serial dilutions are made with methanol for linearity studies. Prepare mixed standard solution to get 20 μg/ml and 50 μg/ml of ofloxacin and ornidazole respectively. Apply 2 μl of each solution.

Sample preparation: Powdered sample equivalent to 100 mg of ofloxacin suspended in methanol, sonicated, diluted to 100 ml, filtered, an aliquot suitably diluted with methanol to get final concentration of 20 μg/ml of ofloxacin and 50 μg/ml of ornidazole. Apply 2 μl for chromatographic evaluation.

Chromatographic equipments:

Sample applicator: Camag Linomat–V

Development chamber: Camag twin-trough glass chamber, 10 × 10 cm

Densitometric scanner: Camag TLC Scanner–III

Chromatographic conditions:

1. Stationary phase: Silica gel $60F_{254}$ pre-coated HPTLC plates, 10 × 10 cm (200 μm) – Merck
2. Mobile phas (MP): Chloroform–methanol–toluene–diethylamine–water (4 : 3 : 5 : 2 : 0.2 v/v)
3. Standard/Sample application:
   Band length: 5 mm Volume applied: 2 μl Spacing: 10 mm
4. Chamber saturation: 20 min (filter paper)
5. RH (%): 55 ± 5
6. Temperature °C: Ambient
7. Separation technique: Ascending
8. Quantity of mobile phase: 14 ml
9. Migration distance: 80 mm
10. Migration time: 12 min

Densitometric evaluation:

Wavelength: UV–304 nm Scanning mode: Reflectance/Absorbance

HRF: Ofloxacin—27; Ornidazole—60

Linearity (ng/band): Ofloxacin—20–100; Ornidazole—50–250

Recovery (%): 95–105 for both the compounds

References: M.G. Pai, Vibhuti Karpe, Rajashree Gude and Sachi Kudchadkar, Abstract No. PA–8, 60th IPC, 2008, Personal communication.

Comments: The method validated for accuracy, precision, linearity, LOD, LOQ, specificity, robustness and ruggedness.

HPTLC : High Performance Thin Layer Chromatography
HPTLC Densitogram

No. 352

Ornidazole

Ofloxacin

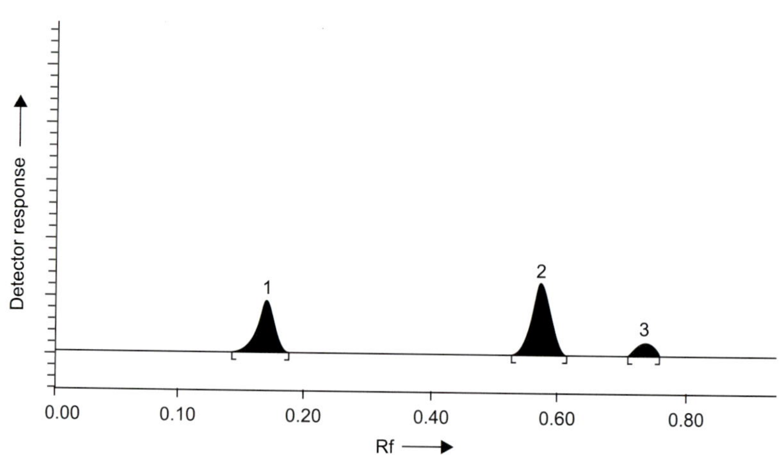

Typical densitogram of the sample containing ofloxacin and ornidazole. For detailed experimental and chromatographic conditions, refer to Protocol No. 352. Peaks identification: 1. Ofloxacin; 2. Ornidazole-I-isomer; 3. Ornidazole-II-isomer.

PROTOCOL FOR HPTLC ANALYSIS OF PHARMACEUTICAL FORMULATION

Protocol No. 352

Formulation: Ofloxacin, Ornidazole
Classification: Alimentary System **Dosage form:** Tablets
Standard preparation: Prepare standard solution of both the drugs in methanol to get 1 mg/ml of ofloxacin and 2.5 mg/ml of ornidazole. Further dilutions were suitably made with methanol. Apply 2–20 µl for linearity studies.
Sample preparation: Powdered sample equivalent to 100 mg of ofloxacin suspended in 50 ml of methanol, sonicated for 10 min, diluted to 100 ml with methanol. Filtered and the filtrate suitably diluted for chromatographic analysis by applying 10 µl of the final solution.
Chromatographic equipments:
Sample applicator: Camag Linomat–V
Development chamber: Camag twin-trough glass chamber, 10 × 10 cm
Densitometric scanner: Camag TLC Scanner–III
Chromatographic conditions:
1. Stationary phase: Silica gel 60F_{254} pre-coated TLC plates, 10 × 10 cm (250 µm) – Merck
2. Mobile phase (MP): (i) Dichloromethane–methanol–25% ammonia (9.5 : 1 : 0.3 v/v); (ii) 1,4-dioxane–ethyl acetate–toluene–glacial acetic acid–water (5 : 5 : 3 : 3 : 2 : 2 v/v)
3. Standard/Sample application:
   Band length: 10 mm Volume applied: 2–20 µl Spacing: 10 mm
4. Chamber saturation: 10 min (MP)
5. RH (%): 55 ± 5
6. Temperature °C: 22 ± 2
7. Separation technique: Ascending
8. Quantity of mobile phase: 10 ml
9. Migration distance: 90 mm
10. Migration time: 20 min

Densitometric evaluation:
Wavelength: UV–318 nm or 287 nm Scanning mode: Reflectance/Absorbance
HRF: Ofloxacin—16; Ornidazole-I (isomer)—56; Ornidazole-II (isomer)—78, 89
Linearity (ng/band): Ofloxacin—50–250; Ornidazole—20–100
Recovery (%): 100.04–100.22 for both the drugs
References: Manisha Puranik, D.V. Bhawsar, Prachi Rathi and P.G. Yeole, *Ind. J. Pharm. Sci.*, **72(4)**, 513–517, 2010, Vipul R. Rohit et al., Abstract No. F-330, 62nd IPC-2010.
Comments:
- The method validated for accuracy, precision, linearity, LOD, LOQ, specificity, robustness and ruggedness.
- The method compared with RP-HPLC method and found to give comparable results.

HPTLC : High Performance Thin Layer Chromatography
HPTLC Densitogram

No. 353

Ofloxacin

Satranidazole

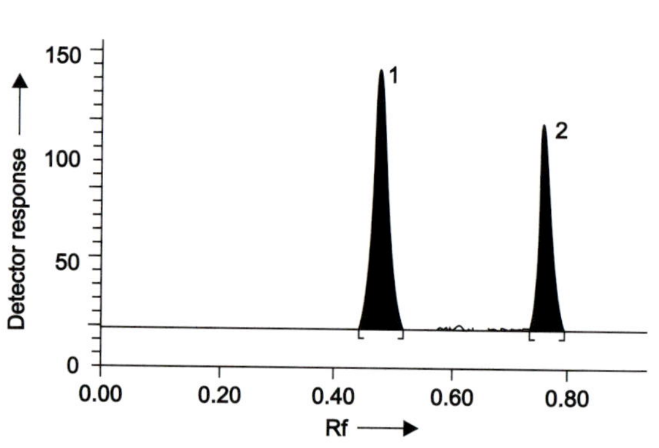

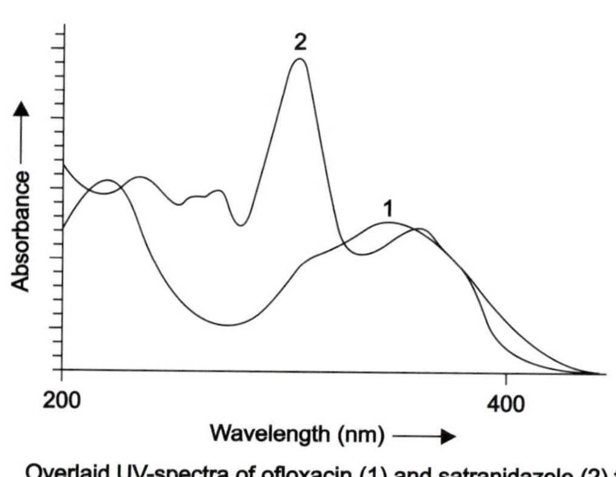

Overlaid UV-spectra of ofloxacin (1) and satranidazole (2) for selection of suitable wavelength for densitometric scanning

Typical densitogram of the sample containing ofloxacin and satranidazole. For detailed experimental and chromatographic conditions, refer to Protocol No. 353. Peaks identification: 1. Ofloxacin; 2. Satranidazole.

PROTOCOL FOR HPTLC ANALYSIS OF PHARMACEUTICAL FORMULATION

Protocol No. 353

Formulation: Ofloxacin, Satranidazole

Classification: Alimentary System **Dosage form:** Tablets

Standard preparation: Prepare standard solution of both the compounds in methanol to get 200 μg/ml of ofloxacin and 300 μg/ml of satranidazole. Further suitable dilutions made for linearity profile.

Sample preparation: Powdered sample equivalent to 200 mg of ofloxacin and 300 mg of satranidazole suspended in 30 ml of methanol, sonicated for 10 min, diluted to 50 ml, filtered through Whatman No. 41 filter paper and filtrate suitably diluted for analysis.

Chromatographic equipments:

Sample applicator: Camag Linomat–V

Development chamber: Camag twin-trough glass chamber, 10 × 10 cm

Densitometric scanner: Camag TLC Scanner–III

Chromatographic conditions:

1. Stationary phase: Silica gel $60F_{254}$ pre-coated HPTLC plates, 10 × 10 cm (200 μm) – Merck
2. Mobile phase (MP): n-butanol–ethanol–25% ammonia (5 : 5 : 4 v/v)
3. Standard/Sample application:
   Band length: 5 mm Volume applied: 10 μl Spacing: 5 mm
4. Chamber saturation: 20 min (MP)
5. RH (%): 55 ± 5
6. Temperature °C: 22 ± 2
7. Separation technique: Ascending
8. Quantity of mobile phase: 14 ml
9. Migration distance: 75 mm
10. Migration time: 30 min

Densitometric evaluation:

Wavelength: UV–320 nm (iso-absorption point)

Scanning mode: Reflectance/Absorbance

HRF: Ofloxacin—48; Satranidazole—77

Linearity (ng/band): Ofloxacin—200–1000; Satranidazole—300–1500

Recovery (%): 99.08–99.85 for both the compounds

References: Godge Rahul, Bhat Leena, Vora Asfak and Damle Mrinalini, *J. Pharm. Res.*, **6(4)**, 233–235, 2007.

Comments: The method validated for accuracy, precision, linearity, LOD, LOQ, specificity, robustness and ruggedness.

HPTLC : High Performance Thin Layer Chromatography
HPTLC Densitogram

No. 354

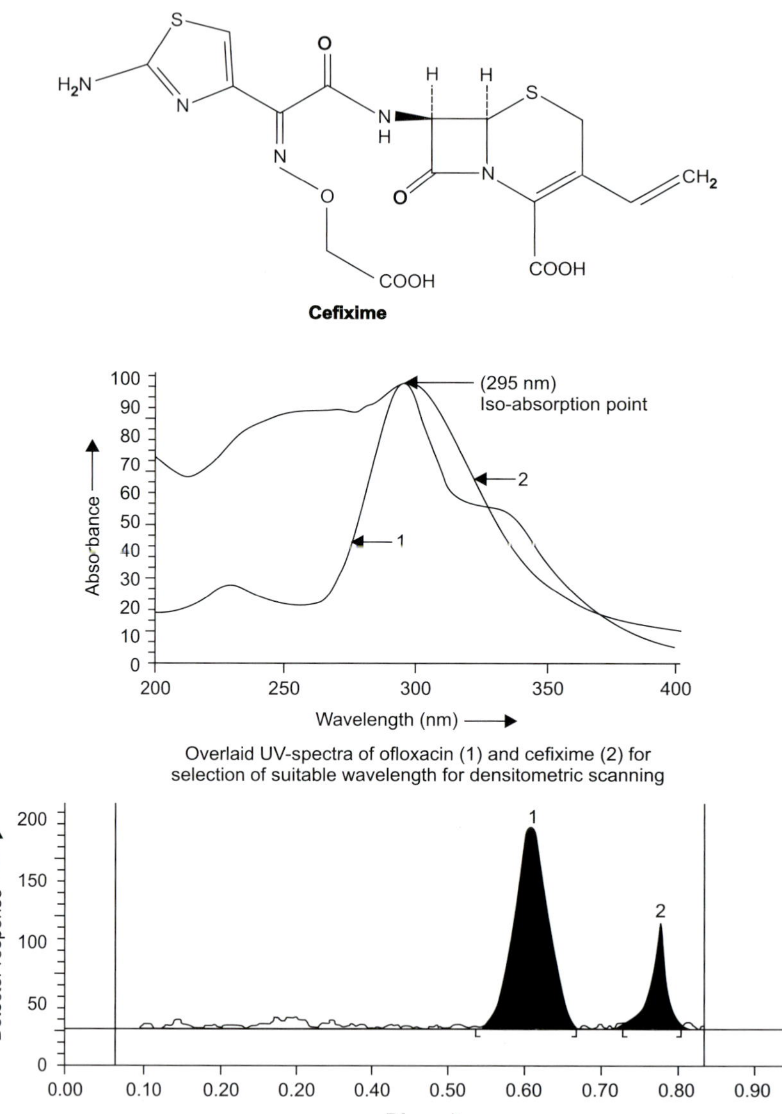

Typical densitogram of the standard containing ofloxacin and cefixime. For detailed experimental and chromatographic conditions, refer to Protocol No. 354. Peaks identification: 1. Ofloxacin; 2. Cefixime.

PROTOCOL FOR HPTLC ANALYSIS OF PHARMACEUTICAL FORMULATION

Protocol No. 354

Formulation: Ofloxacin, Cefixime

Classification: Alimentary System **Dosage form:** Tablets

Standard preparation: Prepare 50 μg/ml solution of each compound in methanol. Apply varying volumes (1–10 μl) for linearity profile.

Sample preparation: Powdered sample equivalent to 5 mg of ofloxacin suspended in 8 ml of methanol, sonicated, diluted and filtered. 1 ml of the filtrate diluted to 10 ml with methanol. Apply 2 μl for chromatographic analysis.

Chromatographic equipments:

Sample applicator: Camag Linomat–V

Development chamber: Camag twin-trough glass chamber, 10 × 10 cm

Densitometric scanner: Camag TLC Scanner–III

Chromatographic conditions:

1. Stationary phase: Silica gel 60F_{254} pre-coated TLC plates, 10 × 10 cm (250 μm) – Merck
2. Mobile phase (MP): Methanol–ethyl acetate–25% ammonia (3.5 : 3.5 : 1.5 v/v)
3. Standard/Sample application:
   Band length: 5 mm Volume applied: 1–10 μl Spacing: 6 mm
4. Chamber saturation: 20 min (MP)
5. RH (%): 55 ± 5
6. Temperature °C: 22 ± 2
7. Separation technique: Ascending
8. Quantity of mobile phase: 17 ml
9. Migration distance: 90 mm
10. Migration time: 20 min

Densitometric evaluation:

Wavelength: UV–295 nm (iso-absorption point)

Scanning mode: Reflectance/Absorbance

HRF: Ofloxacin—61; Cefixime—78

Linearity: 50–500 ng/band for both the compounds

Recovery (%): Ofloxacin—98.34–103.49; Cefixime—99.32–102.20

References: K.S. Khaudagle, S.V. Gandhi, P.B. Deshpande, A.N. Kale and P.R. Deshmukh, *J. Chem and Pharm. Res.*, **2(5)**, 92–96, 2010.

Comments: The method validated for accuracy, precision, linearity, LOD, LOQ, specificity, robustness and ruggedness.

HPTLC : High Performance Thin Layer Chromatography
HPTLC Densitogram

No. 355

Cefixime

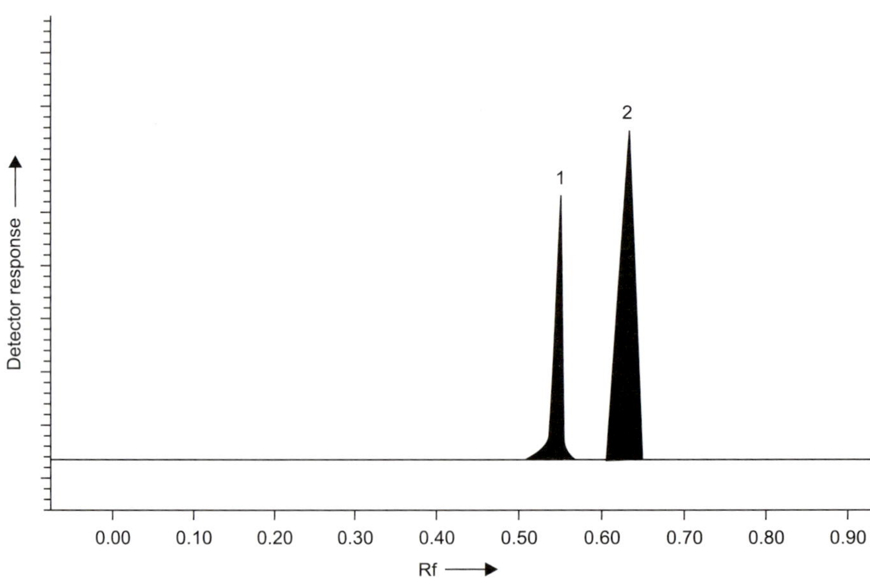

Typical densitogram of the standard containing ofloxacin and cefixime. For detailed experimental and chromatographic conditions, refer to Protocol No. 355. Peaks identification: 1. Cefixime; 2. Ofloxacin.

PROTOCOL FOR HPTLC ANALYSIS OF PHARMACEUTICAL FORMULATION

Protocol No. 355

Formulation: Ofloxacin, Cefixime

Classification: Alimentary System **Dosage form:** Tablets

Standard preparation: Prepare 100 μg/ml solution of both the compounds in methanol. Further dilute suitably to get 30 μg/ml solution. Apply varying volumes (1–6 μl) for linearity profile.

Sample preparation: Powdered sample equivalent to 200 mg of ofloxacin suspended in 60 ml of methanol, sonicated for 45 min, diluted to 100 ml, filtered, the filtrate suitably diluted for assay. Apply 2 μl for chromatographic evaluation.

Chromatographic equipments:

Sample applicator: Camag Linomat–V

Development chamber: Camag twin-trough glass chamber, 20 × 10 cm

Densitometric scanner: Camag TLC Scanner–III

Chromatographic conditions:

1. Stationary phase: Silica gel 60F_{254} pre-coated TLC plates, 20 × 10 cm (250 μm) – Merck
2. Mobile phase (MP): n-butanol–25% ammonia–water–DMSO (8 : 3 : 1 : 2 v/v)
3. Standard/Sample application:
   Band length: 6 mm Volume applied: 1–6 μl Spacing: 6 mm
4. Chamber saturation: 30 min (MP)
5. RH (%): 60 ± 5
6. Temperature °C: 25 ± 2
7. Separation technique: Ascending
8. Quantity of mobile phase: 14 ml
9. Migration distance: 80 mm
10. Migration time: 20 min

Densitometric evaluation:

Wavelength: UV–297 nm Scanning mode: Reflectance/Absorbance

HRF: Cefixime—55; Ofloxacin—65

Linearity: 30–180 ng/band for both the compounds

Recovery (%): 99.74–99.95 for both the compounds

References: Janhavi Rao, Kamini Sethy and Savita Yadav, *Pharmacie Globale (IJCP)*, **2(4)**, 1–4, 2011.

Comments: The method validated for accuracy, precision, linearity, LOD, LOQ, specificity, robustness and ruggedness.

HPTLC : High Performance Thin Layer Chromatography
HPTLC Densitogram

No. 356

Levofloxacin

Ornidazole

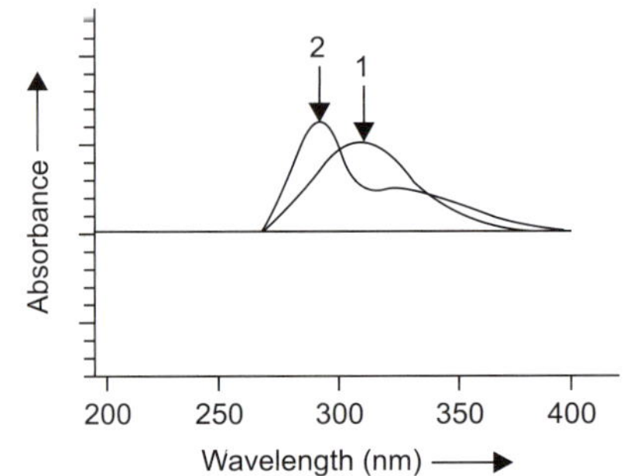

Overlaid UV-spectra of ofloxacin (2) and ornidazole (1) for selection of suitable wavelength for densitometric scanning

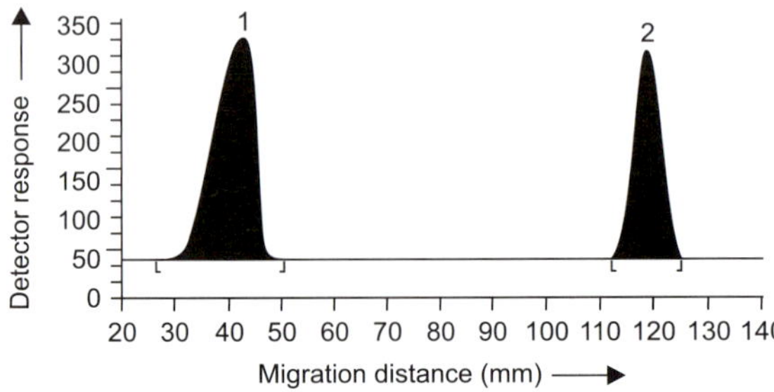

Typical densitogram of the standard containing levofloxacin and ornidazole. For detailed experimental and chromatographic conditions, refer to Protocol No. 356. Peaks identification: 1. Levofloxacin; 2. Ornidazole.

PROTOCOL FOR HPTLC ANALYSIS OF PHARMACEUTICAL FORMULATION

Protocol No. 356

Formulation: Levofloxacin hemihydrate, Ornidazole

Classification: Alimentary System **Dosage form:** Tablets

Standard preparation: Prepare standard solution of both the compounds in methanol to get 12.5 mg/ml (levofloxacin) and 25 mg/ml (ornidazole). Further dilute to get 1250 μg/ml (levofloxacin) and 2500 μg/ml (ornidazole) and use for analysis.

Sample preparation: An appropriate quantity of powdered sample extracted with methanol, filtered through Whatman No. 42 filter paper and suitably diluted with methanol and used for chromatographic analysis.

Chromatographic equipments:

Sample applicator: Camag Linomat–V

Development chamber: Camag twin-trough glass chamber, 10 × 10 cm

Densitometric scanner: Camag TLC Scanner–III

Chromatographic conditions:

1. Stationary phase: Silica gel $60F_{254}$ pre-coated TLC plates, 10 × 10 cm (250 μm) – Merck, pre-washed with methanol, air dried prior to use
2. Mobile phas (MP): n-butanol–water–glacial acetic acid (6 : 2 : 2 v/v)
3. Standard/Sample application:
   Band length: 10 mm Volume applied: 10 μl Spacing: 15 mm
4. Chamber saturation: 10 min (filter paper)
5. RH (%): 55 ± 5
6. Temperature °C: 22 ± 2
7. Separation technique: Ascending
8. Quantity of mobile phase: 10 ml
9. Migration distance: 70 mm
10. Migration time: 20 min

Densitometric evaluation:

Wavelength: UV–366 nm Scanning mode: Reflectance/Absorbance

HRF: Levofloxacin, Ornidazole, see densitogram

Linearity (ng/band): Levofloxacin—1050–1460; Ornidazole—2100–2900

Recovery (%): 99.70–100.45 for both the drug

References: K. Surendra, S.D. Mageswari, R. Maheswari, N. Harikrishnan, C. Roosewelt and V. Gunasekaran, *Asian J. Chem.*, **19(7)**, 5647–5651, 2007.

Comments: The method validated for accuracy, precision, linearity, LOD, LOQ, specificity, robustness and ruggedness.

HPTLC : High Performance Thin Layer Chromatography
HPTLC Densitogram

No. 357

Levofloxacin

Ornidazole

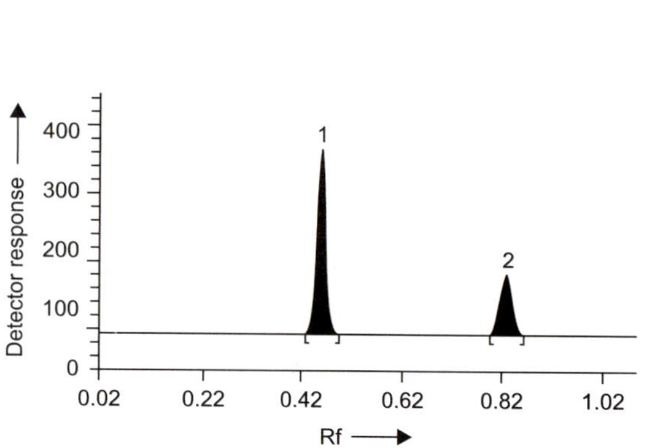

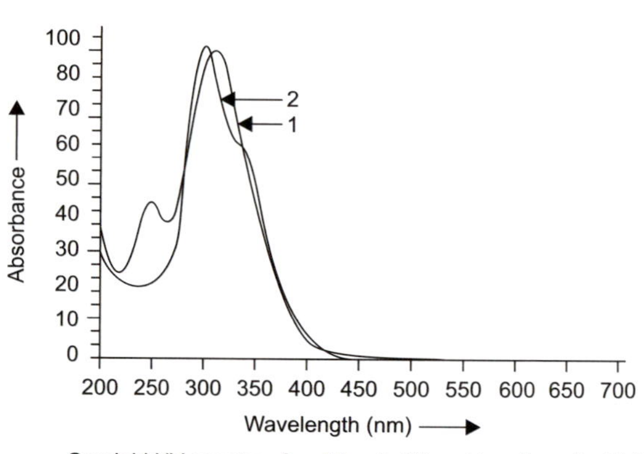

Overlaid UV-spectra of ornidazole (1) and levofloxacin (2) for selection of suitable wavelength for densitometric scanning

Typical densitogram of the sample containing levofloxacin hemihydrate and ornidazole. For detailed experimental and chromatographic conditions, refer to Protocol No. 357. Peaks identification: 1. Levofloxacin; 2. Ornidazole.

PROTOCOL FOR HPTLC ANALYSIS OF PHARMACEUTICAL FORMULATION

Protocol No. 357

Formulation: Levofloxacin hemihydrate, Ornidazole

Classification: Alimentary System **Dosage form:** Tablets

Standard preparation: Prepare mixed standard of both the compounds in methanol to get 100 μg/ml of levofloxacin and 200 μg/ml of ornidazole and apply volume varying from 0.5 to 2.5 μl for linearity.

Sample preparation: Powdered sample equivalent to 10 mg of levofloxacin or 20 mg of ornidazole suspended in methanol, sonicated for 10 min, diluted, filtered and applied 1 μl for assay.

Chromatographic equipments:

Sample applicator: Camag Linomat–V

Development chamber: Camag twin-trough glass chamber, 10 × 10 cm

Densitometric scanner: Camag TLC Scanner–III

Chromatographic conditions:

1. Stationary phase: Silica gel 60F_{254} pre-coated TLC plates, 10 × 10 cm (250 μm) – Merck, pre-washed with methanol, activated (110°C) for 5 min prior to use
2. Mobile phase (MP): n-butanol–methanol–25% ammonia (5 : 1 : 1.5 v/v)
3. Standard/Sample application:
   Band length: 5 mm Volume applied: 0.5–2.5 μl Spacing: 5 mm
4. Chamber saturation: 20 min (MP)
5. RH (%): 55 ± 5
6. Temperature °C: 22 ± 2
7. Separation technique: Ascending
8. Quantity of mobile phase: 15 ml
9. Migration distance: 90 mm
10. Migration time: 40 min

Densitometric evaluation:

Wavelength: UV–298 nm Scanning mode: Reflectance/Absorbance

HRF: Levofloxacin—44; Ornidazole—82

Linearity (ng/band): Levofloxacin—50–250; Ornidazole—100–500

Recovery (%): 99.91–100.08 for both the compounds

References: S.B. Chepurwar, A.A. Shirkhedar, S.B. Bari, R.A. Fursule and S.J. Surana, *J. Chromatogr. Sci.*, **45**, 531–535, 2007.

Comments: The method validated for accuracy, precision, linearity, LOD, LOQ, specificity, robustness and ruggedness.

HPTLC : High Performance Thin Layer Chromatography
HPTLC Densitogram

No. 358

Levofloxacin

Ornidazole

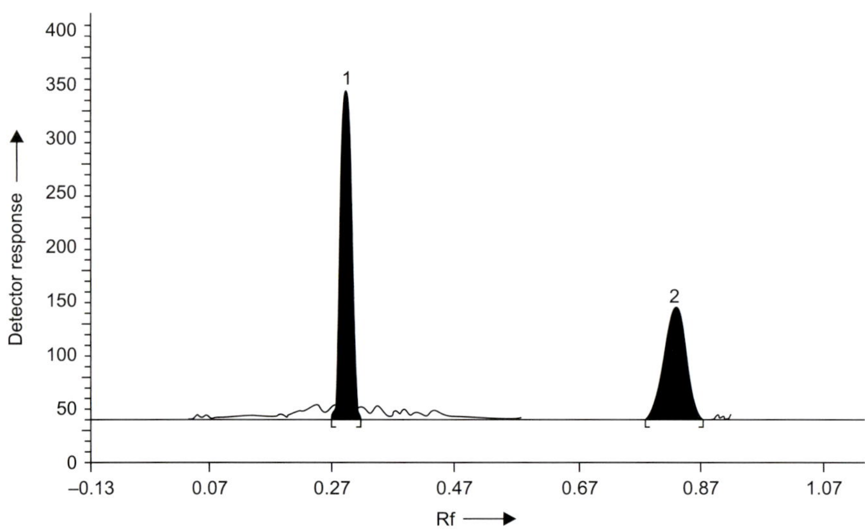

Typical densitogram of the sample containing levofloxacin and ornidazole. For detailed experimental and chromatographic conditions, refer to Protocol No. 358. Peaks identification: 1. Levofloxacin; 2. Ornidazole.

PROTOCOL FOR HPTLC ANALYSIS OF PHARMACEUTICAL FORMULATION

Protocol No. 358

Formulation: Levofloxacin, Ornidazole

Classification: Alimentary System **Dosage form:** Tablets

Standard preparation: Prepare solution of both the compounds separately in methanol to get 100 μg/ml of levofloxacin and 200 μg/ml of ornidazole. Dilute 1 ml of each solution to 10 ml with methanol and apply varying volume of each solution for linearity studies.

Sample preparation: Powdered sample equivalent to 10 mg of levofloxacin suspended in 25 ml of methanol, sonicated for 15 min, dilute to 100 ml with methanol, filtered through nylon filter and 1 ml of the filtrate diluted to 10 ml with methanol. Apply 5 μl of the resulting solution for analysis.

Chromatographic equipments:

Sample applicator: Camag Linomat–V

Development chamber: Camag twin-trough glass chamber, 10 × 10 cm

Densitometric scanner: Camag TLC Scanner–III

Chromatographic conditions:

1. Stationary phase: Silica gel $60F_{254}$ pre-coated HPTLC plates, 10 × 10 cm (200 μm) – Merck, pre-washed with methanol, activated at 50°C for 5 min prior to chromatography
2. Mobile phase (MP): n-butanol–ethanol–8 M ammonia (5 : 0.5 : 1.5 v/v)
3. Standard/Sample application:
   Band length: 6 mm Volume applied: 4–14 μl Spacing: 5 mm
4. Chamber saturation: 30 min (MP)
5. RH (%): 55 ± 5
6. Temperature °C: 22 ± 2
7. Separation technique: Ascending
8. Quantity of mobile phase: 12 ml
9. Migration distance: 80 mm
10. Migration time: 25 min

Densitometric evaluation:

Wavelength: UV–310 nm Scanning mode: Reflectance/Absorbance

HRF: Levofloxacin—31; Ornidazole—83

Linearity (ng/band): Levofloxacin—40–140; Ornidazole—80–280

Recovery (%): Levofloxacin—98.12–100.20; Ornidazole—99.35–101.30

References: Satish A. Patel and Natvarlal J. Patel, *J. Pharma Edu. Res.*, **2(2)**, 78–83, 2011.

Comments: The method validated for accuracy, precision, linearity, LOD, LOQ, specificity, robustness and ruggedness.

HPTLC : High Performance Thin Layer Chromatography
HPTLC Densitogram

No. 359

Ciprofloxacin

Ornidazole

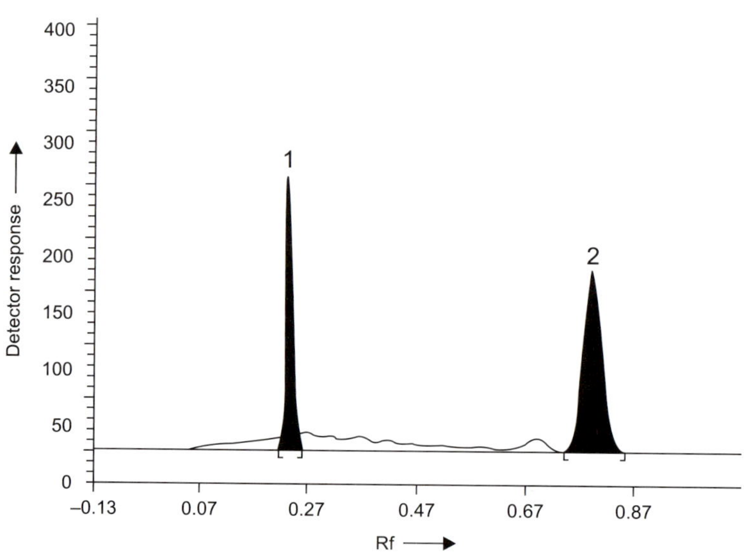

Typical densitogram of the standard containing ciprofloxacin and ornidazole. For detailed experimental and chromatographic conditions, refer to Protocol No. 359. Peaks identification: 1. Ciprofloxacin; 2. Ornidazole.

PROTOCOL FOR HPTLC ANALYSIS OF PHARMACEUTICAL FORMULATION

Protocol No. 359

Formulation: Ciprofloxacin, Ornidazole

Classification: Alimentary System **Dosage form:** Tablets

Standard preparation: Prepare solution of both the compounds in methanol to get 10 μg/ml of ciprofloxacin and 25 μg/ml of ornidazole. Apply varying volumes of each solution (4–14 μl) for linearity profile.

Sample preparation: Powdered sample equivalent to 10 mg of ciprofloxacin suspended in 50 ml of methanol, sonicated for 15 min, diluted to 100 ml. Filtered and 1 ml of the filtrate diluted to 10 ml with methanol and used for chromatographic separation and assay.

Chromatographic equipments:

Sample applicator: Camag Linomat–V

Development chamber: Camag twin-trough glass chamber, 10 × 10 cm

Densitometric scanner: Camag TLC Scanner–III

Chromatographic conditions:

1. Stationary phase: Silica gel $60F_{254}$ pre-coated HPTLC plates, 10 × 10 cm (200 μm) – Merck, pre-washed with methanol, activated at 50°C for 5 min prior to use
2. Mobile phase (MP): n-butanol–ethanol–8M ammonia (5 : 5 : 1.5 v/v)
3. Standard/Sample application:
   Band length: 6 mm Volume applied: 10 μl Spacing: 5 mm
4. Chamber saturation: 30 min (MP)
5. RH (%): 55 ± 5
6. Temperature °C: Ambient
7. Separation technique: Ascending
8. Quantity of mobile phase: 11.5 ml
9. Migration distance: 80 mm
10. Migration time: 20 min

Densitometric evaluation:

Wavelength: UV–315 nm Scanning mode: Reflectance/Absorbance

HRF: Ciprofloxacin—25; Ornidazole—82

Linearity (ng/band): 40–140 for both the compounds

Recovery (%): 99.36–99.96 for both the compounds

References: S.A. Patel and N.J. Patel, *J. Pharm. Research*, **10(4)**, 159–162, 2011.

Comments: The method validated for accuracy, precision, linearity, LOD, LOQ, specificity, robustness and ruggedness.

HPTLC : High Performance Thin Layer Chromatography
HPTLC Densitogram

No. 360

CH_3 N N OCH_3 N F COOH O

Gatifloxacin

OH Cl O_2N N CH_3 N

Ornidazole

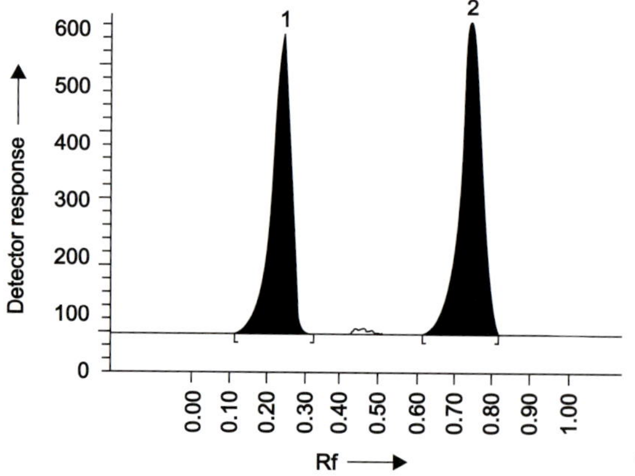

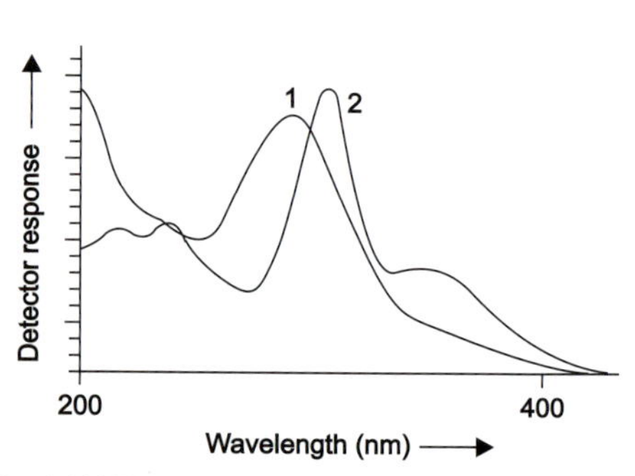

Overlaid UV-spectra of gatifloxacin (1) and ornidazole (2) for selection of optimum wavelength for densitometric scanning

Typical densitogram of the sample containing gatifloxacin and ornidazole. For detailed experimental and chromatographic conditions, refer to Protocol No. 360. Peaks identification: 1. Gatifloxacin; 2. Ornidazole.

PROTOCOL FOR HPTLC ANALYSIS OF PHARMACEUTICAL FORMULATION

Protocol No. 360

Formulation: Gatifloxacin, Ornidazole

Classification: Alimentary System **Dosage form:** Tablets

Standard preparation: Dissolve 10 mg of gatifloxacin and 25 mg of ornidazole in 100 ml of methanol with the aid of sonication (20 min). Dilute 2 ml of the solution to 10 ml to get 20 μg/ml (gatifloxacin) and 50 μg/ml (ornidazole) and use for analysis.

Sample preparation: Powdered sample equivalent to 10 mg of gatifloxacin or 25 mg of ornidazole suspended in 80 ml of methanol, sonicated for 20 min, diluted to 100 ml, filtered and 2 ml of the filtrate diluted to 10 ml with methanol and used for chromatographic application.

Chromatographic equipments:

Sample applicator: Camag Linomat–IV

Development chamber: Camag twin-trough glass chamber, 10 × 10 cm

Densitometric scanner: Camag TLC Scanner–III

Chromatographic conditions:

1. Stationary phase: Silica gel $60F_{254}$ pre-coated TLC plates, 10 × 10 cm (250 μm) – Merck, pre-washed with methanol and air-dried prior to use
2. Mobile phase (MP): (i) n-butanol–methanol–25% ammonia (8 : 1 : 1.5 v/v), (ii) n-butanol–ethanol–8M ammonia (5 : 0.5 : 1.5 v/v)
3. Standard/Sample application:
   Band length: 4 mm Volume applied: 10 μl Spacing: 4 mm
4. Chamber saturation: 45 min (MP)
5. RH (%): 55 ± 5
6. Temperature °C: 25 ± 2
7. Separation technique: Ascending
8. Quantity of mobile phase: 10 ml
9. Migration distance: 45 mm
10. Migration time: 15 min

Densitometric evaluation:

Wavelength: UV–302 nm, 299 nm Scanning mode: Reflectance/Absorbance

HRF: Gatifloxacin—21, 27; Ornidazole—76, 83

Linearity (ng/band): Gatifloxacin—100–500; Ornidazole—250–1250

Recovery (%): Galifloxacin—98.03–100.95; Ornidazole—97.34–101.88

References: B.N. Suhagia, Shailesh A. Shah, I.S. Rathod, Haresh M. Patel, Dinesh R. Shah and Bhavin P. Marolia, *Analytical Science*, **22**, 743–745, 2006; G.N. Oza, S.A. Patel, N.J. Patel, M.R. Patel, Abstract No. 263, 63rd IPC, 2011.

Comments: The method validated for accuracy, precision, linearity, LOD, LOQ, specificity, robustness and ruggedness.

HPTLC : High Performance Thin Layer Chromatography
HPTLC Densitogram

No. 361

Diclofenac sodium

Ornidazole

Gatifloxacin

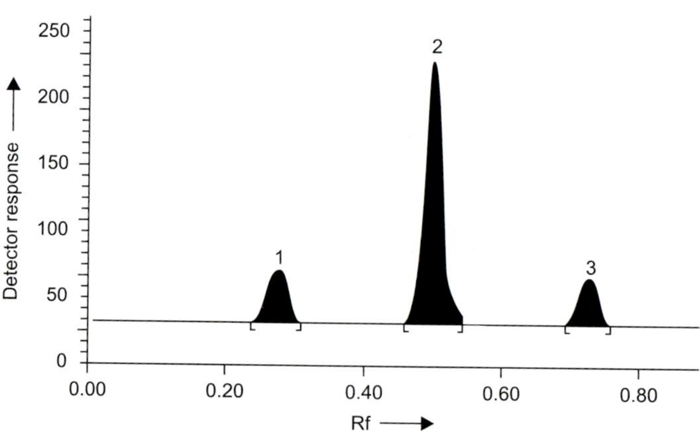

Typical densitogram of the sample containing gatifloxacin and ornidazole. For detailed experimental and chromatographic conditions, refer to Protocol No. 361. Peaks identification: 1. Gatifloxacin; 2. Diclofenac Na^+ (IS); 3. Ornidazole.

PROTOCOL FOR HPTLC ANALYSIS OF PHARMACEUTICAL FORMULATION

Protocol No. 361

Formulation: Gatifloxacin, Ornidazole

Classification: Alimentary System **Dosage form:** Biological sample

Standard preparation: Prepare 1 mg/ml solution of each compound in methanol. Apply varying volumes of each solution for linearity profile.

Sample preparation: After protein precipitation of the plasma, sample extracted with chloroform–formic acid (4 : 0.4 v/v), organic phase separated, evaporated and residue taken up in 1 ml of methanol. Apply 2 μl of reconstituted sample for chromatographic evaluation. Concentration of diclofenac (IS) is constant at 400 ng/band.

Chromatographic equipments:

Sample applicator: Camag Linomat–V

Development chamber: Camag twin-trough glass chamber, 20 × 10 cm

Densitometric scanner: Camag TLC Scanner–III

Chromatographic conditions:

1. Stationary phase: Silica gel $60F_{254}$ pre-coated HPTLC plates, 20 × 10 cm (200 μm) – Merck, pre-washed with methanol and activated at 110°C for 30 min prior to use
2. Mobile phase (MP): (i) Methanol–chloroform–25% ammonia (8.5 : 1 : 0.4); (ii) n-butanol–ethanol–8M ammonia (5 : 0.5 : 1.5 v/v)
3. Standard/Sample application:
   Band length: 6 mm   Volume applied: 2 μl   Spacing: 10 mm
4. Chamber saturation: 20 min (MP)
5. RH (%): 60 ± 5
6. Temperature °C: Ambient
7. Separation technique: Ascending
8. Quantity of mobile phase: 19.8 ml
9. Migration distance: 80 mm
10. Migration time: 15 min

Densitometric evaluation:

Wavelength: UV–297.86 nm (iso-bestic point)

Scanning mode: Reflectance/Absorbance

HRF: Gatifloxacin—28, 27; Diclofenac Na^+ (IS)—50; Ornidazole—77, 83

Linearity: 100–600 ng/band for both the compounds

Recovery (%): 71.79–85.27 for both the compounds

References: Ambadas R. Rote and Prasanna A. Kumbhoje, *J. Chromatography Separation Technique*, 1–4, 2011; and G.N. Oza et al., Abstract No. F-263, 63rd, IPC, 2011.

Comments:

- The method validated for accuracy, precision, linearity, LOD, LOQ, selectivity and extraction efficiency.
- The method is suitable for bioequivalence studies.

HPTLC : High Performance Thin Layer Chromatography
HPTLC Densitogram

No. 362

Cefixime

Ornidazole

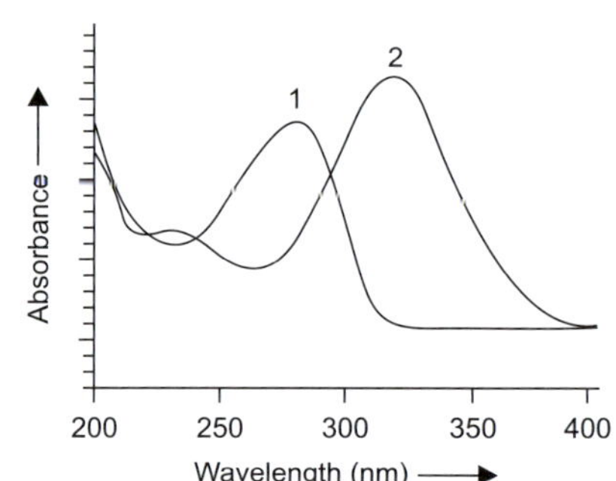

Overlaid UV-spectra of cefixime (1) and ornidazole (2) for selection of suitable wavelength for densitometric scanning

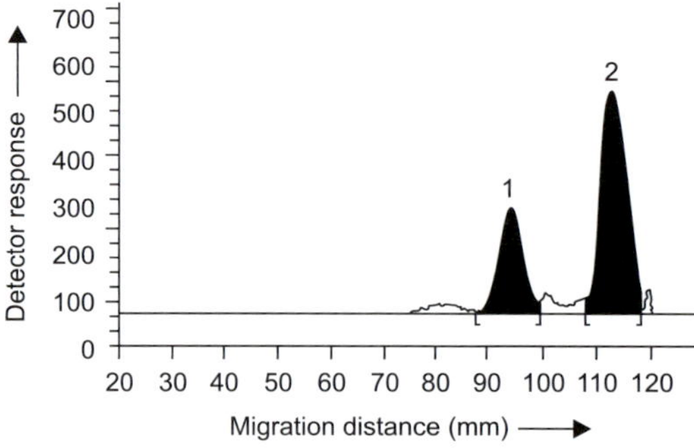

Typical densitogram of the sample containing cefixime and ornidazole. For detailed experimental and chromatographic conditions, refer to Protocol No. 362. Peaks identification: 1. Ornidazole; 2. Cefixime.

PROTOCOL FOR HPTLC ANALYSIS OF PHARMACEUTICAL FORMULATION

Protocol No. 362

Formulation: Ornidazole, Cefixime

Classification: Alimentary System **Dosage form:** Tablets

Standard preparation: Prepare standard solution of both the compounds separately in methanol to get 12.5 mg/ml of ornidazole (ORN) and 5 mg/ml of cefixime (CFX). To get mixed standard, take appropriate volumes of both the solutions and mix to get 250 μg/ml (ORN) and 100 μg/ml (CFX).

Sample preparation: An appropriate weight of the sample is suspended in methanol, sonicated, diluted and filtered. The filtrate suitably diluted for chromatographic application and analysis.

Chromatographic equipments:

Sample applicator: Camag Linomat–IV

Development chamber: Camag twin-trough glass chamber, 10 × 10 cm

Densitometric scanner: Camag TLC Scanner–III

Chromatographic conditions:

1. Stationary phase: Silica gel $60F_{254}$ pre-coated TLC plates, 10 × 10 cm (250 μm) – Merck
2. Mobile phase (MP): Methanol–water (6 : 4 v/v)
3. Standard/Sample application:
   Band length: 10 mm Volume applied: 10 μl Spacing: 16 mm
4. Chamber saturation: 10 min (MP)
5. RH (%): 55 ± 5
6. Temperature °C: 22 ± 2
7. Separation technique: Ascending
8. Quantity of mobile phase: 20 ml
9. Migration distance: 120 mm
10. Migration time: 50 min

Densitometric evaluation:

Wavelength: UV–254 nm Scanning mode: Reflectance/Absorbance

HRF: 1-Ornidazole; 2-Cefixime, see densitogram

Linearity (ng/band): Cefixime—100–900; Ornidazole—250–2500

Recovery (%): 99.06–99.48 for both the compounds

References: N. Sreenath, K. Shivshankar, P. Shanmuga, C. Roosewelt, G. Srinivasa Rao and V. Gunasekaran, *Asian J. Chem.*, **19(5)**, 3621–3626, 2007.

Comments: The method validated for accuracy, precision, linearity, LOD, LOQ, specificity, robustness and ruggedness.

HPTLC : High Performance Thin Layer Chromatography
HPTLC Densitogram

No. 363

Ornidazole

Cefuroxime axetil

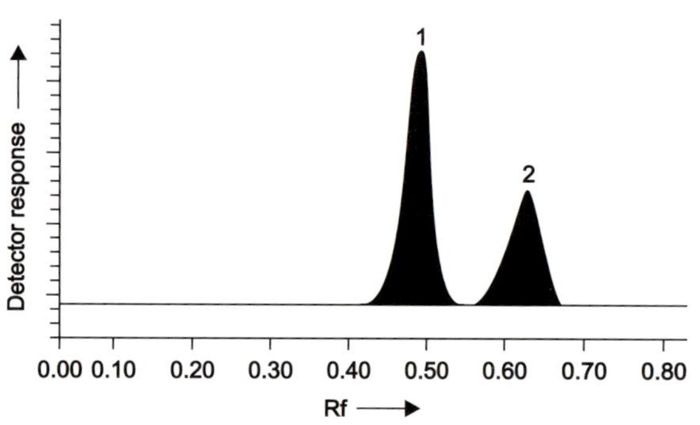

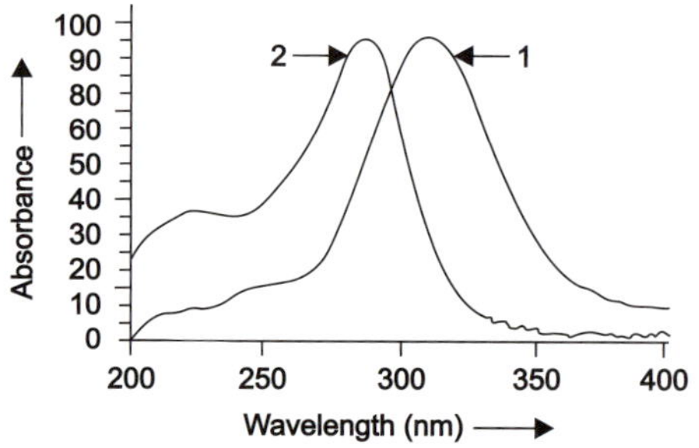

Overlaid UV-spectra of ornidazole (1) and cefuroxime axetil (2) for selection of suitable wavelength for densitometric scanning

Typical densitogram of the sample containing ornidazole and cefuroxime axetil. For detailed experimental and chromatographic conditions, refer to Protocol No. 363. Peaks identification: 1. Ornidazole; 2. Cefuroxime axetil.

PROTOCOL FOR HPTLC ANALYSIS OF PHARMACEUTICAL FORMULATION

Protocol No. 363

Formulation: Ornidazole, Cefuroxime axetil

Classification: Alimentary System **Dosage form:** Tablets

Standard preparation: Prepare 1 mg/ml solution of each compound in methanol. Further serial dilutions made with methanol for linearity studies. Apply 5 µl of each solution.

Sample preparation: Powdered sample equivalent to 50 mg of ornidazole suspended in methanol, sonicated for 5 min, diluted, filtered and further diluted with methanol to get 50 µg/ml (CA) and 100 µg/ml (OR). Apply 4 µl for assay.

Chromatographic equipments:

Sample applicator: Camag Linomat–V

Development chamber: Camag twin-trough glass chamber, 10 × 10 cm

Densitometric scanner: Camag TLC Scanner–III

Chromatographic conditions:

1. Stationary phase: Silica gel $60F_{254}$ pre-coated HPTLC plates, 10 × 10 cm (200 µm) – Merck
2. Mobile phase (MP): Toluene–n-butanol–triethylamine (8.5 : 2 : 0.5 v/v)
3. Standard/Sample application:
   Band length: 5 mm Volume applied: 4 µl Spacing: 5 mm
4. Chamber saturation: 15 min (MP)
5. RH (%): 55 ± 5
6. Temperature °C: 22 ± 2
7. Separation technique: Ascending
8. Quantity of mobile phase: 11 ml
9. Migration distance: 90 mm
10. Migration time: 30 min

Densitometric evaluation:

Wavelength: UV–285 nm Scanning mode: Reflectance/Absorbance

HRF: Ornidazole—50; Cefuroxime axetil—62

Linearity (ng/band): Ornidazole—100–500; Cefuroxime axetil—50–500

Recovery (%): 99.22–101.251 for both the compounds

References: Poonam N. Ranjane, Santosh V. Gandhi, Sayali S. Kadukar and Kailash G. Bothara, *J. Chromatogr. Sci.*, **48(1)**, 26–28, 2010.

Comments: The method validated for accuracy, precision, linearity, LOD, LOQ, specificity, robustness and ruggedness.

HPTLC : High Performance Thin Layer Chromatography
HPTLC Densitogram

No. 364

Pantoprazole sodium

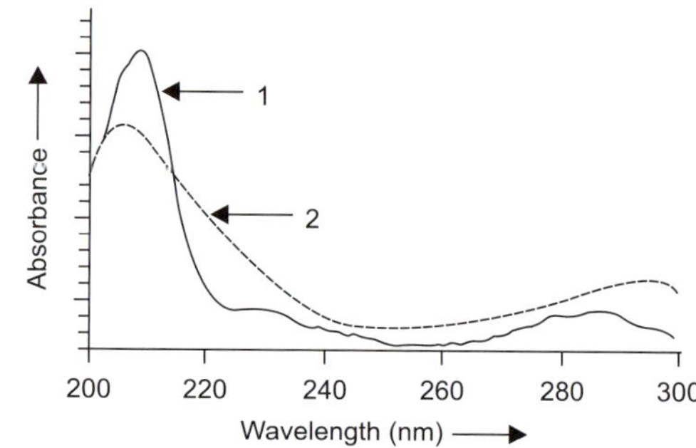

Overlaid UV-spectra of domperidone (1) and pantoprozole (2) for selection of suitable wavelength for densitometric scanning

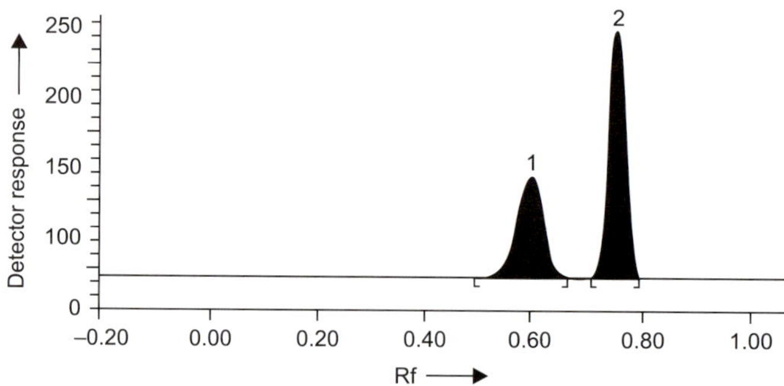

Typical densitogram of the sample containing pantoprazole and domperidone. For detailed experimental and chromatographic conditions, refer to Protocol No. 364. Peaks identification: 1. Domperidone; 2. Pantoprazole sodium.

PROTOCOL FOR HPTLC ANALYSIS OF PHARMACEUTICAL FORMULATION

Protocol No. 364

Formulation: Pantoprazole sodium, Domperidone

Classification: Alimentary System **Dosage form:** Capsules

Standard preparation: Prepare solution of both the compounds in methanol to get 400 μg/ml (pantoprazole) and 300 μg/ml (domperidone). Further dilutions made with methanol to get 80 μg/ml of pantoprazole and 60 μg/ml of domperidone and the resulting solution used for analysis.

Sample preparation: An appropriate weight of the sample suspended in methanol, sonicated for 15 min, diluted, filtered and an appropriate volume spotted for assay.

Chromatographic equipments:

Sample applicator: Camag Linomat–V

Development chamber: Camag twin-trough glass chamber, 10 × 10 cm

Densitometric scanner: Camag TLC Scanner–III

Chromatographic conditions:

1. Stationary phase: Silica gel $60F_{254}$ pre-coated TLC plates, 10 × 10 cm (200 μm) – Merck
2. Mobile phase (MP): Ethyl acetate–methanol (6 : 4 v/v)
3. Standard/Sample application:
   Band length: 6 mm Volume applied: 10 μl Spacing: 8 mm
4. Chamber saturation: 30 min (MP)
5. RH (%): 55 ± 5
6. Temperature °C: 22 ± 2
7. Separation technique: Ascending
8. Quantity of mobile phase: 10 ml
9. Migration distance: 80 mm
10. Migration time: 30 min

Densitometric evaluation:

Wavelength: UV–287 nm Scanning mode: Reflectance/Absorbance

HRF: Domperidone—61; Pantoprazole sodium—76

Linearity (ng/band): Pantoprazole sodium—80–240; Domperidone—60–180

Recovery (%): 99.08–99.35 for both the compounds

References: Bhawesh H. Patel, B.N. Suhagia, M.M. Patel and Jignesh R. Patel, *JAOAC Int.*, **90(1)**, 142–145, 2007.

Comments: The method validated for accuracy, precision, linearity, LOD, LOQ, specificity, robustness and ruggedness.

HPTLC : High Performance Thin Layer Chromatography
HPTLC Densitogram

No. 365

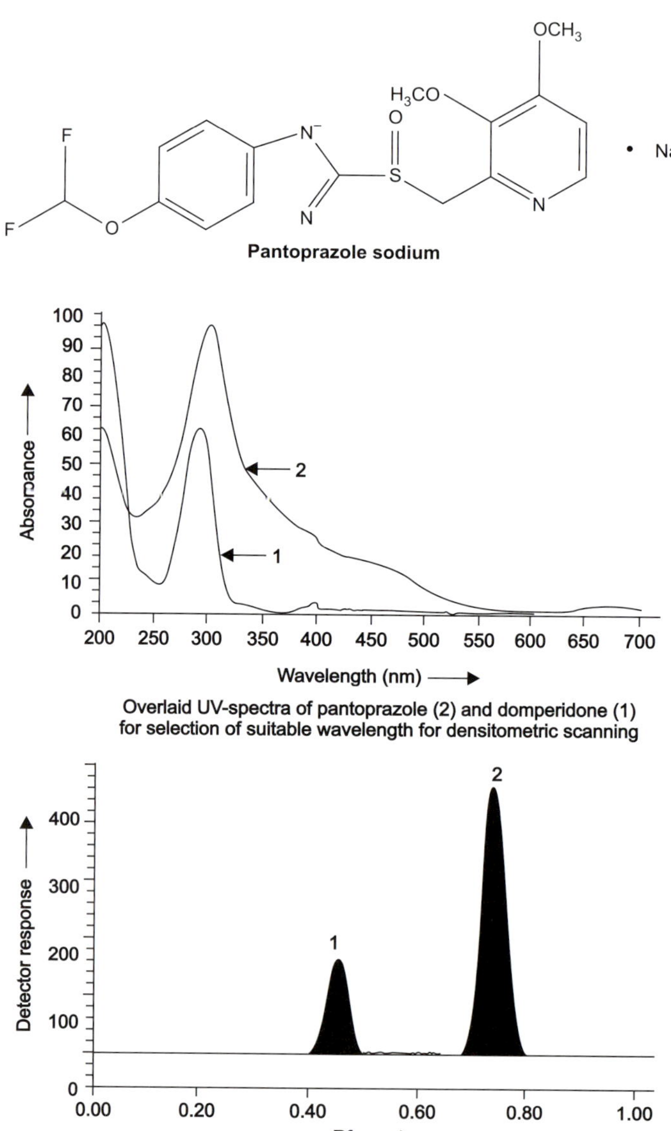

Typical densitogram of the sample containing pantoprazole sodium and domperidone. For detailed experimental and chromatographic conditions, refer to Protocol No. 365. Peaks identification: 1. Domperidone; 2. Pantoprazole Na^+.

PROTOCOL FOR HPTLC ANALYSIS OF PHARMACEUTICAL FORMULATION

Protocol No. 365

Formulation: Pantoprazole sodium, Domperidone

Classification: Alimentary System **Dosage form:** Tablets

Standard preparation: Prepare 1 mg/ml solution of each compound separately in methanol. Further serial dilutions made for linearity profile.

Sample preparation: Powdered sample equivalent to 40 mg of pantoprazole and 10 mg of domperidone suspended in 80 ml of methanol, sonicated for 10 min, diluted and filtered. Apply 6 μl of the resultant solution for assay.

Chromatographic equipments:

Sample applicator: Camag Linomat–V

Development chamber: Camag twin-trough glass chamber, 10 × 20 cm

Densitometric scanner: Camag TLC Scanner–III

Chromatographic conditions:

1. Stationary phase: Silica gel $60F_{254}$ pre-coated HPTLC plates, 10 × 20 cm (200 μm) – Merck, pre-washed with methanol, air dried and stored in desiccator
2. Mobile phase (MP): Methanol–water (5 : 2 v/v), containing 1 g amm. acetate
3. Standard/Sample application:
   Band length: 6 mm Volume applied: 6 μl Spacing: 11.6 mm
4. Chamber saturation: 10 min (MP)
5. RH (%): 55 ± 5
6. Temperature °C: 25 ± 2
7. Separation technique: Ascending
8. Quantity of mobile phase: 15 ml
9. Migration distance: 70 mm
10. Migration time: 20 min

Densitometric evaluation:

Wavelength: UV–286 nm Scanning mode: Reflectance/Absorbance

HRF: Domperidone—42; Pantoprazole Na^+—75

Linearity (μg/band): Pantoprazole—2–10; Domperidone—0.5–2.5

Recovery (%): Pantoprazole Na^+—99.78–99.95; Domperidone—99.64–99.86

References: Seema A. Gosavi, Atul A. Shirkhedkar, Yogini S. Jaiswal and Sanjay J. Surana, *J. Planar Chromatography*, **19(4)**, 302–306, 2006.

Comments: The method validated for accuracy, precision, linearity, LOD, LOQ, specificity, robustness and ruggedness.

HPTLC : High Performance Thin Layer Chromatography
HPTLC Densitogram

No. 366

Domperidone

Pantoprazole sodium

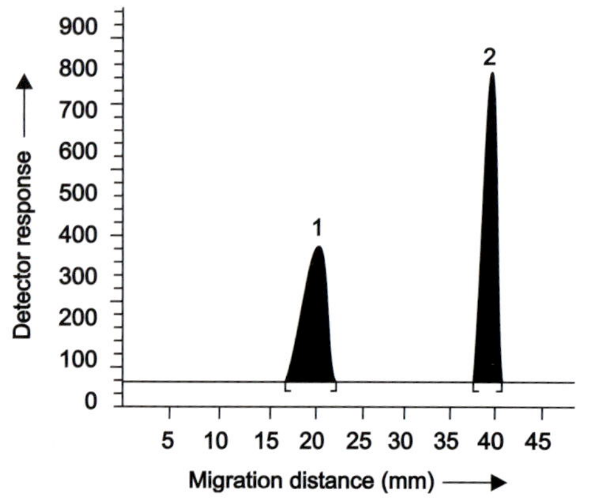

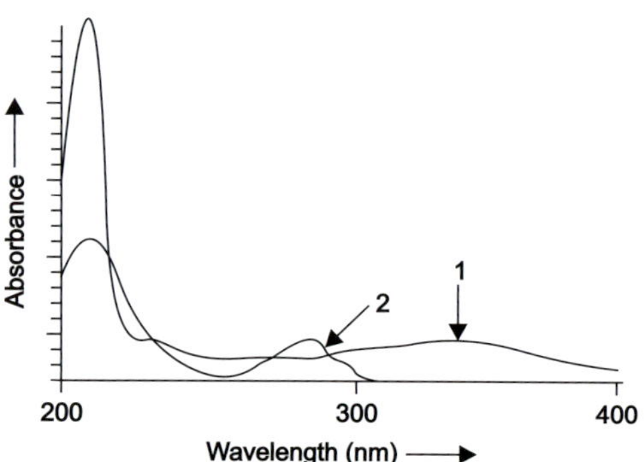

Overlaid UV-spectra of pantoprazole (1) and domperidone (2) for selection of suitable wavelength for densitometric scanning

Typical densitogram of the sample containing pantoprazole Na^{+} and domperidone. For detailed experimental and chromatographic conditions, refer to Protocol No. 366. Peaks identification: 1. Domperidone; 2. Pantoprazole Na^{+}.

PROTOCOL FOR HPTLC ANALYSIS OF PHARMACEUTICAL FORMULATION

Protocol No. 366

Formulation: Pantoprazole sodium, Domperidone

Classification: Alimentary System **Dosage form:** Capsules

Standard preparation: Dissolve separately 20 mg of pantoprazole and 10 mg of domperidone in 50 ml of methanol. Apply 5 μl for chromatographic analysis.

Sample preparation: The sample equivalent to 20 mg of pantoprazole suspended in 30 ml of methanol, shake for 15 min, dilute to 50 ml, filter through Whatman No. 1 filter paper and use the filtrate for analysis.

Chromatographic equipments:

Sample applicator: Camag Linomat–IV

Development chamber: Camag twin-trough glass chamber, 10 × 10 cm

Densitometric scanner: Camag TLC Scanner–III

Chromatographic conditions:

1. Stationary phase: Silica gel $60F_{254}$ pre-coated TLC plates, 10 × 10 cm (250 μm) – Merck
2. Mobile phase (MP): Acetone–toluene–methanol–glacial acetic acid (2 : 8 : 2 : 0.1 v/v)
3. Standard/Sample application:
   Band length: 5 mm Volume applied: 5 μl Spacing: 5 mm
4. Chamber saturation: 15 min (MP)
5. RH (%): 55 ± 5
6. Temperature °C: 25 ± 2
7. Separation technique: Ascending
8. Quantity of mobile phase: 12 ml
9. Migration distance: 70 mm
10. Migration time: 25 min

Densitometric evaluation:

Wavelength: UV–298 nm Scanning mode: Reflectance/Absorbance

HRF: See densitogram

Linearity (μg/ml): Pantoprazole Na^+—2–3.6; Domperidone—1–1.8

Recovery (%): 99.20–100.14 for both the compounds

References: R.B. Kakde, S.N. Gedam and A.V. Kasture, *Asian J. Chem.*, **18(2)**, 1347–1351, 2006.

Comments: The method validated for accuracy, precision, linearity, LOD, LOQ, specificity, robustness and ruggedness.

HPTLC : High Performance Thin Layer Chromatography
HPTLC Densitogram

No. 367

F H$_3$C O NH O N H N Cl O

Mosapride

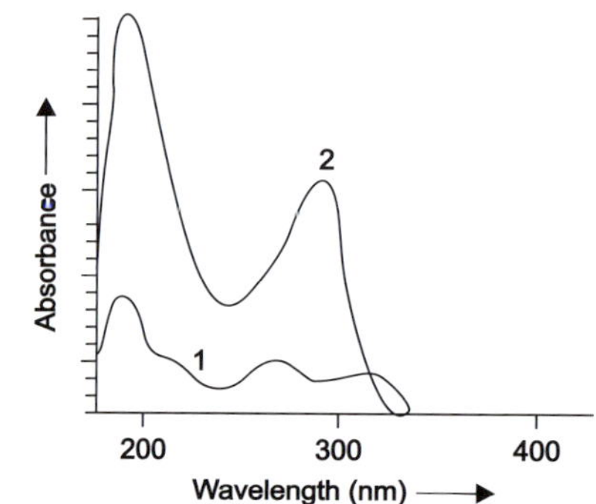

Overlaid UV-spectra of mosapride citrate (1) and pantoprazole Na$^+$ (2) for selection of suitable wavelength for densitometric scanning

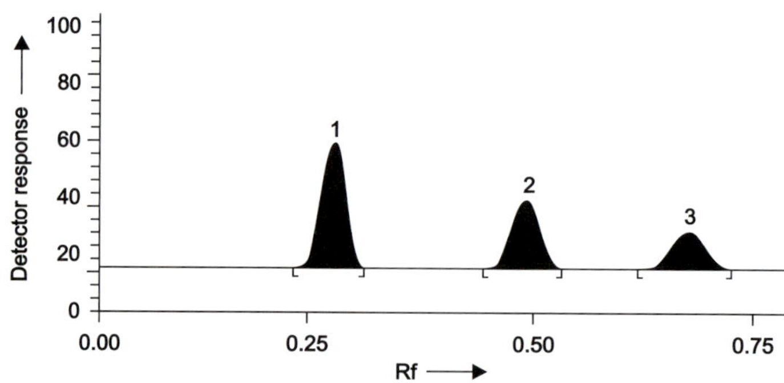

Typical densitogram of the sample containing pantoprazole Na$^+$ and mosapride citrate. For detailed experimental and chromatographic conditions, refer to Protocol No. 367. Peaks identification: 1. Pantoprazole Na$^+$; 2. Mosapride citrate; 3. Loratadine (IS).

PROTOCOL FOR HPTLC ANALYSIS OF PHARMACEUTICAL FORMULATION

Protocol No. 367

Formulation: Pantoprazole sodium, Mosapride citrate

Classification: Alimentary System **Dosage form:** Capsules

Standard preparation: Prepare 100 μg/ml of each compound in methanol. Further dilute with methanol to get 1500 ng/ml of mosapride citrate (MS) and 4000 ng/ml of pantoprazole (PZ). Prepare working standard solution by mixing 1 ml of PZ solution and 1 ml of MS solution, add 1 ml of loratadine solution (500 μg/ml in methanol) as internal standard, dilute to 10 ml with methanol and use for analysis.

Sample preparation: Powdered sample equivalent to 7.5 mg of mosapride citrate suspended in 250 ml of methanol, sonicated for 30 min and diluted to 500 ml. To 1 ml of this solution, add 10 ml of (IS) solution, dilute to 100 ml, filter and apply 10 μl for assay.

Chromatographic equipments:

Sample applicator: Camag Linomat–IV

Development chamber: Camag twin-trough glass chamber, 10 × 10 cm

Densitometric scanner: Camag TLC Scanner–III

Chromatographic conditions:

1. Stationary phase: Silica gel $60F_{254}$ pre-coated HPTLC plates, 10 × 10 cm (200 μm) – Merck, pre-washed with methanol dried (60 min) at 105°C and used
2. Mobile phase (MP): Toluene–acetone–methanol (8 : 2 : 0.5 v/v)
3. Standard/Sample application:
   Band length: 7 mm Volume applied: 10 μl Spacing: 10 mm
4. Chamber saturation: 15 min (MP)
5. RH (%): 55 ± 5
6. Temperature °C: 22 ± 2
7. Separation technique: Ascending
8. Quantity of mobile phase: 10 ml
9. Migration distance: 90 mm
10. Migration time: 40 min

Densitometric evaluation:

Wavelength: UV–254 nm Scanning mode: Reflectance/Absorbance

HRF: Pantoprazole Na^+—26; Mosapride citrate—50; Loratadine (IS)—70

Linearity (μg/ml): Pantoprazole Na^+—0.2–0.6; Mosapride citrate—0.075–225

Recovery (%): Pantoprazole Na^+—99.26–100.75; Mosapride citrate—98.21–100.32

References: N.A. Gomes, V.V. Vaidya, H.S. Karmalkar and G. Gundi, *Indian Drugs*, **44(2)**, 111–116, 2007.

Comments: The method validated for accuracy, precision, linearity, LOD, LOQ, specificity, robustness and ruggedness.

HPTLC : High Performance Thin Layer Chromatography
HPTLC Densitogram

No. 368

Domperidone

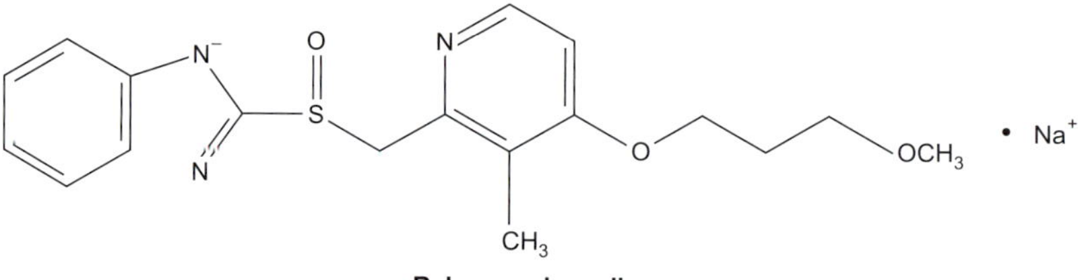

Rabeprazole sodium

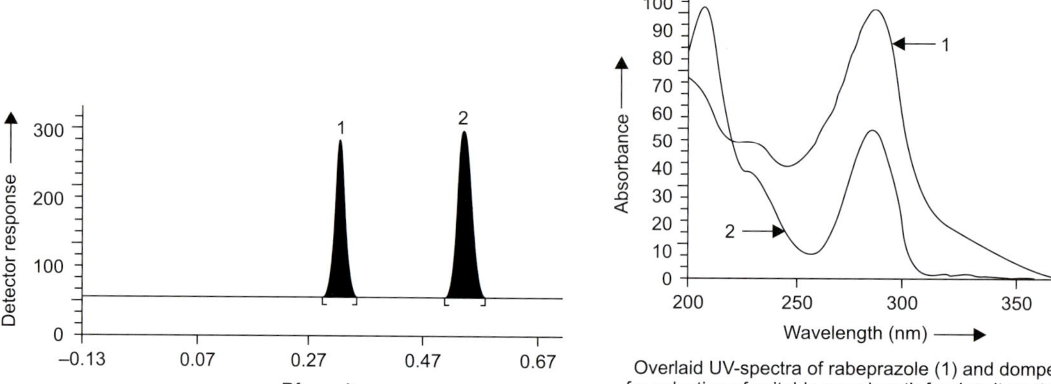

Overlaid UV-spectra of rabeprazole (1) and domperidone (2) for selection of suitable wavelength for densitometric scanning

Typical densitogram of the sample containing rabeprazole Na^+ and domperidone. For detailed experimental and chromatographic conditions, refer to Protocol No. 368. Peaks identification: 1. Domperidone; 2. Rabeprazole Na^+.

PROTOCOL FOR HPTLC ANALYSIS OF PHARMACEUTICAL FORMULATION

Protocol No. 368

Formulation: Rabeprazole sodium, Domperidone

Classification: Alimentary System **Dosage form:** Tablets

Standard preparation: Prepare 1 mg/ml solution of both the compounds in methanol. Further dilutions made to get 100 ng/µl of each solution. Apply varying volumes (0.5–8 µl) for linearity profile.

Sample preparation: Powdered sample equivalent to 20 mg of rabeprazole Na^+ or 10 mg of domperione suspended in 50 ml of methanol, sonicated for 5 min, diluted to 100 ml and filtered through Whatman No. 41 filter paper. The filtrate used for chromatographic separation.

Chromatographic equipments:

Sample applicator: Camag Linomat–V

Development chamber: Camag twin-trough glass chamber, 10 × 10 cm

Densitometric scanner: Camag TLC Scanner–III

Chromatographic conditions:

1. Stationary phase: Silica gel $60F_{254}$ pre-coated TLC plates, 10 × 10 cm (250 µm) – Merck, pre-washed with methanol, activated (110°C) for 5 min, prior to use
2. Mobile phase (MP): Toluene–acetone–methanol (4.5 : 4.5 : 0.5 v/v)
3. Standard/Sample application:
   Band length: 6 mm Volume applied: 0.5–8 µl Spacing: 5 mm
4. Chamber saturation: 5 min (MP)
5. RH (%): 55 ± 5
6. Temperature °C: 22 ± 2
7. Separation technique: Ascending
8. Quantity of mobile phase: 9.5 ml
9. Migration distance: 90 mm
10. Migration time: 15 min

Densitometric evaluation:

Wavelength: UV–285 nm Scanning mode: Reflectance/Absorbance

HRF: Domperidone—32; Rabeprazole Na^+—53

Linearity: 50–800 ng/band for both the drugs

Recovery (%): Rabeprazole Na^+—99.62–100.06; Domperidone—99.78–99.93

References: Santosh V. Gandhi, Samina I. Khan, Rashmi T. Jadhav, Saket S. Jadhav and Gaurav A. Yadhav, *JAOAC Int.*, **92(4)**, 1064, 2009.

Comments: The method validated for accuracy, precision, linearity, LOD, LOQ, specificity, robustness and ruggedness.

HPTLC : High Performance Thin Layer Chromatography
HPTLC Densitogram

No. 369

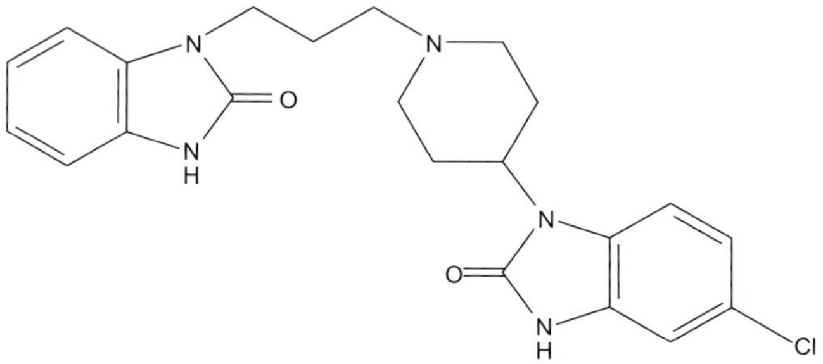

Domperidone

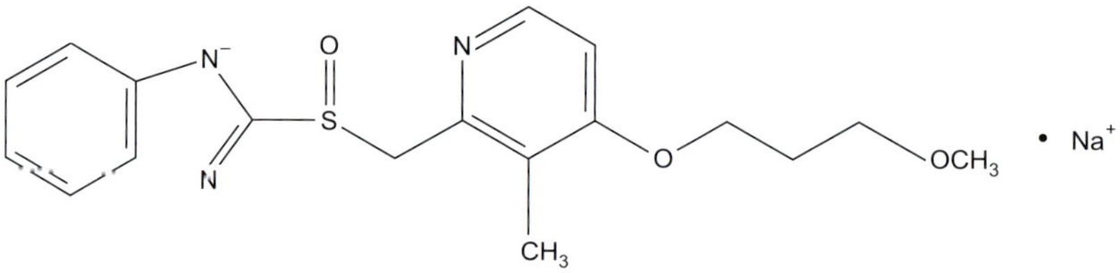

Rabeprazole sodium

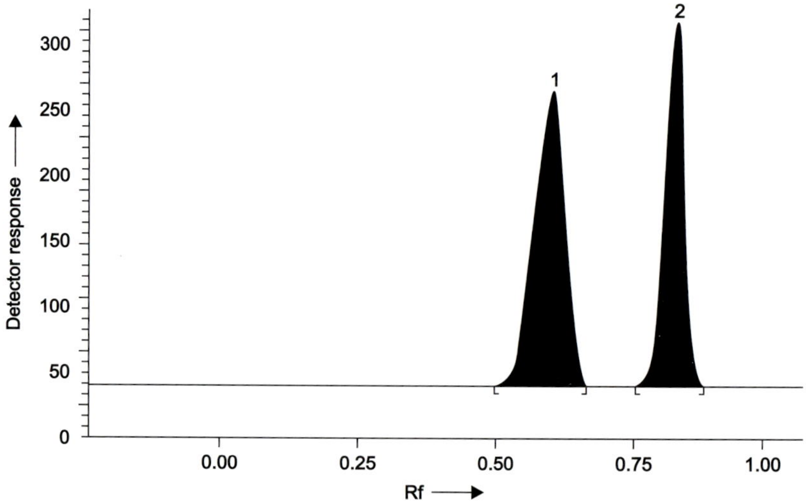

Typical densitogram of the sample containing rabeprazole Na^+ and domperidone. For detailed experimental and chromatographic conditions, refer to Protocol No. 369. Peaks identification: 1. Domperidone; 2. Rabeprazole Na^+.

PROTOCOL FOR HPTLC ANALYSIS OF PHARMACEUTICAL FORMULATION

Protocol No. 369

Formulation: Rabeprazole sodium, Domperidone

Classification: Alimentary System **Dosage form:** Capsules

Standard preparation: Dissolve 200 mg of rabeprazole and 300 mg of domperidone in methanol to produce 100 ml to get 2000 μg/ml (rabeprazole Na^+) and 3000 μg/ml (domperidone). Dilute 1 ml of each solution to 10 ml with methanol and use for HPTLC analysis.

Sample preparation: An appropriate quantity of the sample suspended in 80 ml of methanol, sonicated for 15 min, diluted to 100 ml, filtered through 0.2 μm membrane filter and used for analysis.

Chromatographic equipments:

Sample applicator: Camag Linomat–V

Development chamber: Camag twin-trough glass chamber, 20 × 10 cm

Densitometric scanner: Camag TLC Scanner–III

Chromatographic conditions:

1. Stationary phase: Silica gel $60F_{254}$ pre-coated TLC plates, 20 × 10 cm (250 μm) – Merck, pre-washed with MP, dried (120°C) for 20 min before sample loading
2. Mobile phase (MP): Etylacetate–methanol–benzene–acetonitrile (3 : 2 : 3 : 2 v/v)
3. Standard/Sample application:
   Band length: 6 mm Volume applied: 2–6 μl Spacing: 8 mm
4. Chamber saturation: 30 min (MP)
5. RH (%): 55 ± 5
6. Temperature °C: 22 ± 2
7. Separation technique: Ascending
8. Quantity of mobile phase: 20 ml
9. Migration distance: 80 mm
10. Migration time: 35 min

Densitometric evaluation:

Wavelength: UV–287 nm Scanning mode: Reflectance/Absorbance

HRF: Domperidone—53; Rabeprazole Na^+—78

Linearity (ng/band): Rabeprazole Na^+—400–1200; Domperidone—600–1800

Recovery (%): 99.43–99.82 for both the compounds

References: Bhavesh H. Patel, B.N. Suhagia, M.M. Patel and Jignesh R. Patel, *J. Chromatogr. Sci.*, **46(4)**, 304–307, 2008.

Comments: The method validated for accuracy, precision, linearity, LOD, LOQ, specificity, robustness and ruggedness.

HPTLC : High Performance Thin Layer Chromatography
HPTLC Densitogram

No. 370

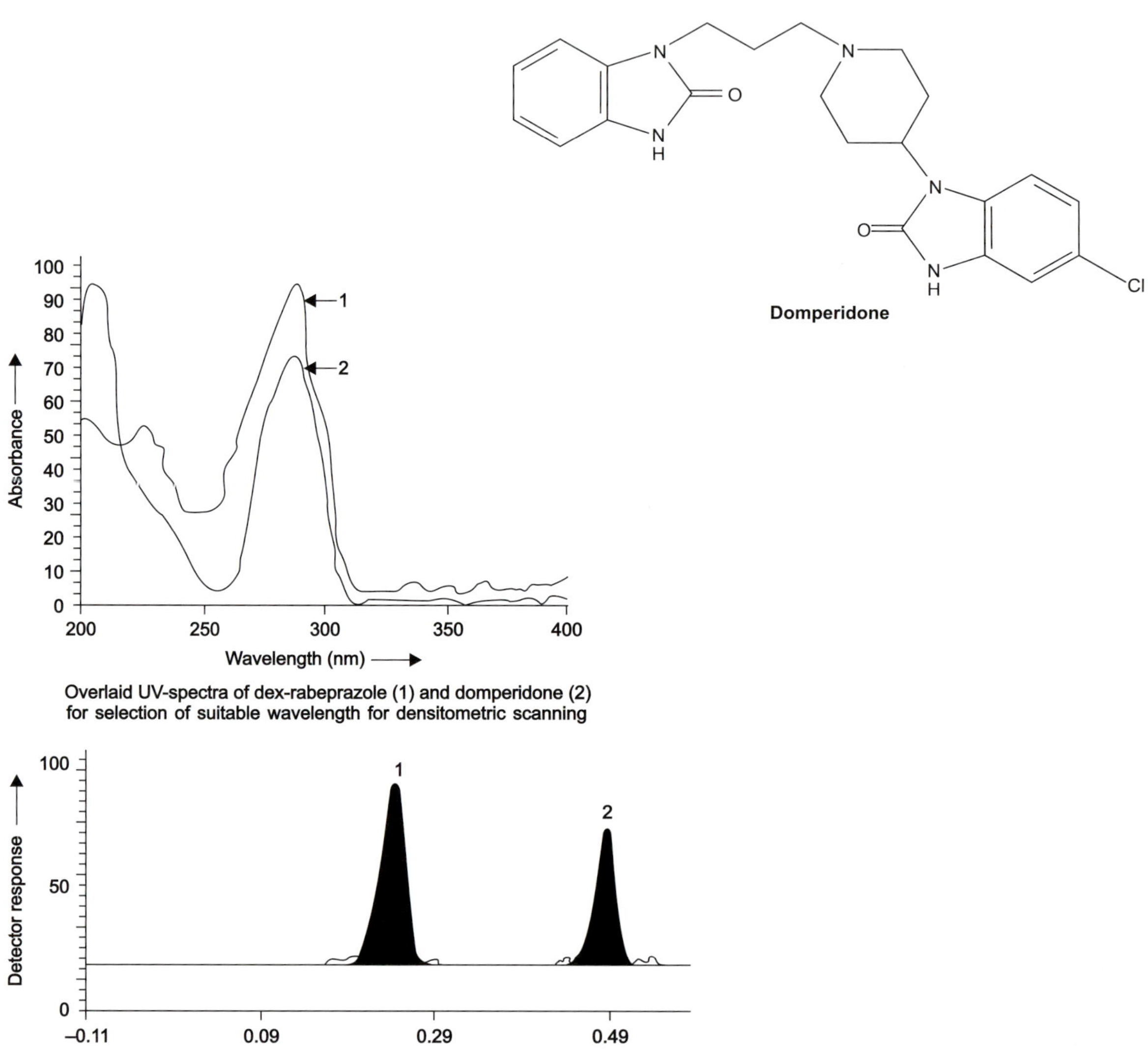

Overlaid UV-spectra of dex-rabeprazole (1) and domperidone (2) for selection of suitable wavelength for densitometric scanning

Typical densitogram of the standard containing domperidone and dex-rabeprazole Na^+. For detailed experimental and chromatographic conditions, refer to Protocol No. 370. Peaks identification: 1. Domperidone; 2. Dex-rabeprazole Na^+.

PROTOCOL FOR HPTLC ANALYSIS OF PHARMACEUTICAL FORMULATION

Protocol No. 370

Formulation: **Dex-Rabeprazole sodium, Domperidone**
Classification: Alimentary System **Dosage form:** Capsules
Standard preparation: Prepare 100 μg/ml solution of each compound separately in methanol. Apply varying volumes of each solution for linearity profile and carry out the chromatographic analysis.
Sample preparation: Powdered sample equivalent to 5 mg of dex-rabeprazole or 15 mg of domperidone suspended in 30 ml of methanol, sonicated for 20 min, diluted to 50 ml with methanol, filtered and the filtrate subjected to chromatographic analysis.
Chromatographic equipments:
Sample applicator: Camag Linomat–V
Development chamber: Camag twin-trough glass chamber, 10 × 10 cm
Densitometric scanner: Camag TLC Scanner–III
Chromatographic conditions:
1. Stationary phase: Silica gel 60F_{254} pre-coated TLC plates, 10 × 10 cm (250 μm) – Merck
2. Mobile phase (MP): Acetone–toluene–methanol (4.5 : 4.5 : 0.5 v/v)
3. Standard/Sample application:
   Band length: 5 mm Volume applied: 0.5–10 μl Spacing: 10 mm
4. Chamber saturation: 30 min (MP)
5. RH (%): 55 ± 5
6. Temperature °C: 22 ± 2
7. Separation technique: Ascending
8. Quantity of mobile phase: 9.5 ml
9. Migration distance: —
10. Migration time: —

Densitometric evaluation:
Wavelength: UV–285 nm Scanning mode: Reflectance/Absorbance
HRF: Domperidone—24; Dex-Rabeprazole—49
Linearity (ng/band): Dex-Rabeprazole—50–350; Domperidone—100–700
Recovery (%): Dex-Rabeprazole—99.29–100.39; Domperidone—100.28–100.67
References: Sohan S. Chitlange, Amir Mulla, Ganesh R. Pawbake and Sagar B. Wankhede, *Preparative Biochem. and Biotechnology*, **40**, 337–346, 2010.
Comments:
- The method validated for accuracy, precision, linearity, LOD, LOQ, specificity, robustness and ruggedness.
- The method is stability indicating (acid, base, oxidative, thermal, photolytic). The degradation products were separated from main compounds.

HPTLC : High Performance Thin Layer Chromatography
HPTLC Densitogram

No. 371

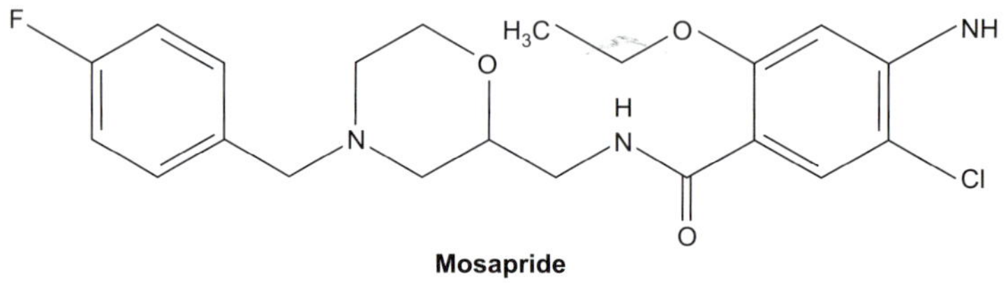

Mosapride

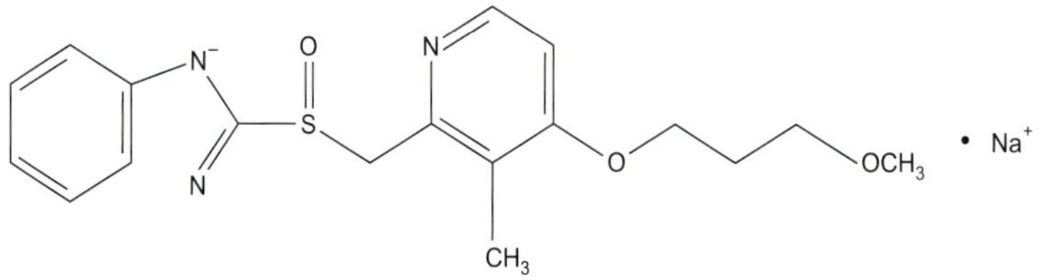

Rabeprazole sodium

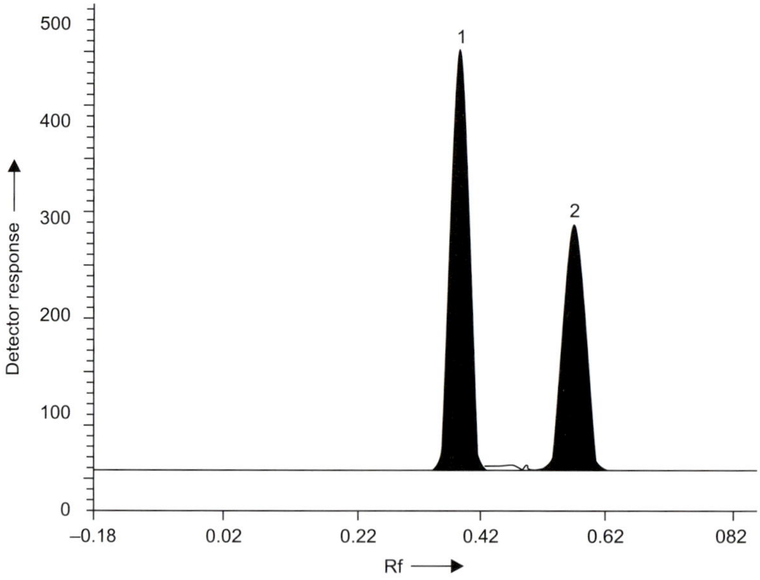

Typical densitogram of the sample containing rabeprazole and mosapride citrate. For detailed experimental and chromatographic conditions, refer to Protocol No. 371. Peaks identification: 1. Rabeprazole; 2. Mosapride citrate.

PROTOCOL FOR HPTLC ANALYSIS OF PHARMACEUTICAL FORMULATION

Protocol No. 371

Formulation: Rabeprazole sodium, Mosapride citrate

Classification: Alimentary System **Dosage form:** Capsules

Standard preparation: Dissolve 20 mg of rabeprazole and 15 mg of mosapride citrate in 50 ml of methanol with the aid of sonication for 20 min. An aliquot (1 ml) was further diluted with methanol to produce 10 ml to get final concentration of 40 μg/ml (rabeprazole) and 30 μg/ml (mosapride). Apply 10 μl for analysis.

Sample preparation: Sample equivalent to 20 mg of rabeprazole and 15 mg of mosapride suspended in 40 ml of methanol, sonicated for 20 min, diluted to 50 ml, filtered through Whatman No. 41 filter paper. 1 ml of the filtrate diluted to 10 ml with methanol and used for chromatographic analysis.

Chromatographic equipments:

Sample applicator: Camag Linomat–V

Development chamber: Camag twin-trough glass chamber, 20 × 20 cm

Densitometric scanner: Camag TLC Scanner–III

Chromatographic conditions:

1. Stationary phase: Silica gel $60F_{254}$ pre-coated TLC plates, 20 × 20 cm (250 μm) – Merck, pre-washed with methanol and air dried prior to use
2. Mobile phase (MP): Ethyl acetate–benzene–methanol (2 : 2.5 : 0.5 v/v)
3. Standard/Sample application:
   Band length: 4 mm Volume applied: 10 μl Spacing: 4 mm
4. Chamber saturation: 45 min (MP)
5. RH (%): —
6. Temperature °C: 25 ± 2
7. Separation technique: Ascending
8. Quantity of mobile phase: 10 ml
9. Migration distance: 75 mm
10. Migration time: 30 min

Densitometric evaluation:

Wavelength: UV–276 nm Scanning mode: Reflectance/Absorbance

HRF: Rabeprazole—41; Mosapride citrate—61

Linearity (ng/band): Rabeprazole—400–1200; Mosapride citrate—300–900

Recovery (%): Rabeprazole—99.18–99.85; Mosapride citrate—99.13–99.63

References: Bhavesh H. Patel, B.N. Suhagia, M.M. Patel and J.R. Patel, *J. Chromatographic Sci.*, **46(1)**, 10–14, 2008.

Comments: The method validated for accuracy, precision, linearity, LOD, LOQ, specificity, robustness and ruggedness.

HPTLC : High Performance Thin Layer Chromatography
HPTLC Densitogram

No. 372

HCl

Itopride hydrochloride

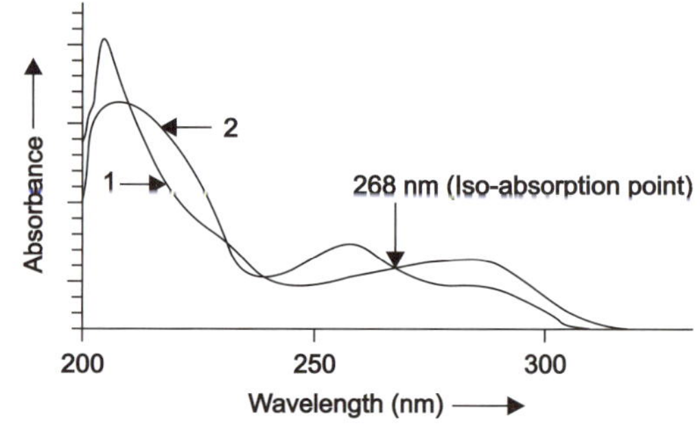

Overlaid UV-spectra of rabeprazole Na^{+} (1) and itopride (2) for selection of suitable wavelength for densitometric scanning

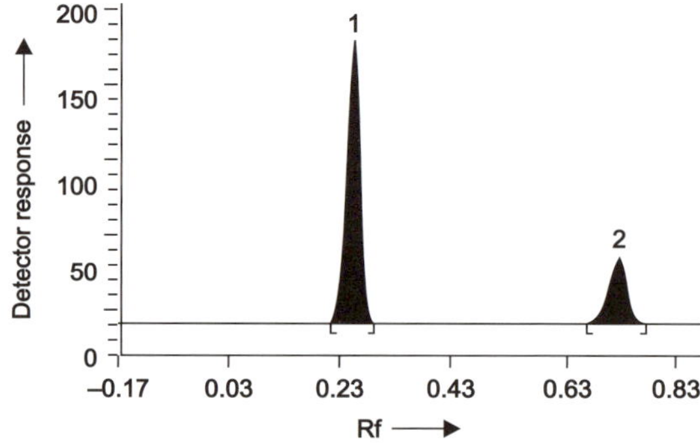

Typical densitogram of the sample containing rabeprazole and itopride HCl. For detailed experimental and chromatographic conditions, refer to Protocol No. 372. Peaks identification: 1. Rabeprazole; 2. Itopride HCl.

PROTOCOL FOR HPTLC ANALYSIS OF PHARMACEUTICAL FORMULATION

Protocol No. 372

Formulation: Rabeprazole sodium, Itopride hydrochloride

Classification: Alimentary System **Dosage form:** Tablets

Standard preparation: The standard solutions of both the compounds were prepared in methanol to get 200 μg/ml (rabeprazole) and 1500 μg/ml (itopride HCl). Further serial dilutions made for linearity profile.

Sample preparation: An appropriate amount of the powdered sample extracted with methanol, filtered through Whatman No. 41 filter paper. 0.8 μl of the solution containing 160 ng of rabeprazole and 1200 ng of itopride HCl was applied to the plate for analysis.

Chromatographic equipments:

Sample applicator: Camag Linomat–V

Development chamber: Camag twin-trough glass chamber, 10 × 10 cm

Densitometric scanner: Camag TLC Scanner–III

Chromatographic conditions:

1. Stationary phase: Silica gel $60F_{254}$ pre-coated TLC plates, 10 × 10 cm (250 μm) – Merck, pre-washed with methanol, activated (110°C) for 30 min, prior to use
2. Mobile phase (MP): n-butanol–toluene–25% ammonia (8.5 : 0.5 : 1 v/v)
3. Standard/Sample application:
   Band length: 6 mm Volume applied: 0.8 μl Spacing: 5 mm
4. Chamber saturation: 30 min (MP)
5. RH (%): 55 ± 5
6. Temperature °C: 22 ± 2
7. Separation technique: Ascending
8. Quantity of mobile phase: 10 ml
9. Migration distance: 85 mm
10. Migration time: 35 min

Densitometric evaluation:

Wavelength: UV–268 nm Scanning mode: Reflectance/Absorbance

HRF: Rabeprazole—24; Itopride HCl—75

Linearity (ng/band): Rabeprazole—40–200; Itopride HCl—300–1500

Recovery (%): Rabeprazole—100.80–101.04; Itopride HCl—99.19–100.61

References: A. Suganthi, Sofiya John and T.K. Ravi, *Ind. J. Pharm Sci.*, **70(3)**, 366–368, 2008.

Comments: The method validated for accuracy, precision, linearity, LOD, LOQ, specificity, robustness and ruggedness.

HPTLC : High Performance Thin Layer Chromatography
HPTLC Densitogram

No. 373

HCl

Itopride hydrochloride

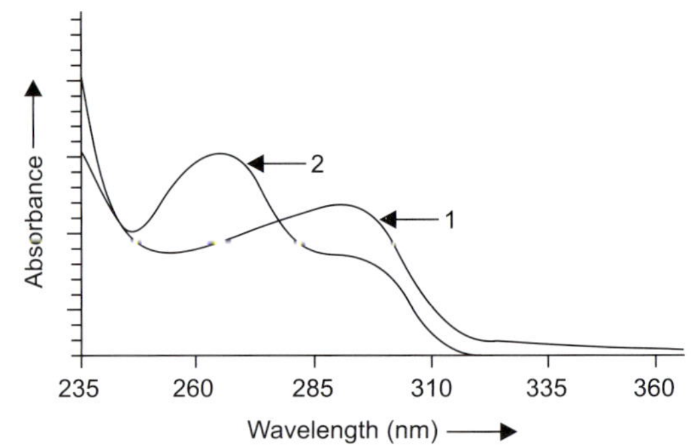

Overlaid UV-spectra of rabeprazole sodium (1) and itopride hydrochloride (2) for selection of suitable wavelength for densitometric scanning

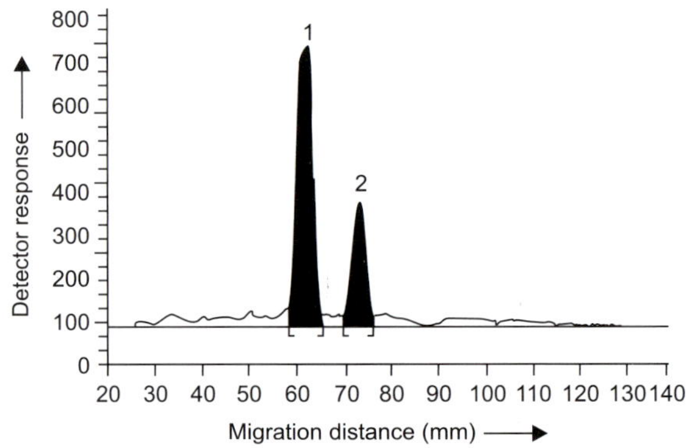

Typical densitogram of the sample containing rabeprazole sodium and itopride hydrochloride. For detailed experimental and chromatographic conditions, refer to Protocol No. 373. Peaks identification: 1. Itopride HCl; 2. Rabeprazole Na^+.

PROTOCOL FOR HPTLC ANALYSIS OF PHARMACEUTICAL FORMULATION

Protocol No. 373

Formulation: Rabeprazole sodium, Itopride hydrochloride

Classification: Alimentary System **Dosage form:** Capsules

Standard preparation: Prepare standard solution of both the compounds in methanol to get 2 mg/ml rabeprazole sodium, 15 mg/ml itopride hydrochloride. Further serial dilutions (900–1900 μg/ml) of itopride HCl and 120–280 μg/ml of rabeprazole Na^+ were prepared in methanol. Apply 10 μl of each solution for linearity profile.

Sample preparation: The sample equivalent to 20 mg of rabeprazole suspended in 80 ml of methanol, sonicated for 15 min, diluted to 100 ml, filtered and used as sample solution for chromatographic analysis.

Chromatographic equipments:

Sample applicator: Camag Linomat–IV

Development chamber: Camag twin-trough glass chamber, 10 × 10 cm

Densitometric scanner: Camag TLC Scanner–III

Chromatographic conditions:

1. Stationary phase: Silica gel $60F_{254}$ pre-coated HPTLC plates, 10 × 10 cm (200 μm) – Merck
2. Mobile phase (MP): Toluene–chloroform–methanol–25% ammonia (5 : 6 : 2 : 0.2 v/v)
3. Standard/Sample application:
   Band length: 10 mm Volume applied: 10 μl Spacing: 19 mm
4. Chamber saturation: 20 min (MP)
5. RH (%): 55 ± 5
6. Temperature °C: 22 ± 2
7. Separation technique: Ascending
8. Quantity of mobile phase: 13 ml
9. Migration distance: 80 mm
10. Migration time: 35 min

Densitometric evaluation:

Wavelength: UV–225 nm Scanning mode: Reflectance/Absorbance

HRF: 1. Itopride HCl; 2. Rabeprazole Na^+; see densitogram

Linearity (ng/band): Rabeprazole Na^+—120–280; Itopride hydrochloride—900–1900

Recovery (%): 98.14–99.35 for both the compounds

References: S.D. Mageswari, K. Surendra, R. Maheswari, N. Hari Krishanan, C. Roosewelt and V. Gunasekaran, *Asian J. Chem.*, **19(7)**, 5634–5638, 2007.

Comments: The method validated for accuracy, precision, linearity, LOD, LOQ, specificity, robustness and ruggedness.

HPTLC : High Performance Thin Layer Chromatography
HPTLC Densitogram

No. 374

Rabeprazole sodium

Ondansetron

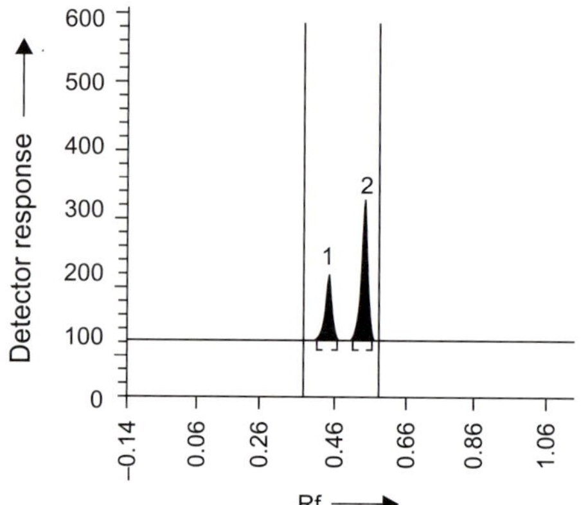

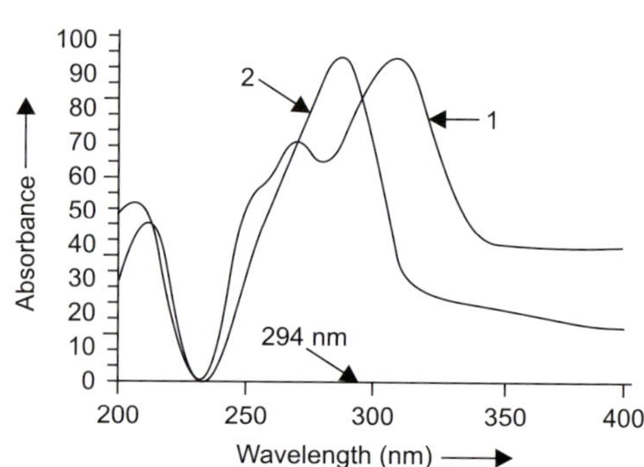

Overlaid UV-spectra of rabeprazole (1) and ondansetron (2) for selection of suitable wavelength for densitometric scanning

Typical densitogram of the sample containing rabeprazole and ondansetron. For detailed experimental and chromatographic conditions, refer to Protocol No. 374. Peaks identification: 1. Ondansetron; 2. Rabeprazole Na^{+}.

PROTOCOL FOR HPTLC ANALYSIS OF PHARMACEUTICAL FORMULATION

Protocol No. 374

Formulation: Rabeprazole sodium, Ondansetron

Classification: Alimentary System **Dosage form:** Capsules

Standard preparation: Standard solution of both the compounds prepared in methanol to get 500 μg/ml of each. Further dilutions made to get 0.05 μg/ml for rabeprazole and 0.015 μg/ml for ondansetron and used for analysis.

Sample preparation: Powdered sample equivalent to 20 mg of rabeprazole or 6 mg of ondansetron suspended in methanol, sonicated for 15 min, diluted, filtered and filtrate suitably diluted to get final concentration of 0.5 μg/ml (rabeprazole) and 0.015 μg/ml (ondansetron). Apply 6 μl for assay.

Chromatographic equipments:

Sample applicator: Camag Linomat–V

Development chamber: Camag twin-trough glass chamber, 10 × 20 cm

Densitometric scanner: Camag TLC Scanner–III

Chromatographic conditions:

1. Stationary phase: Silica gel $60F_{254}$ pre-coated HPTLC plates, 10 × 20 cm (200 μm) – Merck, pre-washed with methanol, activated prior to use
2. Mobile phase (MP): Dichloromethane–methanol (9 : 1 v/v)
3. Standard/Sample application:
   Band length: 5 mm Volume applied: 6 μl Spacing: 14.1 mm
4. Chamber saturation: 20 min (MP)
5. RH (%): 55 ± 5
6. Temperature °C: 22 ± 2
7. Separation technique: Ascending
8. Quantity of mobile phase: 20 ml
9. Migration distance: 80 mm
10. Migration time: 35 min

Densitometric evaluation:

Wavelength: UV–294 nm Scanning mode: Reflectance/Absorbance

HRF: Ondansetron—41; Rabeprazole Na^+—51

Linearity: 100–500 ng/band for both the compounds

Recovery (%): 99.83–99.96 for both the compounds

References: P.B. Raval Manisha Puranik, S.J. Wadher and P.G. Yeole, *Ind. J. Pharm. Sci.*, **70(3)**, 386–390, 2008.

Comments: The method validated for accuracy, precision, linearity, LOD, LOQ, specificity, robustness and ruggedness.

HPTLC : High Performance Thin Layer Chromatography
HPTLC Densitogram

No. 375

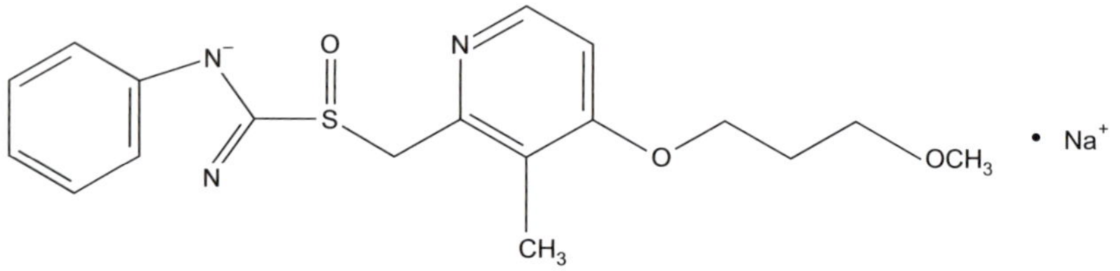

Rabeprazole sodium

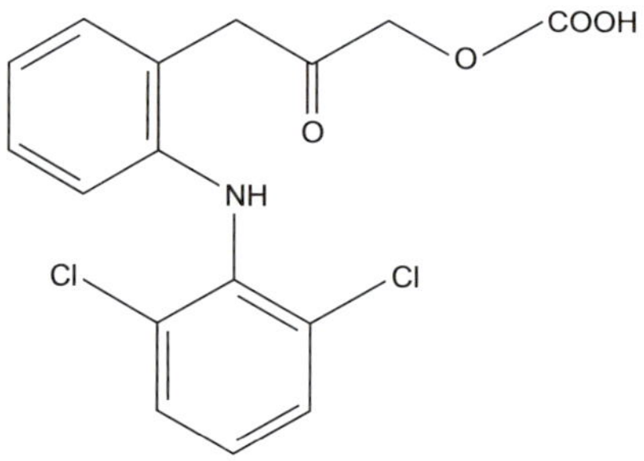

Aceclofenac

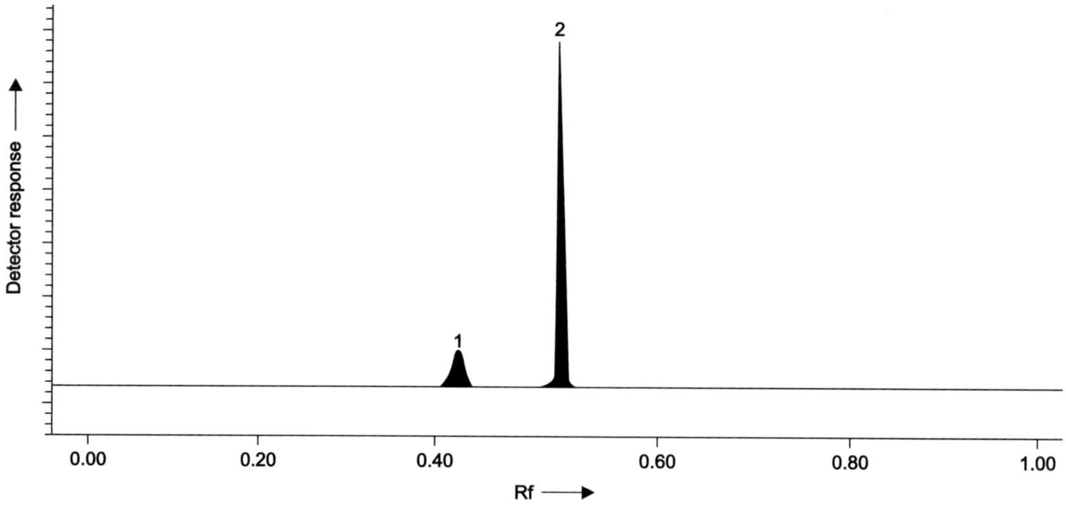

Typical densitogram of the standard containing rabeprazole sodium and aceclofenac. For detailed experimental and chromatographic conditions, refer to Protocol No. 375. Peaks identification: 1. Rabeprazole sodium; 2. Aceclofenac.

PROTOCOL FOR HPTLC ANALYSIS OF PHARMACEUTICAL FORMULATION

Protocol No. 375

Formulation: Rabeprazole sodium, Aceclofenac

Classification: Alimentary System **Dosage form:** Capsules

Standard preparation: Prepare 100 μg/ml solution of each compound in methanol. Apply varying amounts of each solution for linearity profile.

Sample preparation: The sample equivalent to 20 mg of rabeprazole or 200 mg of aceclofenac suspended in methanol, sonicated for 30 min, suitably diluted, filtered and the filtrage further suitably diluted for chromatographic analysis.

Chromatographic equipments:

Sample applicator: Camag Linomat–V

Development chamber: Camag twin-trough glass chamber, 20 × 10 cm

Densitometric scanner: Camag TLC Scanner–III

Chromatographic conditions:

1. Stationary phase: Silica gel 60F_{254} pre-coated TLC plates, 20 × 10 cm (250 μm) – Merck, pre-washed with methanol, activated at 110°C for 5 min, prior to use glacial acetic acid
2. Mobile phase (MP): Toluene–ethyl acetate–methanol (6 : 4 : 1 : 0.2 v/v)
3. Standard/Sample application:
   Band length: 6 mm Volume applied: — Spacing: 6 mm
4. Chamber saturation: 30 min (MP)
5. RH (%): 65 ± 5
6. Temperature °C: 25 ± 2
7. Separation technique: Ascending
8. Quantity of mobile phase: 22 ml
9. Migration distance: 80 mm
10. Migration time: 20 min

Densitometric evaluation:

Wavelength: UV–279 nm Scanning mode: Reflectance/Absorbance

HRF: Rabeprazole sodium—43; Aceclofenac—57

Linearity (ng/band): Rabeprazole sodium—100–200; Aceclofenac—1000–200

Recovery (%): Rabeprazole sodium—98.32–99.53; Aceclofenac—99.87–100.16

References: Vishal V. Bharekar, Toufik S. Mulla, Savita S. Yadav, Milind P. Rajput and Janhavi R. Rao, *Int. J. Comprehensive Pharmacy*, 2011.

Comments: The method validated for accuracy, precision, linearity, LOD, LOQ, specificity, robustness and ruggedness.

HPTLC : High Performance Thin Layer Chromatography
HPTLC Densitogram

No. 376

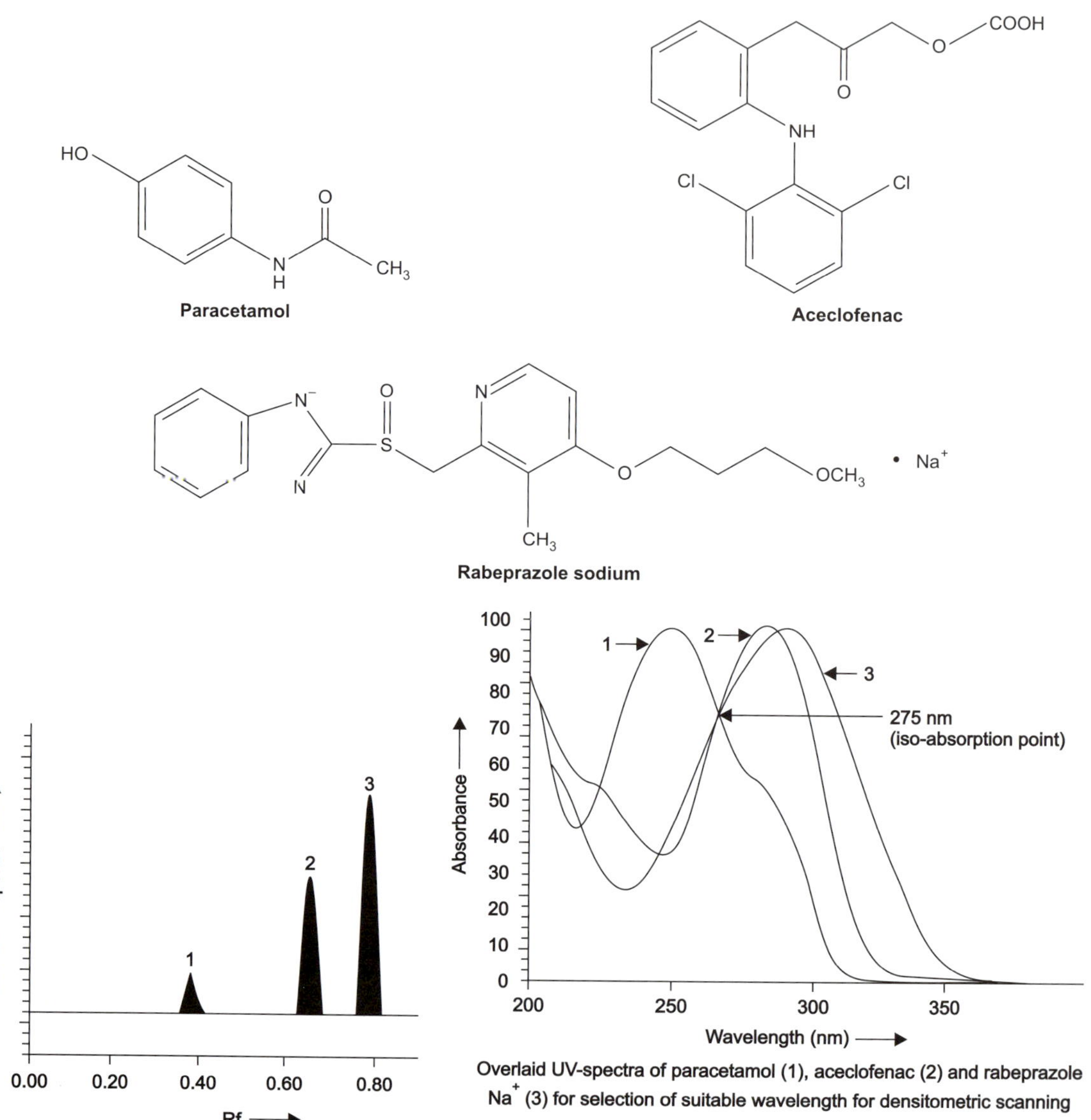

Overlaid UV-spectra of paracetamol (1), aceclofenac (2) and rabeprazole Na^{+} (3) for selection of suitable wavelength for densitometric scanning

Typical densitogram of the standard containing paracetamol, aceclofenac and rabeprazole. For detailed experimental and chromatographic conditions, refer to Protocol No. 376. Peaks identification: 1. Rabeprazole sodium; 2. Aceclofenac; 3. Paracetamol.

PROTOCOL FOR HPTLC ANALYSIS OF PHARMACEUTICAL FORMULATION

Protocol No. 376

Formulation: **Rabeprazole sodium, Aceclofenac, Paracetamol**

Classification: Alimentary System **Dosage form:** Tablets

Standard preparation: Prepare solution of each compound separately in methanol to get 50 mg/ml of paracetamol, 10 mg/ml of aceclofenac and 1 mg/ml of rabeprazole. These solutions further diluted to get 100–500 μg/ml of paracetamol, 20–100 μg/ml of aceclofenac and 2–10 μg/ml of rabeprazole. Apply 0.2–1 μl of each solution for linearity profile.

Sample preparation: Powdered sample equivalent to 50 mg of aceclofenac suspended in 40 ml of methanol, sonicated for 5 min, diluted to 50 ml with methanol, filtered and used for chromatographic evaluation.

Chromatographic equipments:

Sample applicator: Camag Linomat–V

Development chamber: Camag twin-trough glass chamber, 20 × 10 cm

Densitometric scanner: Camag TLC Scanner–III

Chromatographic conditions:

1. Stationary phase: Silica gel $60F_{254}$ pre-coated HPTLC plates, 20 × 10 cm (200 μm) – Merck
2. Mobile phase (MP): Ethyl acetate–methanol–glacial acetic acid (9 : 1 : 0.1 v/v)
3. Standard/Sample application:
   Band length: 6 mm Volume applied: 0.2–1 μl Spacing: 10 mm
4. Chamber saturation: 10 min (MP)
5. RH (%): 55 ± 5
6. Temperature °C: 25 ± 2
7. Separation technique: Ascending
8. Quantity of mobile phase: 20 ml
9. Migration distance: 80 mm
10. Migration time: 20 min

Densitometric evaluation:

Wavelength: UV–275 nm (iso-absorption point)

Scanning mode: Reflectance/Absorbance

HRF: Rabeprazole sodium—39; Aceclofenac—63; Paracetamol—79

Linearity (ng/band): Paracetamol—100–500; Aceclofenac—20–100; Rabeprazole—2–10

Recovery (%): Paracetamol—98.89–101.04; Aceclofenac—99.88–100.08; Rabeprazole—98.98–99.22

References: Mallikarjuna Rao N. and Gowri Sankar D., *Int. J. Pharm. Tech. Res.*, **3(2)**, 909–918, 2011.

Comments: The method validated for accuracy, precision, linearity, LOD, LOQ, specificity, robustness and ruggedness.

HPTLC : High Performance Thin Layer Chromatography
HPTLC Densitogram

No. 377

Rabeprazole sodium

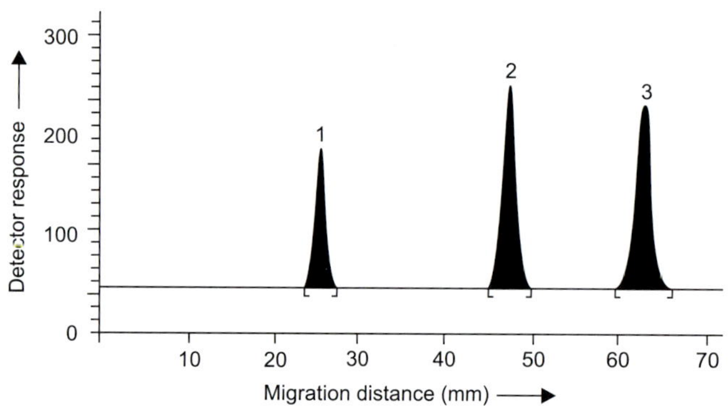

Typical densitogram of the drug and its degradation products.
Peaks identification : 1 and 3 – degradation products, 2. Rabeprazole

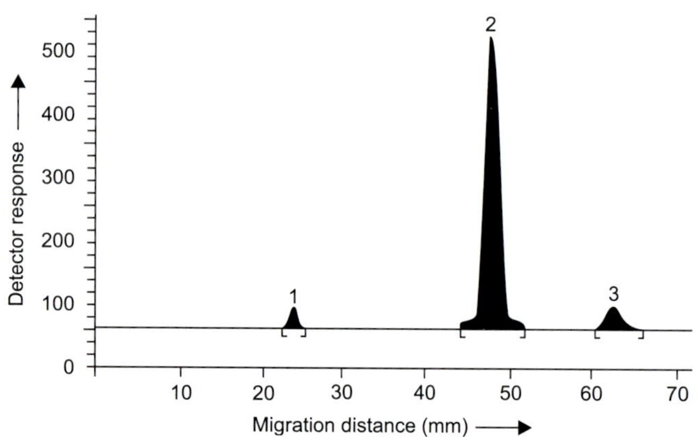

Typical densitogram of the expired tablet sample.
Peaks identification : 2. Rabeprazole; 1 and 3 – degradation products

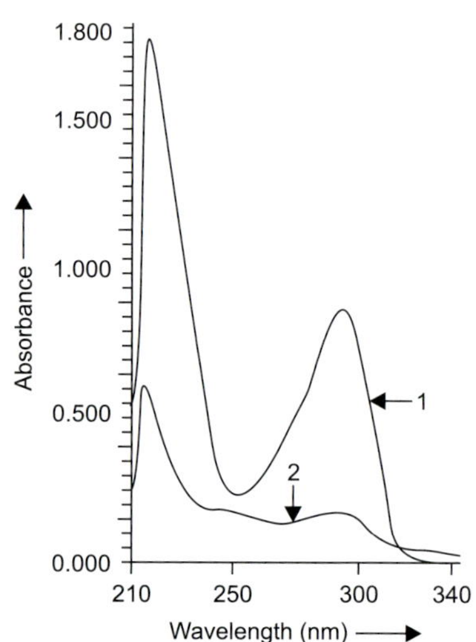

Overlaid UV-spectra of rabeprazole (1) and degradation product (2) for selection of suitable wavelength for densitometric scanning

For detailed experimental and chromatographic conditions refer to Protocol No. 377.

PROTOCOL FOR HPTLC ANALYSIS OF PHARMACEUTICAL FORMULATION

Protocol No. 377

Formulation: Rabeprazole sodium and its degradation products

Classification: Alimentary System **Dosage form:** Tablets

Standard preparation: Standard solution of the drug (1 mg/ml) was prepared in methanol. Further serial dilutions made for linearity profile.

Sample preparation: Powdered sample equivalent to 15 mg of rabeprazole suspended in methanol, sonicated for 10 min, filtered and suitably diluted. Apply 10 μl of the filtrate for chromatographic separation and degradation profile.

Chromatographic equipments:

Sample applicator: Camag Linomat–V

Development chamber: Camag twin-trough glass chamber, 20 × 10 cm

Densitometric scanner: Camag TLC Scanner–III

Chromatographic conditions:

1. Stationary phase: Silica gel $60F_{254}$ pre-coated HPTLC plates, 20 × 20 cm (200 μm) – Merck
2. Mobile phase (MP): Toluene–acetone–methanol (9 : 9 : 0.6 v/v)
3. Standard/Sample application:
   Band length: 4 mm Volume applied: 10 μl Spacing: 8 mm
4. Chamber saturation: 30 min (MP)
5. RH (%): 55 ± 5
6. Temperature °C: 22 ± 2
7. Separation technique: Ascending
8. Quantity of mobile phase: 18 ml
9. Migration distance: 80 mm
10. Migration time: 25 min

Densitometric evaluation:

Wavelength: UV–284 nm Scanning mode: Reflectance/Absorbance

HRF: Rabeprazole – see densitogram

Linearity: Rabeprazole—0.5–2.5 μg/band

Recovery (%): 99.1–100.8

References: Alaa El-Gindy, Fawzy El-Yazy El-Yazby and Moustafa M. Maher, *J. Pharm. Biomed. Anal.*, **31**, 229–242, 2003.

Comments:

- The method validated for accuracy, precision, linearity, LOD, LOQ, specificity, robustness and ruggedness.
- The method is stability indicating (acid, base, oxidative, thermolytic, photolytic). The degradation products were separated from main compound.

HPTLC : High Performance Thin Layer Chromatography
HPTLC Densitogram

No. 378

Rabeprazole sodium

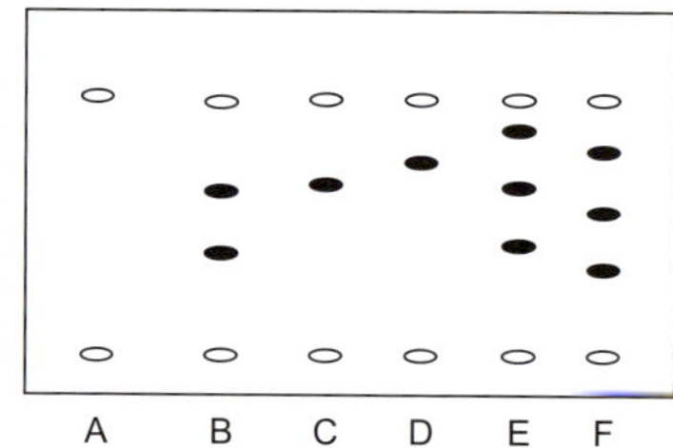

Degradation products (DP) of rabeprazole sodium from acid, base, oxidation, dry heat and photo degradation. (A) Standard rabeprazole sodium; (B) Rabeprazole sodium + 0.1 N HCl; (C) Rabeprazole sodium + 0.1 N NaOH; (D) Rabeprazole sodium + 10% H_2O_2; (E) Rabeprazole sodium exposed to dry heat; (F) Rabeprazole sodium exposed to light heat

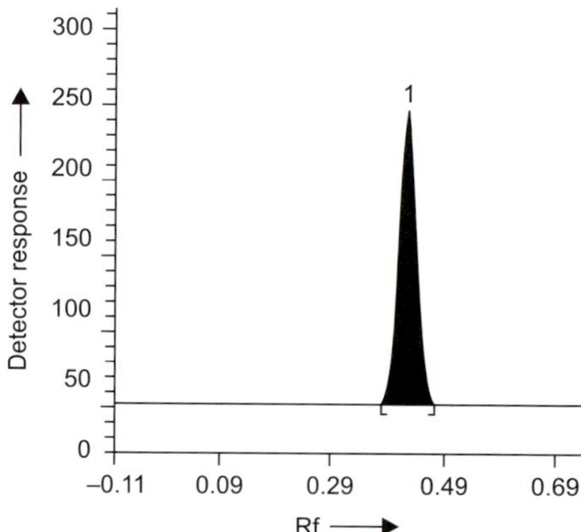

Typical densitogram of the sample containing rabeprazole sodium. For detailed experimental and chromatographic conditions, refer to Protocol No. 378. Peaks identification: 1. Rabeprazole.

PROTOCOL FOR HPTLC ANALYSIS OF PHARMACEUTICAL FORMULATION

Protocol No. 378

Formulation: Rabeprazole sodium and its degradation products

Classification: Alimentary System **Dosage form:** Tablets

Standard preparation: Prepare 1 mg/ml solution of the substance in methanol. Further serial dilutions made with methanol for linearity range. Apply 0.4–2.4 µl of the stock solution for degradation profile.

Sample preparation: Powdered sample equivalent to 10 mg of rabeprazole suspended in methanol, sonicated, diluted to 100 ml with methanol, filtered through 0.45 µm membrane filter. Apply 10 µl (1000 ng) for chromatographic separation and analysis.

Chromatographic equipments:

Sample applicator: Camag Linomat–V

Development chamber: Camag twin-trough glass chamber, 20 × 10 cm

Densitometric scanner: Camag TLC Scanner–III

Chromatographic conditions:

1. Stationary phase: Silica gel 60 RP-18F$_{2545}$ pre-coated HPTLC plates, 20 × 10 cm Merck
2. Mobile phase (MP): Acetone–water (7 : 3 v/v)
3. Standard/Sample application:
   Band length: 10 mm Volume applied: 10 µl Spacing: 15.4 mm
4. Chamber saturation: 30 min (MP)
5. RH (%): 60 ± 5
6. Temperature °C: 25 ± 2
7. Separation technique: Ascending
8. Quantity of mobile phase: 20 ml
9. Migration distance: 80 mm
10. Migration time: 25 min

Densitometric evaluation:

Wavelength: UV–284 nm Scanning mode: Reflectance/Absorbance

HRF: Rabeprazole—45

Linearity: 400–2400 ng/band

Recovery (%): 99.56–101.04

References: Atul A. Shir Khedkar and Sanjay J. Surana, *Eurasian J. Anal. Chem.*, **4(1)**, 87–97, 2009.

Comments:

- The method validated for accuracy, precision, linearity, LOD, LOQ, specificity, robustness and ruggedness.
- The method is stability indicating (acid, base, oxidative, thermal, photolytic). The degradation products were separated from main compounds.

HPTLC : High Performance Thin Layer Chromatography
HPTLC Densitogram

No. 379

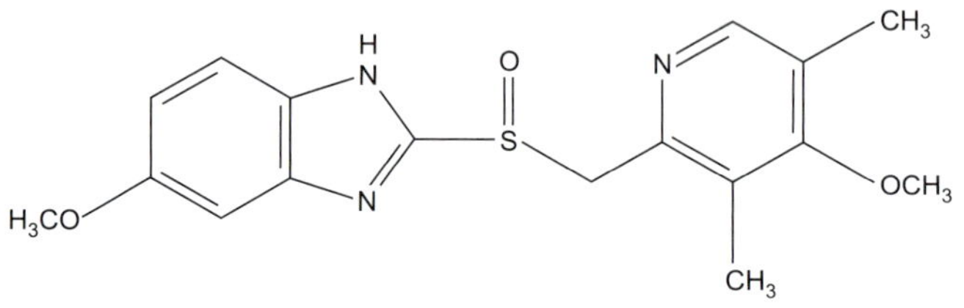

Omeprazole

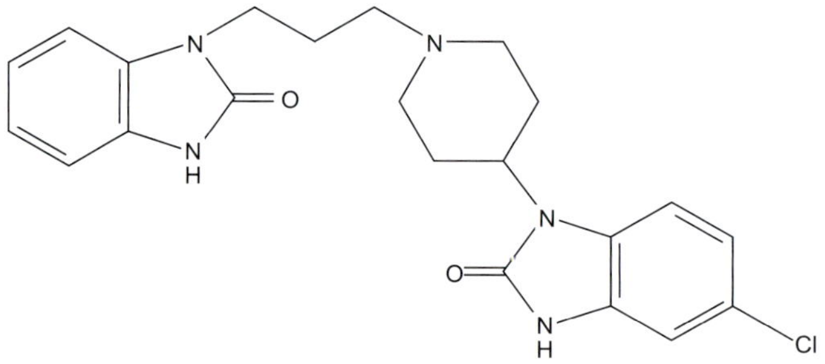

Domperidone

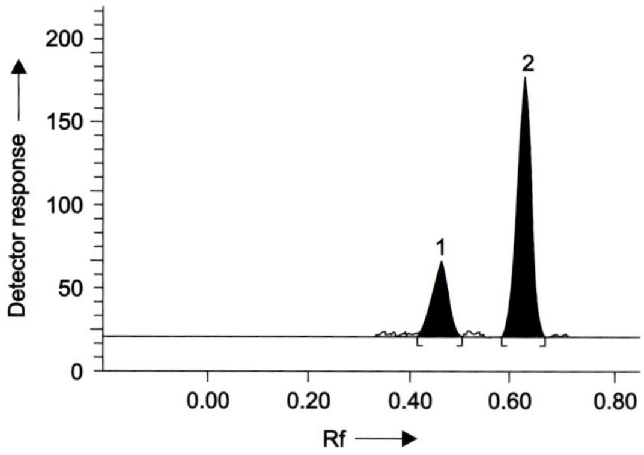

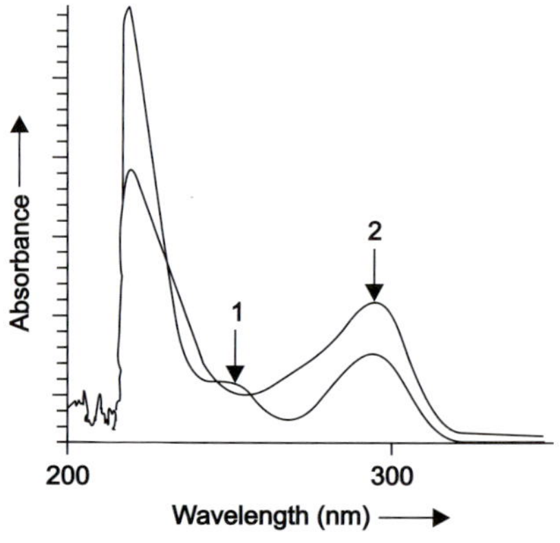

Overlaid UV-spectra of domperidone (1) and omeprazole (2) for selection of suitable wavelength for densitometric scanning

Typical densitogram of the sample containing omeprazole and domperidone. For detailed experimental and chromatographic conditions, refer to Protocol No. 379. Peaks identification: 1. Domperidone; 2. Omeprazole.

PROTOCOL FOR HPTLC ANALYSIS OF PHARMACEUTICAL FORMULATION

Protocol No. 379

Formulation: Omeprazole, Domperidone

Classification: Alimentary System **Dosage form:** Capsules

Standard preparation: Prepare 100 µg/ml solution of each compound in methanol and use for chromatographic analysis.

Sample preparation: The sample equivalent to 10 mg of omperazole suspended in 80 ml of methanol, sonicated for 15 min, diluted to 100 ml, filtered through 0.2 µm nylon membrane filter. Apply 10 µl for assay.

Chromatographic equipments:

Sample applicator: Camag Linomat–V

Development chamber: Camag twin-trough glass chamber, 20 × 10 cm

Densitometric scanner: Camag TLC Scanner–III

Chromatographic conditions:

1. Stationary phase: Silica gel $60F_{254}$ pre-coated HPTLC plates, 20 × 10 cm (200 µm) – Merck, pre-washed with methanol and air dried
2. Mobile phase (MP): Ethyl acetate–methanol–benzene (4 : 2 : 4 v/v)
3. Standard/Sample application:
   Band length: 4 mm Volume applied: 10 µl Spacing: 4 mm
4. Chamber saturation: 30 min (MP)
5. RH (%): 55 ± 5
6. Temperature °C: 25 ± 2
7. Separation technique: Ascending
8. Quantity of mobile phase: 10 ml
9. Migration distance: 80 mm
10. Migration time: 35 min

Densitometric evaluation:

Wavelength: UV–295 nm Scanning mode: Reflectance/Absorbance

HRF: Domperidone—45; Omeprazole—63

Linearity: 120–360 ng/band for both the drugs

Recovery (%): 99.37–100.97 for both the compounds

References: Bhavesh Patel, Madhubhai Patel and Jignesh Patel, *J. Liq. Chromatogr. and Related Tech.*, **30**, 1749–1762, 2007.

Comments: The method validated for accuracy, precision, linearity, LOD, LOQ, specificity, robustness and ruggedness.

HPTLC : High Performance Thin Layer Chromatography
HPTLC Densitogram

No. 380

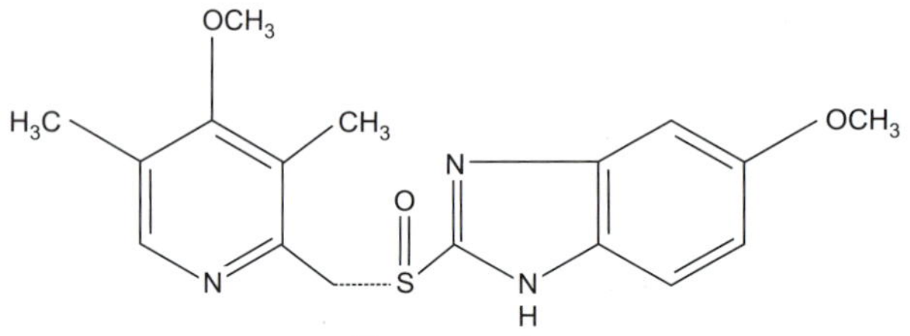

OCH_3, H_3C, CH_3, N, O, S, N, H, OCH_3

Esomeprazole

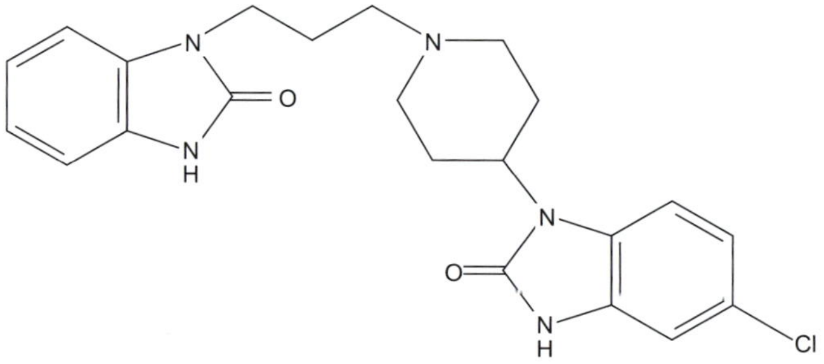

N, O, N, H, N, N, O, N, H, Cl

Domperidone

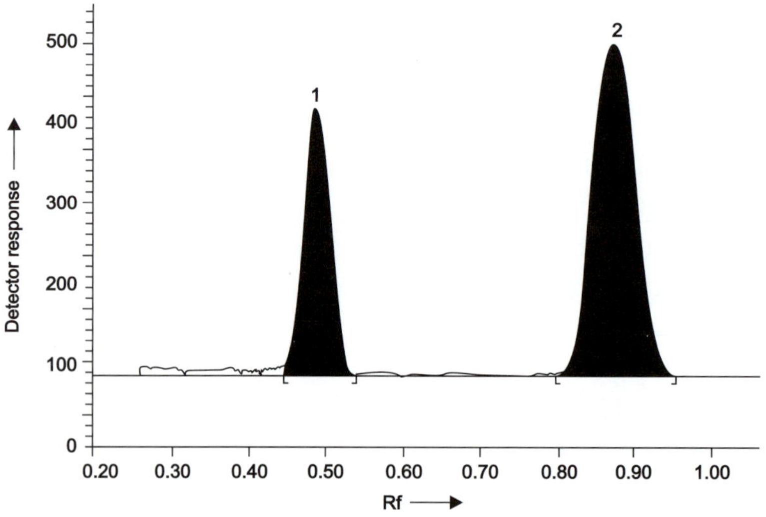

Detector response ⟶ 0, 100, 200, 300, 400, 500

1, 2

0.20 0.30 0.40 0.50 0.60 0.70 0.80 0.90 1.00

Rf ⟶

Typical densitogram of the sample containing esomeprazole and domperidone. For detailed experimental and chromatographic conditions, refer to Protocol No. 380. Peaks identification: 1. Domperidone; 2. Esomeprazole.

PROTOCOL FOR HPTLC ANALYSIS OF PHARMACEUTICAL FORMULATION

Protocol No. 380

Formulation: Esomeprazole, Domperidone

Classification: Alimentary System **Dosage form:** Tablets

Standard preparation: Prepare solution of each compound separately in solvent to get 20 mg/ml of esomeprazole and 10 mg/ml of domperidone. Further serial dilutions are made with the solvent for linearity studies. Apply 10 μl of each solution.

Solvent: Mixture of chloroform–methanol (1 : 1).

Sample preparation: Accurately weighed quantity of the powdered sample equivalent to 10 mg of domperidone suspended in methanol, sonicated, diluted to 10 ml with methanol, filtered. Apply 10 μl of this solution for assay.

Chromatographic equipments:

Sample applicator: Camag Linomat–IV

Development chamber: Camag twin-trough glass chamber, 10 × 10 cm

Densitometric scanner: Camag TLC Scanner–III

Chromatographic conditions:

1. Stationary phase: Silica gel $60F_{254}$ pre-coated, 10 × 10 cm (200 μm) – Merck
2. Mobile phase (MP): Chloroform–acetonitrile–25% ammonia (5 : 10 : 0.25 v/v)
3. Standard/Sample application:
   Band length: 16 mm Volume applied: 10 μl Spacing: 10 mm
4. Chamber saturation: 10 min (MP)
5. RH (%): 55 ± 5
6. Temperature °C: 20 ± 5
7. Separation technique: Ascending
8. Quantity of mobile phase: 15 ml
9. Migration distance: 100 mm
10. Migration time: 30 min

Densitometric evaluation:

Wavelength: UV–222 nm Scanning mode: Reflectance/absorbance

HRF: Domperidone—48; Esomeprazole—0.89

Linearity (μg/ml): Domperidone—600–1400; Esomeprazole—12–2800

Recovery (%): 99.64–100.68 for both the compounds

References: C. Roosewelt, A.R. Magesh, A.G. Sheeja Rekha, P. Shanmuga Pandian and V. Gunasekaran, *Asian J. Chem.*, **19(4)**, 2955–2960, 2007.

Comments: The method validated for accuracy, precision, linearity, LOD, LOQ, specificity, robustness and ruggedness.

HPTLC : High Performance Thin Layer Chromatography
HPTLC Densitogram

No. 383

Domperidone

Lansoprazole

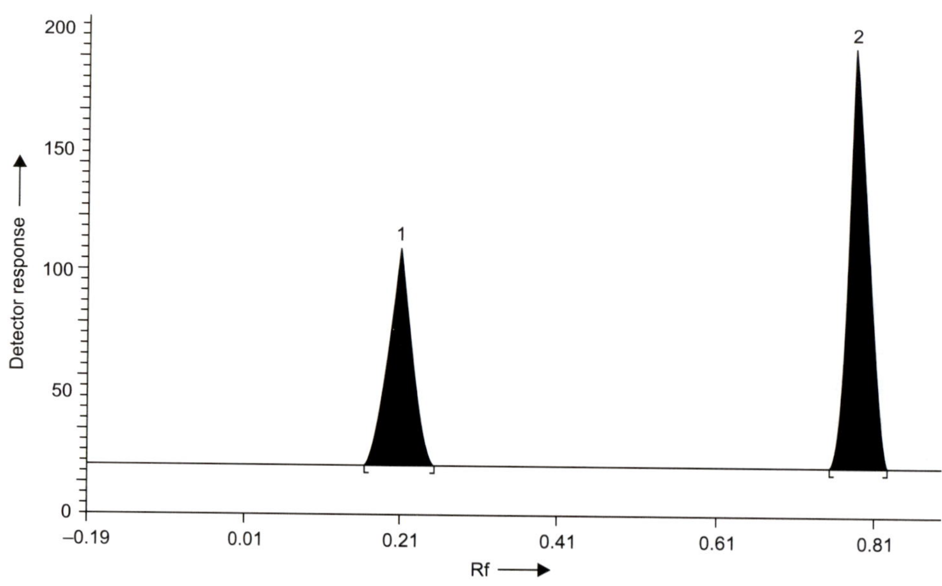

Typical densitogram of the sample containing lansoprazole and domperidone. For detailed experimental and chromatographic conditions, refer to Protocol No. 383. Peaks identification: 1. Domperidone; 2. Lansoprazole.

PROTOCOL FOR HPTLC ANALYSIS OF PHARMACEUTICAL FORMULATION

Protocol No. 383

Formulation: **Lansoprazole, Domperidone**

Classification: Alimentary System **Dosage form:** Tablets

Standard preparation: 100 μg/ml solution of each compound was prepared in methanol. Apply 1–5 μl of each solution for linearity profile.

Sample preparation: Powdered sample equivalent to 10 mg of lansoprazole or domperidone suspended in 60 ml of methanol, sonicated for 10 min, diluted to 100 ml with methanol, filtered and used for chromatographic analysis.

Chromatographic equipments:

Sample applicator: Camag Linomat–V

Development chamber: Camag twin-trough glass chamber, 10 × 10 cm

Densitometric scanner: Camag TLC Scanner–III

Chromatographic conditions:

1. Stationary phase: Silica gel $60F_{254}$ pre-coated plates 10 × 10 cm (250 μm)
2. Mobile phase (MP): n-butanol–glacial acetic acid–water (9.3 : 0.25 : 0.5 v/v)
3. Standard/Sample application:
   Band length: 6 mm Volume applied: 1–5 μl Spacing: 10 mm
4. Chamber saturation: 25 min (MP)
5. RH (%): 55 ± 5
6. Temperature °C: 22 ± 2
7. Separation technique: Ascending
8. Quantity of mobile phase: 10 ml
9. Migration distance: 85 mm
10. Migration time: 35 min

Densitometric evaluation:

Wavelength: UV–288 nm Scanning mode: Reflectance/Absorbance

HRF: Domperidone—21; Lansoprazole—78

Linearity (ng/band): Lansoprazole—100–500; Domperidone—100–500

Recovery (%): Lansoprazole—98.47–101.35; Domperidone—98.21–98.82

References: J.V. Susheel, M. Lekha and T.K. Ravi, *Ind. J. Pharm. Sci.*, **69(5)**, 684–686, 2007.

Comments: The method validated for accuracy, precision, linearity, LOD, LOQ, specificity, robustness and ruggedness.

HPTLC : High Performance Thin Layer Chromatography
HPTLC Densitogram

No. 384

H_3C N CH_3 O S H N H N CH_3 NO_2

Ranitidine

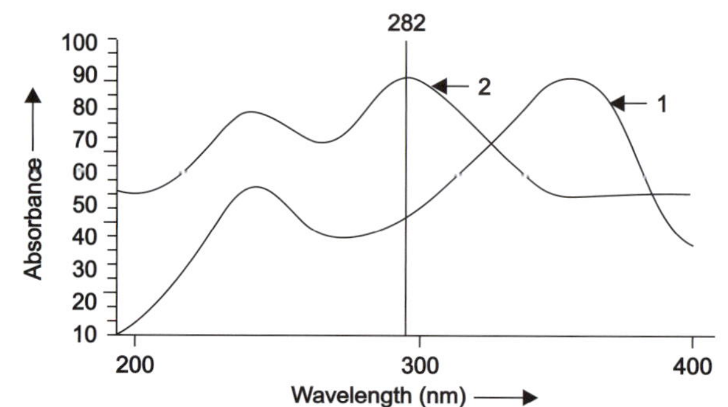

Overlaid UV-spectra of ranitidine (1) and domperidone (2) for selection of suitable wavelength for densitometric scanning

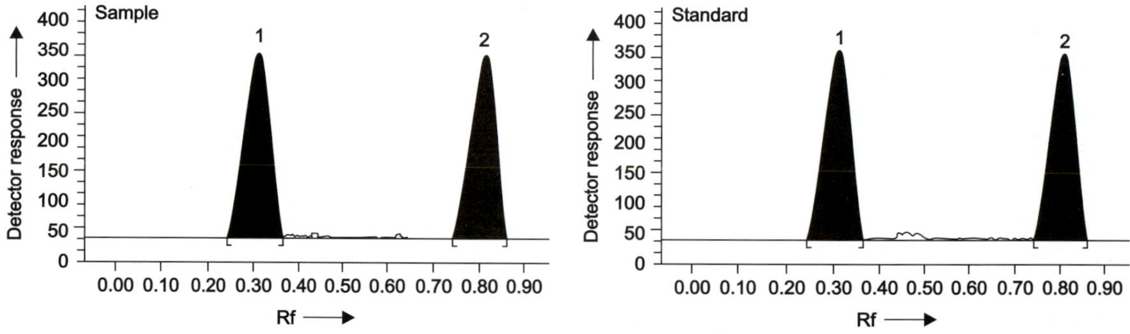

Typical densitogram of the sample and standard containing ranitidine and domperidone. For detailed experimental and chromatographic conditions, refer to Protocol No. 384. Peaks identification: 1. Domperidone; 2. Ranitidine HCl.

PROTOCOL FOR HPTLC ANALYSIS OF PHARMACEUTICAL FORMULATION

Protocol No. 384

Formulation: **Ranitidine hydrochloride, Domperidone**

Classification: Alimentary System **Dosage form:** Tablets

Standard preparation: Prepare 1 mg/ml solution of each compound separately in methanol. Further serial dilutions made for linearity studies.

Sample preparation: Powdered sample equivalent to 25 mg of ranitidine hydrochloride suspended in methanol, sonicated for 10 min, diluted to 25 ml, filtered and the solution further diluted suitably for assay. Apply 10 μl.

Chromatographic equipments:

Sample applicator: Camag Linomat–IV

Development chamber: Camag twin-trough glass chamber, 10 × 10 cm

Densitometric scanner: Camag TLC Scanner–III

Chromatographic conditions:

1. Stationary phase: Silica gel $60F_{254}$ pre-coated HPTLC plates, 10 × 10 cm (200 μm) – Merck
2. Mobile phase (MP): Methanol–1,4-dioxane (4 : 6 v/v)
3. Standard/Sample application:
   Band length: 6 mm Volume applied: 2–12 μl Spacing: 5 mm
4. Chamber saturation: 10 min (MP)
5. RH (%): 55 ± 5
6. Temperature °C: 22 ± 2
7. Separation technique: Ascending
8. Quantity of mobile phase: 10 ml
9. Migration distance: 70 mm
10. Migration time: 25 min

Densitometric evaluation:

Wavelength: UV–282 nm Scanning mode: Reflectance/Absorbance

HRF: Domperidone—30; Ranitidine HCl—80

Linearity (μg/ml): Ranitidine HCl—3–50; Domperidone—0.2–3.5

Recovery (%): Ranitidine HCl—100.25–100.78; Domperidone—99.54–100.29

References: Manoj S. Charde, Sanjay G. Walode, Madhukar R. Tajne and Avinash V. Kasture, *Asian J. Chem.*, **17(4)**, 2402–2410, 2005.

Comments:

- The method validated for accuracy, precision, linearity, LOD, LOQ, specificity, robustness and ruggedness.
- The method is stability indicating (acid, base, oxidative, thermal, photolytic). The degradation products were separated from main compounds.

HPTLC : High Performance Thin Layer Chromatography
HPTLC Densitogram

No. 386

Ranitidine

Dicyclomine hydrochloride

Overlaid UV-spectra of ranitidine HCl (1) and dicyclomine HCl (2) for selection of suitable wavelength for densitometric scanning

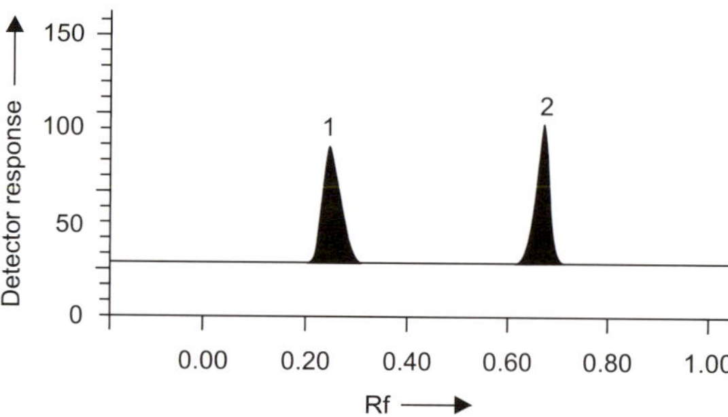

Typical densitogram of the standard containing ranitidine HCl and dicyclomine HCl. For detailed experimental and chromatographic conditions, refer to Protocol No. 386. Peaks identification: 1. Ranitidine HCl; 2. Dicyclomine HCl.

PROTOCOL FOR HPTLC ANALYSIS OF PHARMACEUTICAL FORMULATION

Protocol No. 386

Formulation: Ranitidine hydrochloride, Dicyclomine hydrochloride
Classification: Alimentary System **Dosage form:** Tablets
Standard preparation: Prepare 100 μg/ml solution of dicyclomine hydrochloride and 150 μg/ml of ranitidine hydrochloride, both in methanol. Apply 1–6 μl of ranitidine HCl and 4–24 μl of dicyclomine HCl for linearity studies of both the compounds.
Sample preparation: Weigh powdered sample equivalent to 10 mg of dicyclomine HCl, suspend in methanol, sonicate, make up to 10 ml with methanol. Centrifuge and filter. 1 ml of this solution diluted to 10 ml with methanol for assay of dicyclomine HCl. 1 ml of the solution further diluted for assay of ranitidine HCl. Apply 4 μl of each solution for chromatographic analysis.
Chromatographic equipments:
Sample applicator: Camag Linomat–V
Development chamber: Camag twin-trough glass chamber, 20 × 10 cm
Densitometric scanner: Camag TLC Scanner–III
Chromatographic conditions:
1. Stationary phase: Silica gel $60F_{254}$ pre-coated HPTLC plates, 20 × 10 cm (250 μm) – Merck, pre-washed with methanol activated at 105°C for 20 min, prior to use
2. Mobile phase (MP): Methanol–water–acetic acid (8 : 2 : 0.1 v/v)
3. Standard/Sample application:
Band length: 8 mm Volume applied: 4 μl Spacing: 12.1 mm
4. Chamber saturation: 30 min (MP)
5. RH (%): 55 ± 5
6. Temperature °C: 22 ± 2
7. Separation technique: Ascending
8. Quantity of mobile phase: 20 ml
9. Migration distance: 150 mm
10. Migration time: 20 min

Densitometric evaluation:
Wavelength: UV–410 nm Scanning mode: Reflectance/Absorbance
HRF: Ranitidine HCl—27; Dicyclomine HCl—67
Linearity (ng/band): Ranitidine HCl—150–9000; Dicyclomine HCl—400–2400
Recovery (%): Ranitidine HCl—98.50–99.15; Dicyclomine HCl—98.81–100.57
References: R.K. Nanda, S.E. Potawale, V.V. Bhagwat, R.S. Deshmukh and P.B. Deshpande, *J. Pharm. Res.*, **3(8)**, 2010.
Comments:
- The method validated for accuracy, precision, linearity, LOD, LOQ, specificity, robustness and ruggedness.
- After development, the plate dried in stream of dry air and dipped in the reagent for 2 s and scanned at 410 nm.
Reagent: Dissolve 0.8 g of KI and 0.8 g of iodine in 40 ml of ethyl alcohol, add 10 ml of HCl.

HPTLC : High Performance Thin Layer Chromatography
HPTLC Densitogram

No. 387

Famotidine

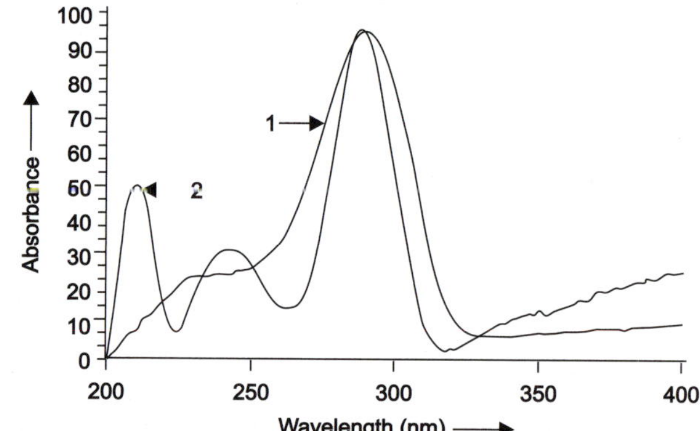

Overlaid UV-spectra of famotidine (1) and domperidone (2) for selection of suitable wavelength for densitometric scanning

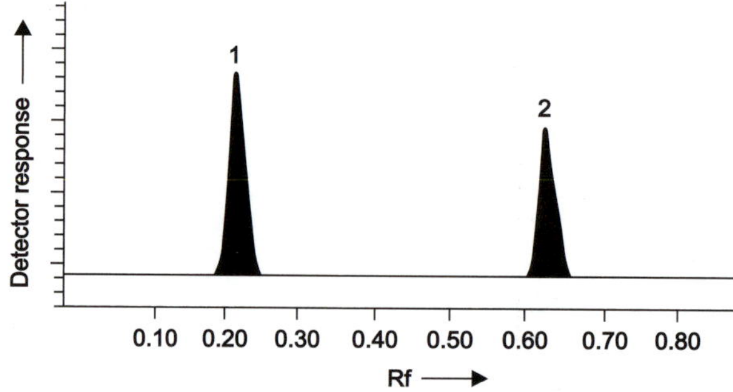

Typical densitogram of the standard containing famotidine and domperidone. For detailed experimental and chromatographic conditions, refer to Protocol No. 387. Peaks identification: 1. Famotidine; 2. Domperidone.

PROTOCOL FOR HPTLC ANALYSIS OF PHARMACEUTICAL FORMULATION

Protocol No. 387

Formulation: Domperidone, Famotidine

Classification: Alimentary System **Dosage form:** Tablets

Standard preparation: Prepare 1 mg/ml solution of each compound in methanol. Further dilute 0.5 ml of each solution to 10 ml with methanol (50 μg/ml) and apply varying volumes for linearity studies.

Sample preparation: Powdered sample equivalent to 10 mg of domperidone suspended in 5 ml of methanol, sonicated for 5 min, diluted to 10 ml with methanol. Filtered and 0.5 ml of filtrate diluted to 10 ml with methanol. Apply 2 μl for assay.

Chromatographic equipments:

Sample applicator: Camag Linomat–V

Development chamber: Camag twin-trough glass chamber, 10 × 10 cm

Densitometric scanner: Camag TLC Scanner–III

Chromatographic conditions:

1. Stationary phase: Silica gel $60F_{254}$ pre-coated HPTLC plates, 10 × 10 cm (250 μm) – Merck, pre-washed with methanol, activated at 110°C for 5 min, prior to use
2. Mobile phase (MP): Toluene–methanol–triethylamine (6 : 3 : 0.5 v/v)
3. Standard/Sample application:
   Band length: 6 mm Volume applied: 2–10 μl Spacing: 5 mm
4. Chamber saturation: 15 min (MP)
5. RH (%): 55 ± 5
6. Temperature °C: 22 ± 2
7. Separation technique: Ascending
8. Quantity of mobile phase: 9.5 ml
9. Migration distance: 90 mm
10. Migration time: 15 min

Densitometric evaluation:

Wavelength: UV–290 nm Scanning mode: Reflectance/Absorbance

HRF: Famotidine—23; Domperidone—67

Linearity: 100–500 ng/band for both the compounds

Recovery (%): Famotidine—99.89–100.06; Domperidone—98.73–99.98

References: Padmanabh Deshpande, Santhosh V. Gandhi, Vandana Bhavnani, Raviraj Bandewar, Abhijeet Diware and Virushali Diwale, *Res. J. Pharmaceutical, Biological and Chemical Sciences*, **1(4)**, 354–359, 2010.

Comments: The method validated for accuracy, precision, linearity, LOD, LOQ, specificity, robustness and ruggedness.

HPTLC : High Performance Thin Layer Chromatography
HPTLC Densitogram

No. 388

Famotidine

Domperidone

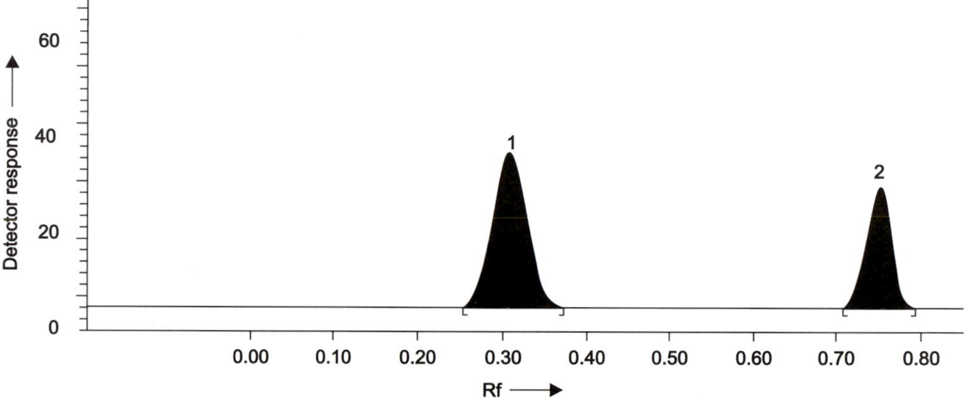

Typical densitogram of the standard containing famotidine and domperidone. For detailed experimental and chromatographic conditions, refer to Protocol No. 388. Peaks identification: 1. Famotidine; 2. Domperidone.

PROTOCOL FOR HPTLC ANALYSIS OF PHARMACEUTICAL FORMULATION

Protocol No. 388

Formulation: Domperidone, Famotidine

Classification: Alimentary System **Dosage form:** Tablets

Standard preparation: Prepare 1 mg/ml solution of each compound in methanol. Further dilute 0.5 ml of each solution to 10 ml with methanol (50 μg/ml) and apply varying volumes for linearity studies.

Sample preparation: Powdered sample equivalent to 10 mg of domperidone suspended in 5 ml of methanol, sonicated for 5 min, diluted to 10 ml with methanol. Filtered and 0.5 ml of filtrate diluted to 10 ml with methanol. Apply 2 μl for assay.

Chromatographic equipments:

Sample applicator: Camag Linomat–V

Development chamber: Camag twin-trough glass chamber, 10 × 10 cm

Densitometric scanner: Camag TLC Scanner–III

Chromatographic conditions:

1. Stationary phase: Silica gel $60F_{254}$ pre-coated HPTLC plates, 10 × 10 cm (250 μm) – Merck, pre-washed with methanol and activated at 110°C for 20 min, prior to use
2. Mobile phase (MP): Ethyl acetate–methanol–toluene–25% ammonia (8 : 3 : 4 : 0.4 v/v)
3. Standard/Sample application:
   Band length: 4 mm Volume applied: 5 μl Spacing: 6 mm
4. Chamber saturation: 15 min (MP)
5. RH (%): 55 ± 5
6. Temperature °C: 22 ± 2
7. Separation technique: Ascending
8. Quantity of mobile phase: 15 ml
9. Migration distance: 80 mm
10. Migration time: 20 min

Densitometric evaluation:

Wavelength: UV–285 nm Scanning mode: Reflectance/Absorbance

HRF: Famotidine—32; Domperidone—75

Linearity: 100–600 ng/band for both the compounds

Recovery (%): Famotidine—97.28–104.74; Domperidone—99.02–100.71

References: M.G. Pai, Vibhuti Karpe and Rajashree Gude, Personal communication.

Comments: The method validated for accuracy, precision, linearity, LOD, LOQ, specificity, robustness and ruggedness.

HPTLC : High Performance Thin Layer Chromatography
HPTLC Densitogram

No. 389

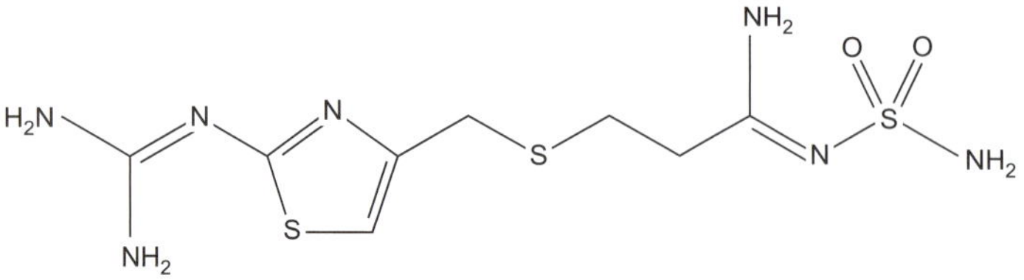

Famotidine

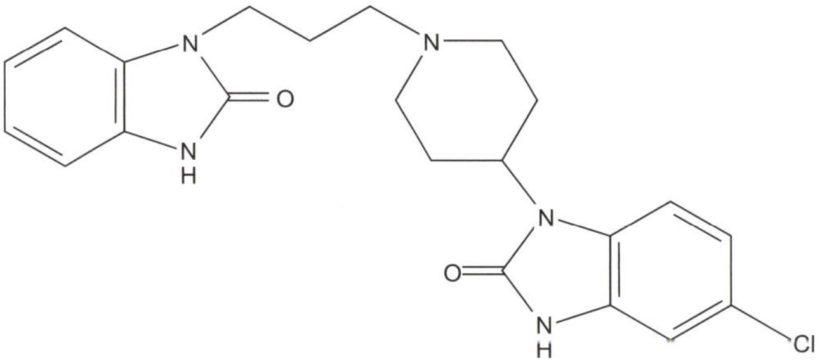

Domperidone

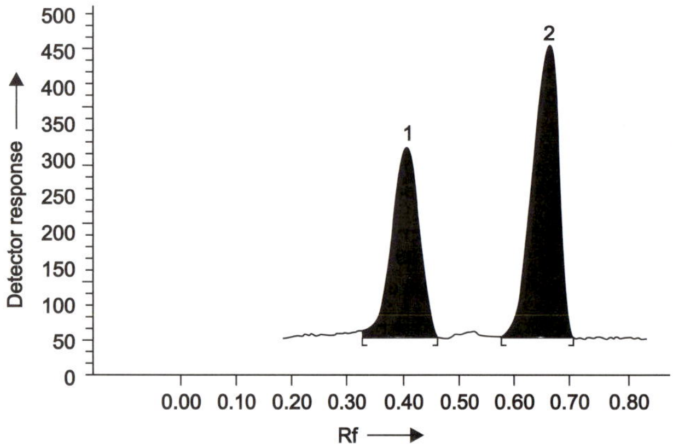

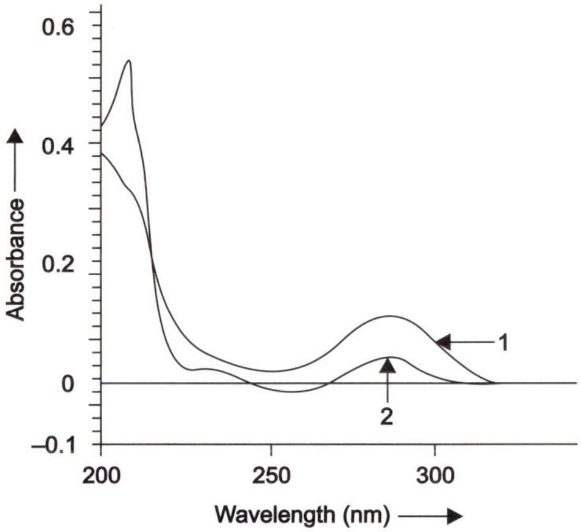

Overlaid UV-spectra of domperidone (1) and famotidine (2) for selection of suitable wavelength for densitometric scanning

Typical densitogram of the sample containing domperidone and famotidine. For detailed experimental and chromatographic conditions, refer to Protocol No. 389. Peaks identification: 1. Famotidine; 2. Domperidone.

PROTOCOL FOR HPTLC ANALYSIS OF PHARMACEUTICAL FORMULATION

Protocol No. 389

Formulation: Domperidone, Famotidine

Classification: Alimentary System **Dosage form:** Tablets

Standard preparation: Prepare 1 mg/ml solution of both the compounds in methanol. Further serial dilutions are made for linearity profile. Apply 10 μl of each solution for linearity profile.

Sample preparation: Powdered sample equivalent to 20 mg of famotidine or 10 mg of domperidone suspended in 40 ml of methanol, sonicated, diluted, centrifuged and the solution suitably diluted for chromatographic analysis.

Chromatographic equipments:

Sample applicator: Camag Linomat–V

Development chamber: Camag twin-trough glass chamber, 20 × 10 cm

Densitometric scanner: Camag TLC Scanner–III

Chromatographic conditions:

1. Stationary phase: Silica gel 60F_{254} pre-coated TLC plates, 20 × 10 cm (250 μm) – Merck, pre-washed with methanol, activated at 110°C for 5 min prior to use
2. Mobile phase (MP): Ethyl acetate–methanol–water (8 : 1.5 : 0.3 v/v)
3. Standard/Sample application:
   Band length: 6 mm Volume applied: 10 μl Spacing: 5 mm
4. Chamber saturation: 30 min (MP)
5. RH (%): 60 ± 5
6. Temperature °C: 25 ± 2
7. Separation technique: Ascending
8. Quantity of mobile phase: 19 ml
9. Migration distance: 80 mm
10. Migration time: 15 min

Densitometric evaluation:

Wavelength: UV–288 nm Scanning mode: Reflectance/Absorbance

HRF: Famotidine—42; Domperidone—67

Linearity (ng/band): Domperidone—300–700; Famotidine—1200–2800

Recovery (%): 98.26–98.88 for both the compounds

References: Sathiyanarayanan L., P.V. Kulkarni, Ajinkya R. Nikam and K.R. Mahadik, *Der Pharma Chemica*, **3(1)**, 134–143, 2011.

Comments: The method validated for accuracy, precision, linearity, LOD, LOQ, specificity and robustness.

HPTLC : High Performance Thin Layer Chromatography
HPTLC Densitogram

No. 390

Famotidine

Domperidone

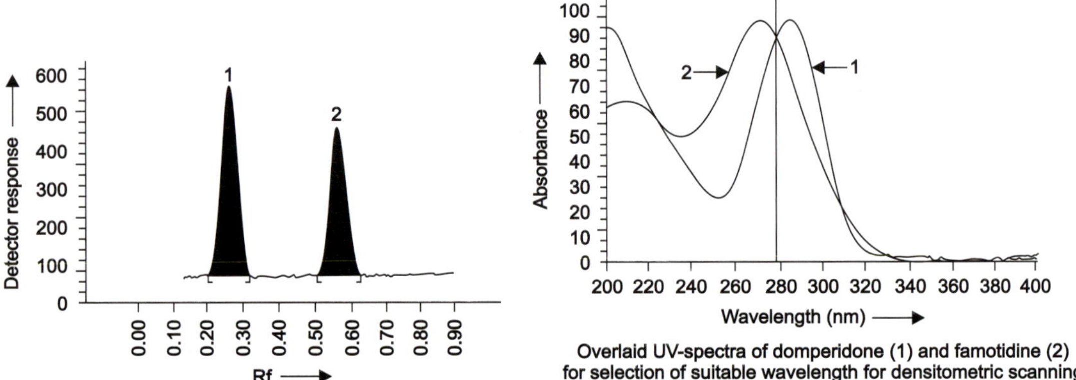

Overlaid UV-spectra of domperidone (1) and famotidine (2) for selection of suitable wavelength for densitometric scanning

Typical densitogram of the standard containing famotidine and domperidone. For detailed experimental and chromatographic conditions, refer to Protocol No. 390. Peaks identification: 1. Famotidine; 2. Domperidone.

PROTOCOL FOR HPTLC ANALYSIS OF PHARMACEUTICAL FORMULATION

Protocol No. 390

Formulation: Domperidone, Famotidine

Classification: Alimentary System **Dosage form:** Tablets

Standard preparation: Prepare 100 μg/ml solution of domperidone and 200 μg/ml solution of famotidine, both in methanol. Further dilutions are made suitably with methanol for linearity profile.

Sample preparation: Powdered sample equivalent to 10 mg of domperidone suspended in 20 ml of methanol, sonicated for 30 min, diluted, centrifuged (3000 rpm) for 5 min. Supernatant suitably diluted with methanol. Apply 2 μl of the resulting solution for chromatographic evaluation.

Chromatographic equipments:

Sample applicator: Camag Linomat–V

Development chamber: Camag twin-trough glass chamber, 10 × 10 cm

Densitometric scanner: Camag TLC Scanner–III

Chromatographic conditions:

1. Stationary phase: Silica gel $60F_{254}$ pre-coated TLC plates, 10 × 10 cm (250 μm) – Merck, pre-washed with methanol, activated at 110°C for 5 min prior to use
2. Mobile phase (MP): n-butanol–water (6 : 1 v/v)
3. Standard/Sample application:
   Band length: 6 mm Volume applied: 1–6 μl Spacing: 5 mm
4. Chamber saturation: 30 min (MP)
5. RH (%): 60 ± 5
6. Temperature °C: 25 ± 2
7. Separation technique: Ascending
8. Quantity of mobile phase: 14 ml
9. Migration distance: 80 mm
10. Migration time: 20 min

Densitometric evaluation:

Wavelength: UV–280 nm (iso-absorption point)

Scanning mode: Reflectance/Absorbance

HRF: Famotidine—27; Domperidone—58

Linearity (ng/band): Domperidone—100–600; Famotidine—200–1200

Recovery (%): Domperidone—95.11–97.27; Famotidine—95.30–98.65

References: S.M. Pawar, B.S. Patel and R.Y. Patel, *Int. J. Advances in Pharmaceutical Sci.*, **1(1)**, 54–59, 2010.

Comments: The method validated for accuracy, precision, linearity, LOD, LOQ, specificity and robustness.

HPTLC : High Performance Thin Layer Chromatography
HPTLC Densitogram

No. 391

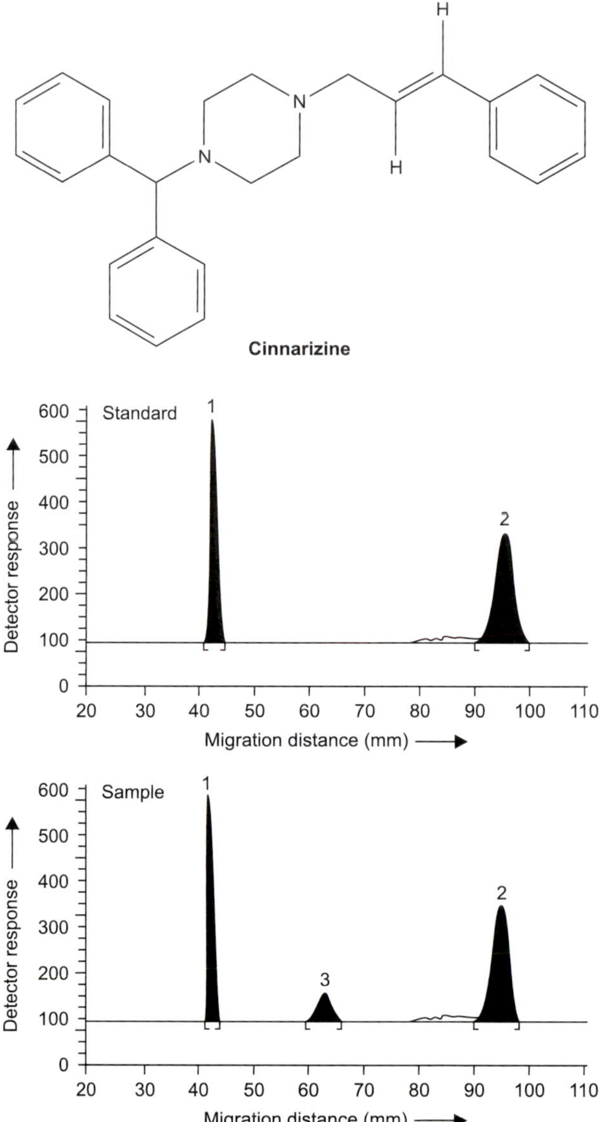

Typical densitogram of the sample and standard containing domperidone and cinnarizine. For detailed experimental and chromatographic conditions, refer to Protocol No. 391. Peaks identification: 1. Domperidone; 2. Cinnarizine; 3. Excipient.

PROTOCOL FOR HPTLC ANALYSIS OF PHARMACEUTICAL FORMULATION

Protocol No. 391

Formulation: Domperidone, Cinnarizine

Classification: Alimentary System **Dosage form:** Tablets

Standard preparation: Prepare solution of both the compounds in methanol to get 750 μg/ml of domperidone and 1000 μg/ml of cinnarizine. Further dilutions made to get different concentrations ranging for 100–600 μg/ml of cinnarizine and 75–450 μg/ml of domperidone. Apply 10 μl of each solution for analysis.

Sample preparation: Powdered sample equivalent to 25 mg of cinnarizine suspended in 20 ml of MP, sonicated to dissolve, dilute to 25 ml, filter, dilute 10 ml of the filtrate to 25 ml with MP and use 10 μl for application to chromatoplate for analysis.

Chromatographic equipments:

Sample applicator: Camag Linomat–IV

Development chamber: Camag twin-trough glass chamber, 10 × 10 cm

Densitometric scanner: Camag TLC Scanner–III

Chromatographic conditions:

1. Stationary phase: Silica gel 60F_{254} pre-coated TLC plates, 10 × 10 cm (200 μm) – Merck
2. Mobile phase (MP): Toluene–ethyl acetate–methanol (7.0 : 5.0 : 2.5 v/v)
3. Standard/Sample application:
   Band length: 6 mm Volume applied: 10 μl Spacing: 15 mm
4. Chamber saturation: 30 min (MP)
5. RH (%): 55 ± 5
6. Temperature °C: 22 ± 2
7. Separation technique: Ascending
8. Quantity of mobile phase: 14 ml
9. Migration distance: 110 mm
10. Migration time: 60 min

Densitometric evaluation:

Wavelength: UV–271 nm Scanning mode: Reflectance/Absorbance

HRF: Domperidone—40; Cinnarizine—85

Linearity (μg/ml): Domperidone—75–450; Cinnarizine—100–600

Recovery (%): Domperidone—98.93–100.25; Cinnarizine—99.02–99.90

References: Vinodhini C., Kalidoss, A.S., and Vaidhyalingam V., *Indian Drugs*, **42(9)**, 600–603, 2005.

Comments: The method validated for accuracy, precision, linearity, LOD, LOQ, specificity, robustness and ruggedness.

HPTLC : High Performance Thin Layer Chromatography
HPTLC Densitogram

No. 392

Cinnarizine

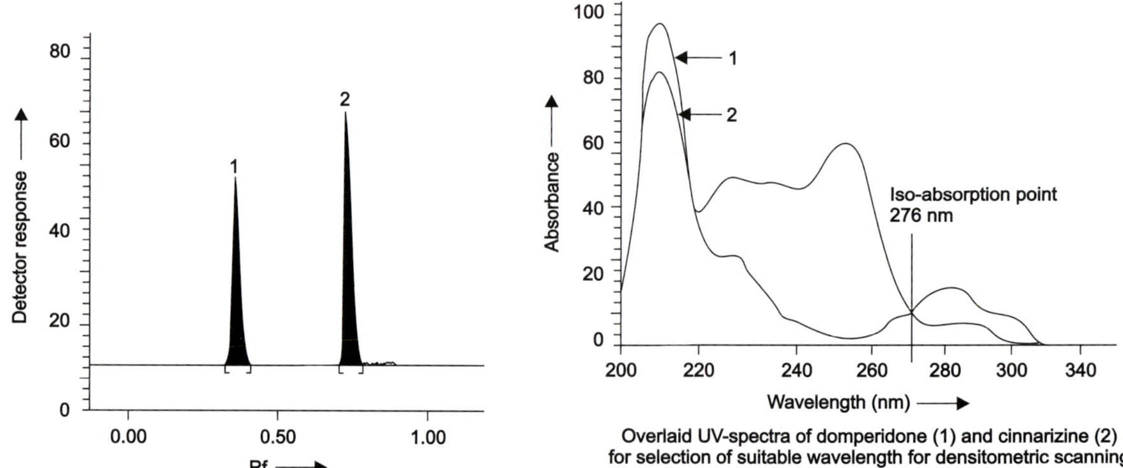

Overlaid UV-spectra of domperidone (1) and cinnarizine (2) for selection of suitable wavelength for densitometric scanning

Typical densitogram of the sample containing domperidone and cinnarizine. For detailed experimental and chromatographic conditions, refer to Protocol No. 392. Peaks identification: 1. Cinnarizine; 2. Domperidone.

PROTOCOL FOR HPTLC ANALYSIS OF PHARMACEUTICAL FORMULATION

Protocol No. 392

Formulation: Domperidone maleate, Cinnarizine

Classification: Alimentary System **Dosage form:** Tablets

Standard preparation: Prepare 1 mg/ml solution of each compound in methanol. Further serial dilutions made with methanol. Apply 1 µl of each solution for linearity profile.

Sample preparation: An appropriate quantity of powdered sample suspended in methanol, sonicated, filtered and diluted suitably to get 500 ng/µl of cinnarizine and 375 ng/µl domperidone. Apply 1 µl of the solution for assay.

Chromatographic equipments:

Sample applicator: Camag Linomat–IV

Development chamber: Camag twin-trough glass chamber, 10 × 10 cm

Densitometric scanner: Camag TLC Scanner–II

Chromatographic conditions:

1. Stationary phase: Silica gel $60F_{254}$ pre-coated HPTLC plates, 10 × 10 cm (200 µm) – Merck
2. Mobile phase (MP): Methanol–dichloromethane–formic acid (1 : 9 : 0.05 v/v)
3. Standard/Sample application:
   Band length: 8 mm Volume applied: 1 µl Spacing: 5 mm
4. Chamber saturation: 10 min (MP)
5. RH (%): 55 ± 5
6. Temperature °C: 22 ± 2
7. Separation technique: Ascending
8. Quantity of mobile phase: 10 ml
9. Migration distance: 70 mm
10. Migration time: 20 min

Densitometric evaluation:

Wavelength: UV–276 nm (iso-absorption point)

Scanning mode: Reflectance/Absorbance

HRF: Cinnarizine—48; Domperidone—80

Linearity (ng/µl): Domperidone—50–1000; Cinnarizine—60–1000

Recovery (%): Domperidone—97.67–91.80; Cinnarizine—97.0–99.78

References: A.P. Argekar and S.G. Powar, *J. Planar Chromatography*, **12(4)**, 272–274, 1999.

Comments: The method validated for accuracy, precision, linearity, LOD, LOQ, specificity, robustness and ruggedness.

HPTLC : High Performance Thin Layer Chromatography
HPTLC Densitogram

No. 393

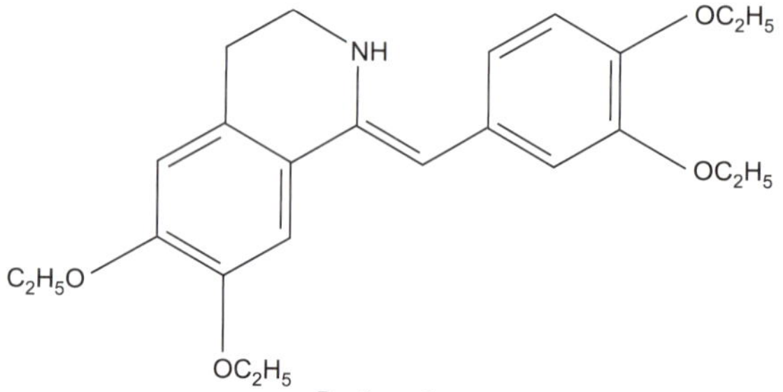

Drotaverine

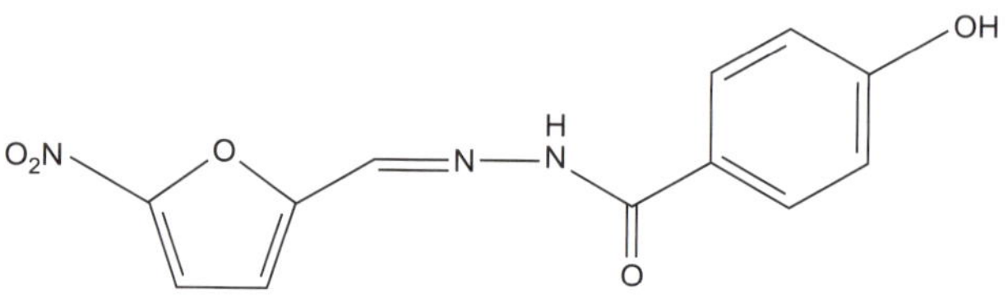

Nifuroxazide

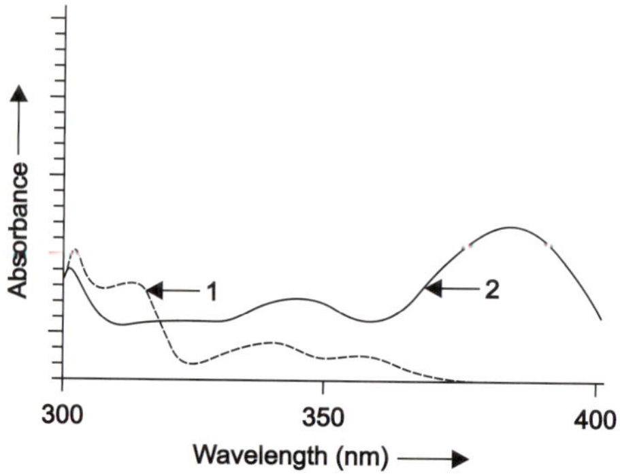

Overlaid UV-spectra of drotaverine HCl (1) and nifuroxazide (2) for selection of suitable wavelength for densitometric scanning

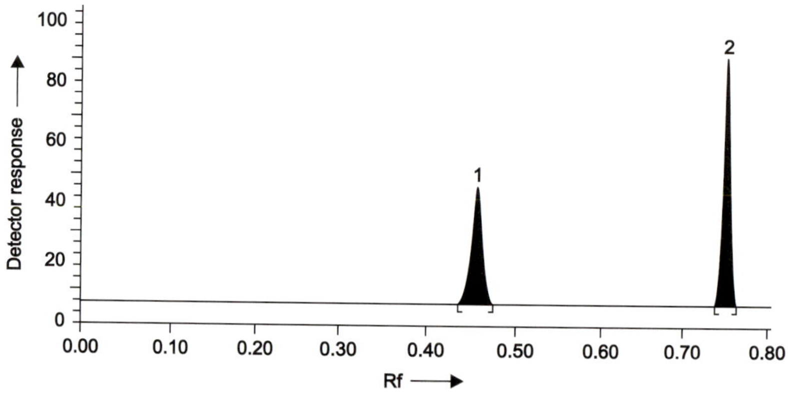

Typical densitogram of the sample containing drotaverine hydrochloride and nifuroxazide. For detailed experimental and chromatographic conditions, refer to Protocol No. 393. Peaks identification: 1. Drotaverine HCl; 2. Nifuroxazide.

PROTOCOL FOR HPTLC ANALYSIS OF PHARMACEUTICAL FORMULATION

Protocol No. 393

Formulation: Drotaverine hydrochloride, Nifuroxazide

Classification: Alimentary System **Dosage form:** Tablets

Standard preparation: Prepare 500 µg/ml solution of each compound in absolute alcohol (protected from light due to photosensitivity). Further dilute 20 ml to 100 ml with absolute alcohol (100 µg/ml). Apply 1–10 µl for linearity profile.

Sample preparation: Weigh appropriate quantity of the sample, extract with absolute alcohol (protect from light), dilute, filter, further dilute and apply 6 µl of the resulting solution for assay.

Chromatographic equipments:

Sample applicator: Camag Linomat–IV

Development chamber: Camag twin-trough glass chamber, 20 × 20 cm

Densitometric scanner: Camag TLC Scanner–III

Chromatographic conditions:

1. Stationary phase: Silica gel $60F_{254}$ pre-coated TLC plates, 20 × 20 cm (250 µm) – Merck
2. Mobile phase (MP): Chloroform–acetone–methanol–glacial acetic acid (6 : 3 : 0.9 : 0.1 v/v)
3. Standard/Sample application:
   Band length: 10 mm Volume applied: 1–10 µl Spacing: 10 mm
4. Chamber saturation: 20 min (MP)
5. RH (%): 55 ± 5
6. Temperature °C: 22 ± 2
7. Separation technique: Ascending
8. Quantity of mobile phase: 20 ml
9. Migration distance: 70 mm
10. Migration time: 25 min

Densitometric evaluation:

Wavelength: UV–365 nm Scanning mode: Reflectance/Absorbance

HRF: Drotaverine HCl—46; Nifuroxazide—75

Linearity: 0.2–1 µg/band for both the compounds

Recovery (%): 100.11–100.59 for both the compounds

References: Fadia H. Metwally, Mohammed Abdelkawy and Ibrahim A. Nagub, *JAOAC Int.*, **89(1)**, 78–87, 2006.

Comments: The method validated for accuracy, precision, linearity, LOD, LOQ, specificity, robustness and ruggedness.

HPTLC : High Performance Thin Layer Chromatography
HPTLC Densitogram

No. 394

Sulpiride

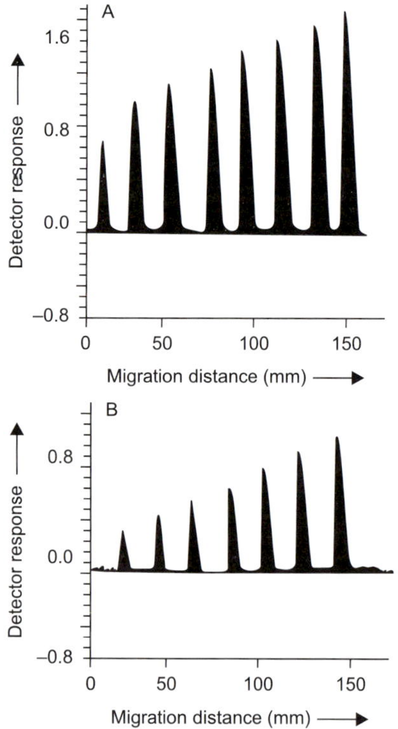

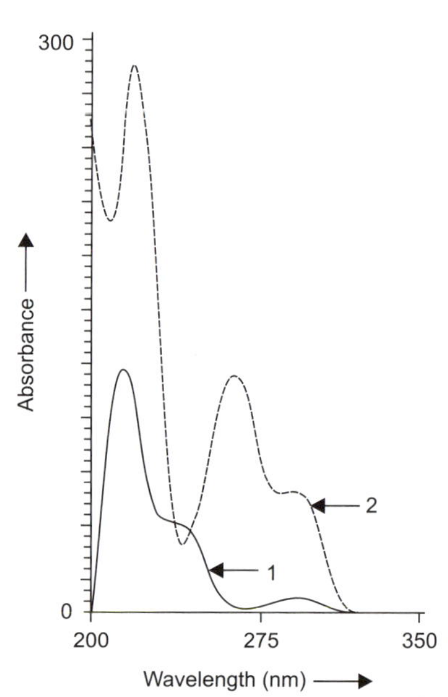

Overlaid UV-spectra of mebeverine HCl (1) and sulpiride (2) for selection of suitable wavelength for densitometric scanning

A. Linearity profile of mebeverine HCl.

B. Linearity profile of sulpiride.

For detailed experimental and chromatographic conditions, refer to Protocol No. 394.

PROTOCOL FOR HPTLC ANALYSIS OF PHARMACEUTICAL FORMULATION

Protocol No. 394

Formulation: Mebeverine hydrochloride, Sulpiride
Classification: Alimentary System **Dosage form:** Tablets
Standard preparation: Prepare 1 mg/ml solution of each compound in methanol. Further serial dilutions made with methanol for linearity studies. Apply 10 μl of each solution.
Sample preparation: Powdered sample equivalent to 100 mg of mebeverine HCl suspended in 80 ml of methanol, shaken for 10 min, diluted to 100 ml, filtered through methanol wetted filter paper. The filtrate suitably diluted for assay.
Chromatographic equipments:
Sample applicator: 10 μl Hamilton microsyringe
Development chamber: Flat-bottom glass chamber, 20 × 20 cm
Densitometric scanner: Shimadzu dual wavelength flying spot scanner
Chromatographic conditions:
1. Stationary phase: Silica gel $60F_{254}$ pre-coated TLC plates, 20 × 20 cm (250 μm) – Merck
2. Mobile phase (MP): Ethanol–diethylether–triethylamine (70 : 30 : 1 v/v)
3. Standard/Sample application:
   Band length: 10 mm Volume applied: 10 μl Spacing: 10 mm
4. Chamber saturation: 20 min. (MP)
5. RH (%): 55 ± 5
6. Temperature °C: 22 ± 2
7. Separation technique: Ascending
8. Quantity of mobile phase: 20 ml
9. Migration distance: 160 mm
10. Migration time: —

Densitometric evaluation:
Wavelength: UV–240 nm (Sulpiride); UV–262 nm (Mebeverine)
Scanning mode: Reflectance/Absorbance
HRF: Sulpiride—29; Mebeverine hydrochloride—45
Linearity (μg/ml): Mebeverine HCl—4–12; Sulpiride—2–8
Recovery (%): 99.95–100.57 for both the drugs
References: Abdel Fattah M. El Walily, Alaa El Gindy and Mohamed F. Bedair, *J. Pharm. Biomed. Anal.*, **21**, 535–548, 1999.
Comments:
- The method validated for accuracy, precision, linearity, LOD, LOQ, specificity, robustness and ruggedness.
- The method is stability indicating (acid, base, oxidative, thermal, photolytic). The degradation products were separated from main compounds.

HPTLC : High Performance Thin Layer Chromatography
HPTLC Densitogram

No. 395

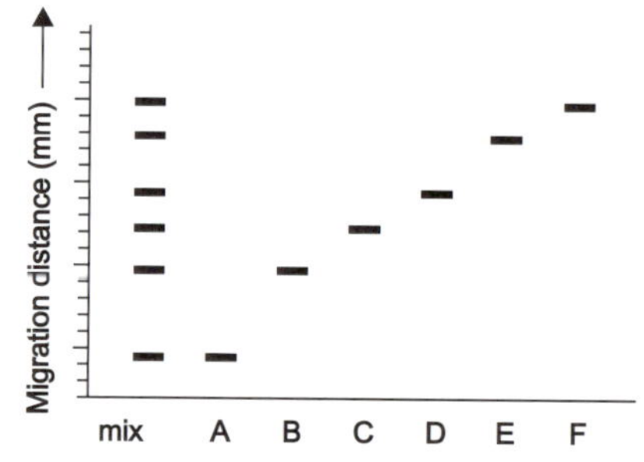

Mebeverine hydrochloride

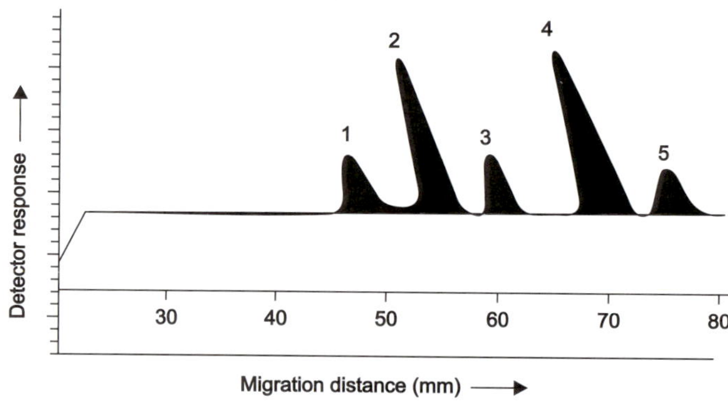

C = Sulpiride; E = Mebeverine HCl
Other spots correspond to degradation products and impurities

Typical densitogram of the synthetic mixture containing mebeverine HCl and sulpiride along with impurities and degradation products. For detailed experimental and chromatographic conditions, refer to Protocol No. 395. Peaks identification: 2. Sulpiride; 4. Mebeverine HCl 1, 3 and 5 are impurities and degradation products.

PROTOCOL FOR HPTLC ANALYSIS OF PHARMACEUTICAL FORMULATION

Protocol No. 395

Formulation: Mebeverine hydrochloride, Sulpiride

Classification: Alimentary System **Dosage form:** Tablets

Standard preparation: Prepare 1 mg/ml solution of each compound in methanol. Further dilutions suitably made for linearity profile.

Sample preparation: Each tablet containing 100 mg of mebeverine hydrochloride and 25 mg of sulpiride was suitably processed for assay.

Chromatographic equipments:

Sample applicator: Camag Linomat–IV

Development chamber: Camag twin-trough glass chamber, 20 × 10 cm

Densitometric scanner: Camag TLC Scanner–III

Chromatographic conditions:

1. Stationary phase: Silica gel $60F_{254}$ pre-coated HPTLC plates, 10 × 10 cm (200 μm)
2. Mobile phase (MP): Absolute ethanol–methylene chloride–triethylamine (7 : 3 : 0.2 v/v)
3. Standard/Sample application:
   Band length: 6 mm Volume applied: 1–10 μl Spacing: 5 mm
4. Chamber saturation: 20 min (MP)
5. RH (%): 60 ± 5
6. Temperature °C: 25 ± 2
7. Separation technique: Ascending
8. Quantity of mobile phase: 20 ml
9. Migration distance: —
10. Migration time: —

Densitometric evaluation:

Wavelength: UV–221 nm Scanning mode: Reflectance/Absorbance

HRF: Sulpiride—42; Mebeverine HCl—62

Linearity (μg/band): Sulpiride—0.4–1.4; Mebeverine HCl—0.2–1.6

Recovery (%): 99.79–99.87 for both the compounds

References: Ibrahim A. Naguib and Mohammed Abdelkawy E., *J. Med. Chem.*, **45**, 3719–3725, 2010.

Comments:

- The method validated for accuracy, precision, linearity, LOD, LOQ, specificity, robustness and ruggedness.
- The method is stability indicating (acid, base, oxidative, thermal, photolytic). The degradation products were separated from main compounds.
- Analytical results were comparable with HPLC method.

HPTLC : High Performance Thin Layer Chromatography
HPTLC Densitogram

No. 396

Hyoscine (Scopolamine)

Hyoscyamine (Atropine)

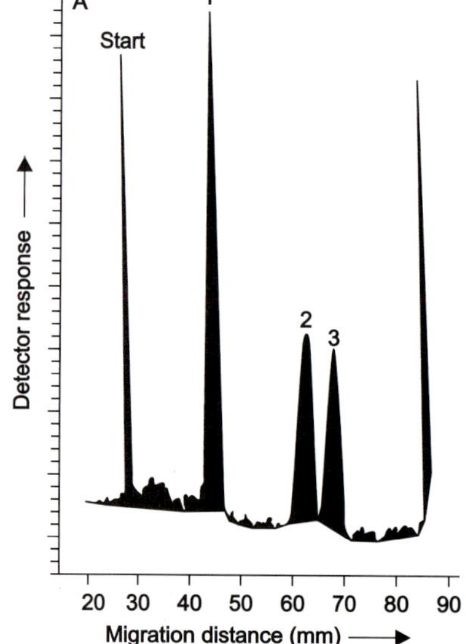

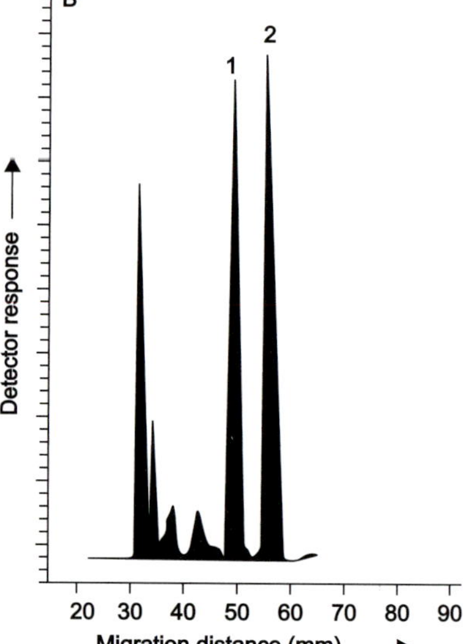

Typical densitogram (A) of the sample containing atropine sulphate and scopolamine. For detailed experimental and chromatographic conditions, refer to Protocol No. 396. Peaks identification: 1. Atropine sulphate; 2. Scopolamine.

Densitogram B. Using silica gel $60F_{254}$ TLC plates as stationary phase and mixture of trichloroethane–diethylamine (9 : 1 v/v) as mobile; detection by spraying with PDAB reagent and scanning at 270 nm. HRf: 1. Atropine sulphate—23; 2. Scopolamine—31. (No reversal of retention factor).

PROTOCOL FOR HPTLC ANALYSIS OF PHARMACEUTICAL FORMULATION

Protocol No. 396

Formulation: Atropine sulphate (Hyoscyamine), Scopolamine (Hyoscine)

Classification: Alimentary System **Dosage form:** Tablets

Standard preparation: Prepare 10 μg/ml solution of each compound in methanol and use for analysis.

Sample preparation: Extract the powdered sample with methanol with the aid of sonication, dilute, filter and use for estimation. The final solution contains 10 μg/ml of each compound.

Chromatographic equipments:

Sample applicator: Camag Linomat–IV

Development chamber: Flat bottom glass chamber, 20 × 20 cm

Densitometric scanner: Camag TLC Scanner–II

Chromatographic conditions:

1. Stationary phase: Silica gel 60 RP–18F$_{254s}$ pre-coated HPTLC plates, 10 × 10 cm (200 μm) – Merck
2. Mobile phase (MP): Acetone–0.5 M sodium chloride (40 : 60 v/v)
3. Standard/Sample application:
   Band length: 5 mm Volume applied: 10 μl Spacing: 5 mm
4. Chamber saturation: 15 min (MP)
5. RH (%): 55 ± 5
6. Temperature °C: 22 ± 2
7. Separation technique: Ascending
8. Quantity of mobile phase: 20 ml
9. Migration distance: 70 mm
10. Migration time: 40 min

Densitometric evaluation:

Wavelength: UV–254 nm Scanning mode: Reflectance/Absorbance

HRF: Atropine sulphate—70; Scopolamine—80

Linearity: 5–50 ng for both the compounds

Recovery (%): —

References: Application notes on HPLC/HPTLC; E. Merck, p. 138.

Comments: Both the compound could be separated, by NP-chromatography and visualized by PDAB reagent-see densitogram B.

HPTLC : High Performance Thin Layer Chromatography
HPTLC Densitogram

No. 397

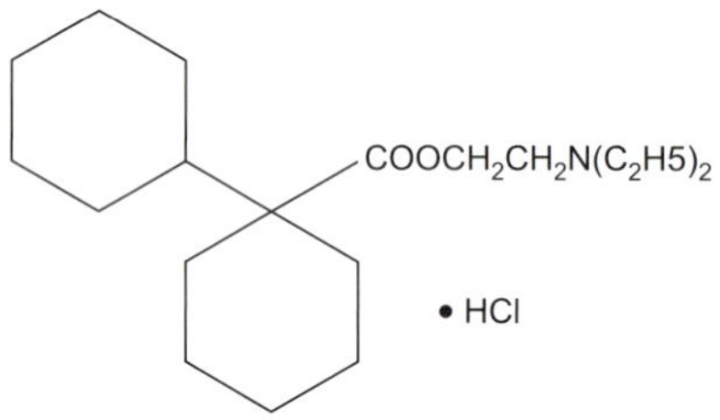
COOCH2CH2N(C2H5)2
• HCl

Dicyclomine hydrochloride

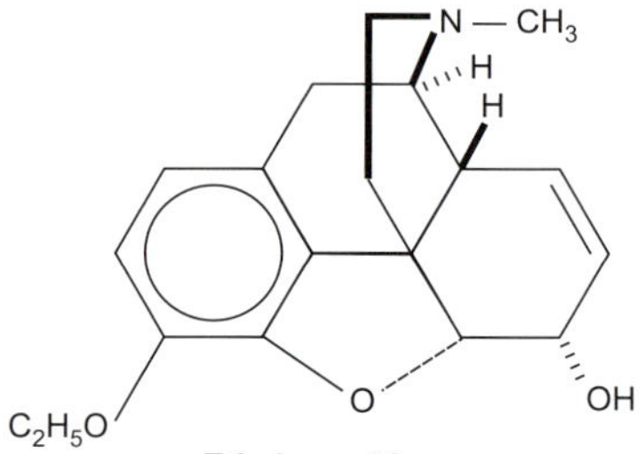
N — CH3
H
H
OH
O
C2H5O

Ethylmorphine

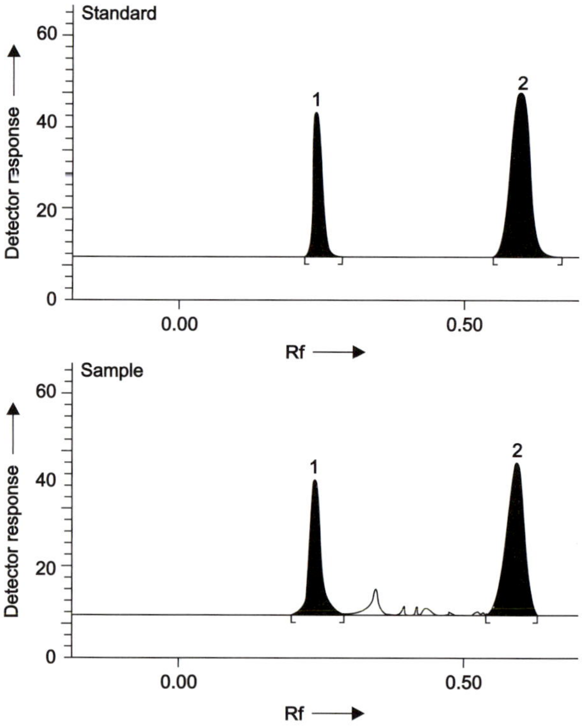
Standard
Detector response
60
40
20
0
1
2
0.00
0.50
Rf
Sample
Detector response
60
40
20
0
1
2
0.00
0.50
Rf

Typical densitogram of the sample and the standard containing ethylmorphine and dicyclomine hydrochloride. For detailed experimental and chromatographic conditions, refer to Protocol No. 397. Peaks identification: 1. Ethylmorphine; 2. Dicyclomine HCl.

PROTOCOL FOR HPTLC ANALYSIS OF PHARMACEUTICAL FORMULATION

Protocol No. 397

Formulation: Ethylmorphine, Dicylomine hydrochloride
Classification: Alimentary System **Dosage form:** Tablets
Standard preparation: Prepare 1 mg/ml solution of dicylomine hydrochloride (DH) and ethylmorphine (EM) in methanol. Mix 3.3 ml of solution (EM) and 6 ml of solution (DH) and dilute to 10 ml with methanol and use for analysis.
Sample preparation: Powdered sample equivalent to 15 mg of dicyclomine hydrochloride suspended in 15 ml of methanol, sonicated for 10 min, diluted to 25 ml with methanol, filtered and used for chromatographic application.
Chromatographic equipments:
Sample applicator: Camag Linomat–IV
Development chamber: Camag twin-trough glass chamber, 10 × 10 cm
Densitometric scanner: Camag TLC Scanner–II
Chromatographic conditions:
1. Stationary phase: Silica gel $60F_{254}$ pre-coated HPTLC plates, 10 × 10 cm (200 μm) – Merck
2. Mobile phase (MP): Toluene–acetone–methanol–25% ammonia (7 : 2 : 1 : 0.05 v/v)
3. Standard/Sample application:
   Band length: 10 mm Volume applied: 15 μl Spacing: 10 mm
4. Chamber saturation: 20 min (MP)
5. RH (%): 55 ± 5
6. Temperature °C: 22 ± 2
7. Separation technique: Ascending
8. Quantity of mobile phase: 10 ml
9. Migration distance: 50 mm
10. Migration time: 14 min

Densitometric evaluation:
Wavelength: Vis: 623 nm Scanning mode: Reflectance/Absorbance
HRF: Ethylmorphine—25; Dicyclomine HCl—60
Linearity: Ethylmorphine—1–10 μg; Dicyclomine HCl—5–25 μg
Recovery (%): 97.55–98.45 for both the compounds
References: P. Parimoo, M. Mounisswamy, A. Bharathi, N. Lakshmi, *Indian Drugs*, **31(5)**, 211–214, 1994.
Comments:
- After development, the plate was dipped in diluted reagent, air dried and scanned at 623 nm within 20 min.
- Reagent: Dissolve 6.06 of pot. thiocyanate, 50 g of $CoCl_2$ and 3.4 g of sod. acetate in 20 ml of water, add 2.5 ml of 1M HCl, dilute to 25 ml with water; 20 ml of the reagent further diluted to 250 ml with methanol (diluted reagent).

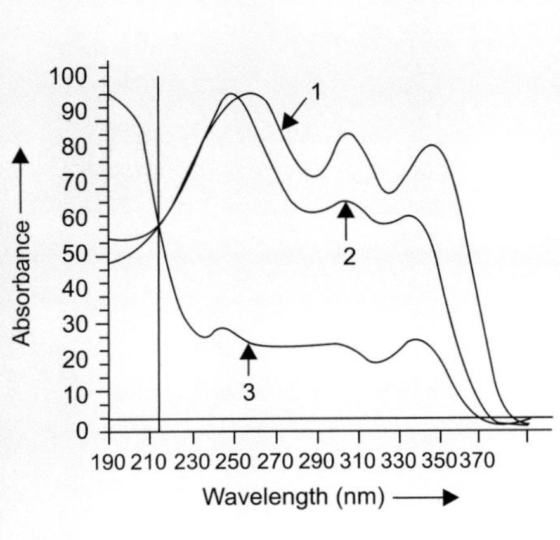

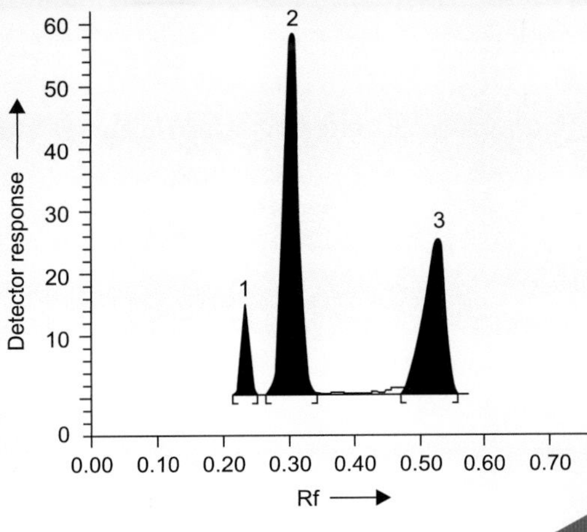

8

Central Nervous System

- Sedatives and tranquillisers
- Anti-emetics and antinauseants
- Antimigraines

Protocols and Densitograms from 398 to 432

Learn by experience or from experienced.

HPTLC : High Performance Thin Layer Chromatography
HPTLC Densitogram

No. 398

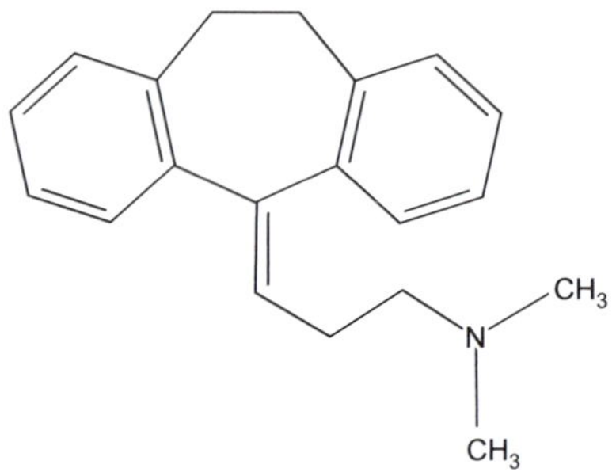

Amitriptyline

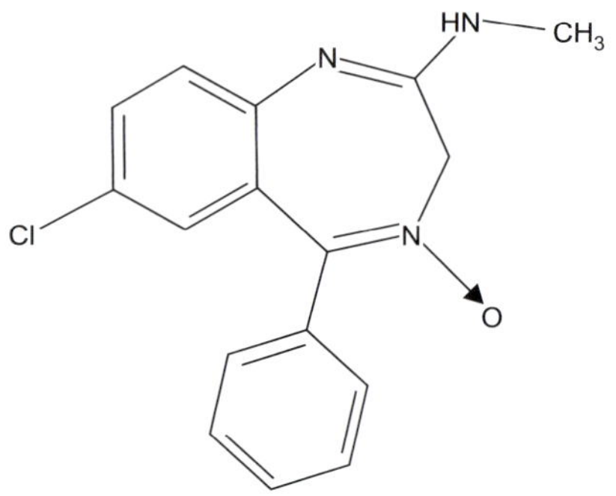

Chlordiazepoxide

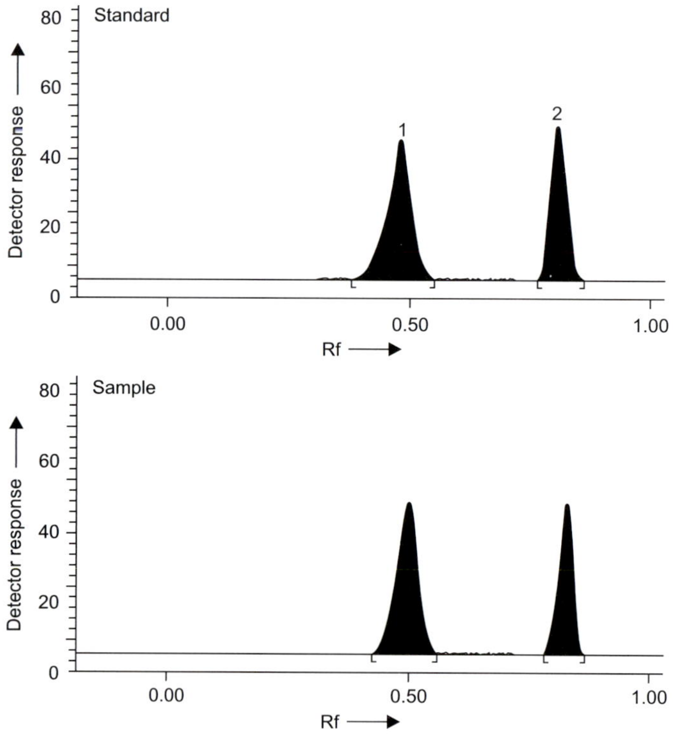

Standard

Sample

Typical densitogram of the standard and the sample containing amitriptyline hydrochloride and chlordiazepoxide. For detailed experimental and chromatographic conditions, refer to Protocol No. 398. Peaks identification: 1. Amitriptyline HCl; 2. Chlordiazepoxide.

PROTOCOL FOR HPTLC ANALYSIS OF PHARMACEUTICAL FORMULATION

Protocol No. 398

Formulation: **Amitriptyline hydrochloride, Chlordiazepoxide**

Classification: Central Nervous System **Dosage form:** Tablets

Standard preparation: Dissolve about 25 mg of amitriptyline and 10 mg of chlordiazepoxide accurately weighted in 25 ml of methanol. Dilute 0.25 to 10 ml with methanol and use for analysis.

Sample preparation: Weigh finely powdered sample equivalent to 10 mg of chlordiazepoxide, add 10–15 ml of methanol, sonicate and dilute to 25 ml, filter and dilute 0.25 ml of filtrate to 10 ml with methanol and use for analysis.

Chromatographic equipments:

Sample applicator: Camag Linomat–IV

Development chamber: Camag twin-trough glass chamber, 10 × 10 cm

Densitometric scanner: Camag TLC Scanner–III

Chromatographic conditions:

1. Stationary phase: Silica gel 60F_{254} pre-coated HPTLC plates, 10 × 10 cm (200 μm) – Merck
2. Mobile phase (MP): Ethyl acetate–methanol–diethylamine (9.5 : 0.5 : 0.05 v/v)
3. Standard/Sample application:
   Band length: 5 mm Volume applied: 4 μl Spacing: 5 mm
4. Chamber saturation: 5 min (MP)
5. RH (%): 55 ± 5
6. Temperature °C: 22 ± 2
7. Separation technique: Ascending
8. Quantity of mobile phase: 10 ml
9. Migration distance: 50 mm
10. Migration time: 15 min

Densitometric evaluation:

Wavelength: UV–245 nm Scanning mode: Reflectance/Absorbance

HRF: Amitriptyline HCl—49; Chlordiazepoxide—78

Linearity (ng/band): Amitriptyline HCl—50–250; Chlordiazepoxide—10–100

Recovery (%): 100.80–102.0 for both the compounds

References: P.P. Shirke, M.K. Patel, V.A. Tamhane, V.B. Tirodkar, *Eastern Pharmacist*, **37**, 179–180, 1994.

Comments:

- The method validated for accuracy, precision, linearity, LOD, LOQ, specificity, robustness and ruggedness.
- Several market samples of similar composition were analysed by the proposed method with reproducible results.

HPTLC : High Performance Thin Layer Chromatography
HPTLC Densitogram

No. 399

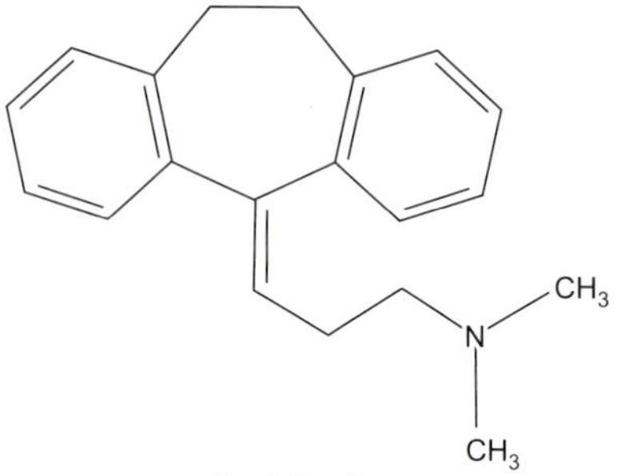

Amitriptyline

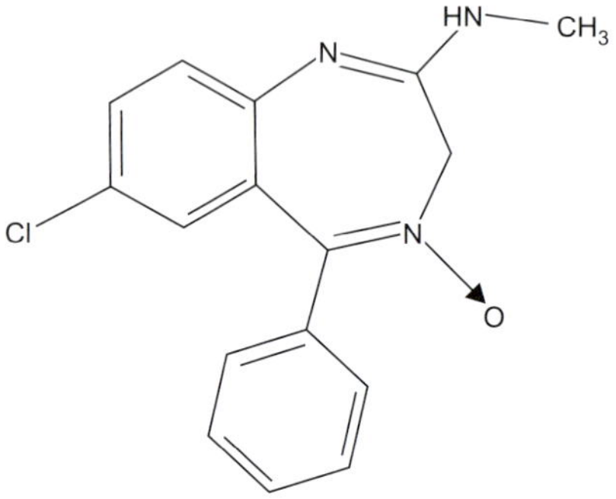

Chlordiazepoxide

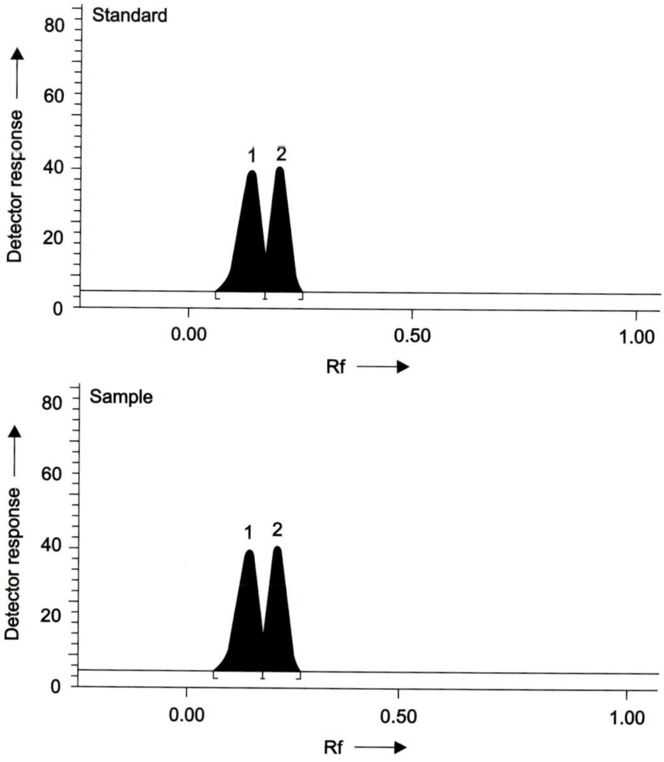

Standard

Sample

Typical densitogram of the standard and sample containing amitriptyline hydrochloride and chlordiazepoxide. For detailed experimental and chromatographic conditions, refer to Protocol No. 399. Peaks identification: 1. Amitriptyline HCl; 2. Chlordiazepoxide.

PROTOCOL FOR HPTLC ANALYSIS OF PHARMACEUTICAL FORMULATION

Protocol No. 399

Formulation: Amitriptyline hydrochloride, Chlordiazepoxide

Classification: Central Nervous System **Dosage form:** Tablets

Standard preparation: Prepare 1 mg/ml solution of amitriptyline hydrochloride in methanol (A). Prepare 40 μg/ml solution of chlordiazepoxide in methanol (B). Mix 0.25 ml each of solutions A and B and dilute to 1 ml with methanol to use for analysis.

Sample preparation: Powdered sample equivalent to 10 mg of chlordiazepoxide suspended in 15 ml of methanol, sonicated for 5 min, diluted to 25 ml, filtered and 0.25 ml of the filtrate diluted to 10 ml with methanol to use for chromatographic analysis.

Chromatographic equipments:

Sample applicator: Camag Linomat–IV

Development chamber: Camag twin-trough glass chamber, 10 × 10 cm

Densitometric scanner: Camag TLC Scanner–II

Chromatographic conditions:

1. Stationary phase: Silica gel 60 RP–18_{254s} pre-coated HPTLC plates, 10 × 10 cm (200 μm) – Merck
2. Mobile phase (MP): 0.5 M sodium chloride–methanol–acetonitrile–glacial acetic acid (5 : 2 : 3 : 0.1 v/v)
3. Standard/Sample application:
   Band length: 5 mm Volume applied: 4 μl Spacing: 5 mm
4. Chamber saturation: 30 min (MP)
5. RH (%): 55 ± 5
6. Temperature °C: 22 ± 2
7. Separation technique: Ascending
8. Quantity of mobile phase: 10 ml
9. Migration distance: 50 mm
10. Migration time: 20 min

Densitometric evaluation:

Wavelength: UV–245 nm Scanning mode: Reflectance/Absorbance

HRF: Amitriptyline HCl—12; Chlordiazepoxide—19

Linearity (ng/band): Amitriptyline HCl—50–200; Chlordiazepoxide—10–80

Recovery (%): 99.15–99.75 for both the compounds

References: —

Comments:

- The method was optimized and analytical work carried out at **Anchrom's HPTLC Application Laboratory**, Mumbai, India.
- Several market samples of similar composition were analysed by the proposed method with reproducible results.

HPTLC : High Performance Thin Layer Chromatography
HPTLC Densitogram

No. 400

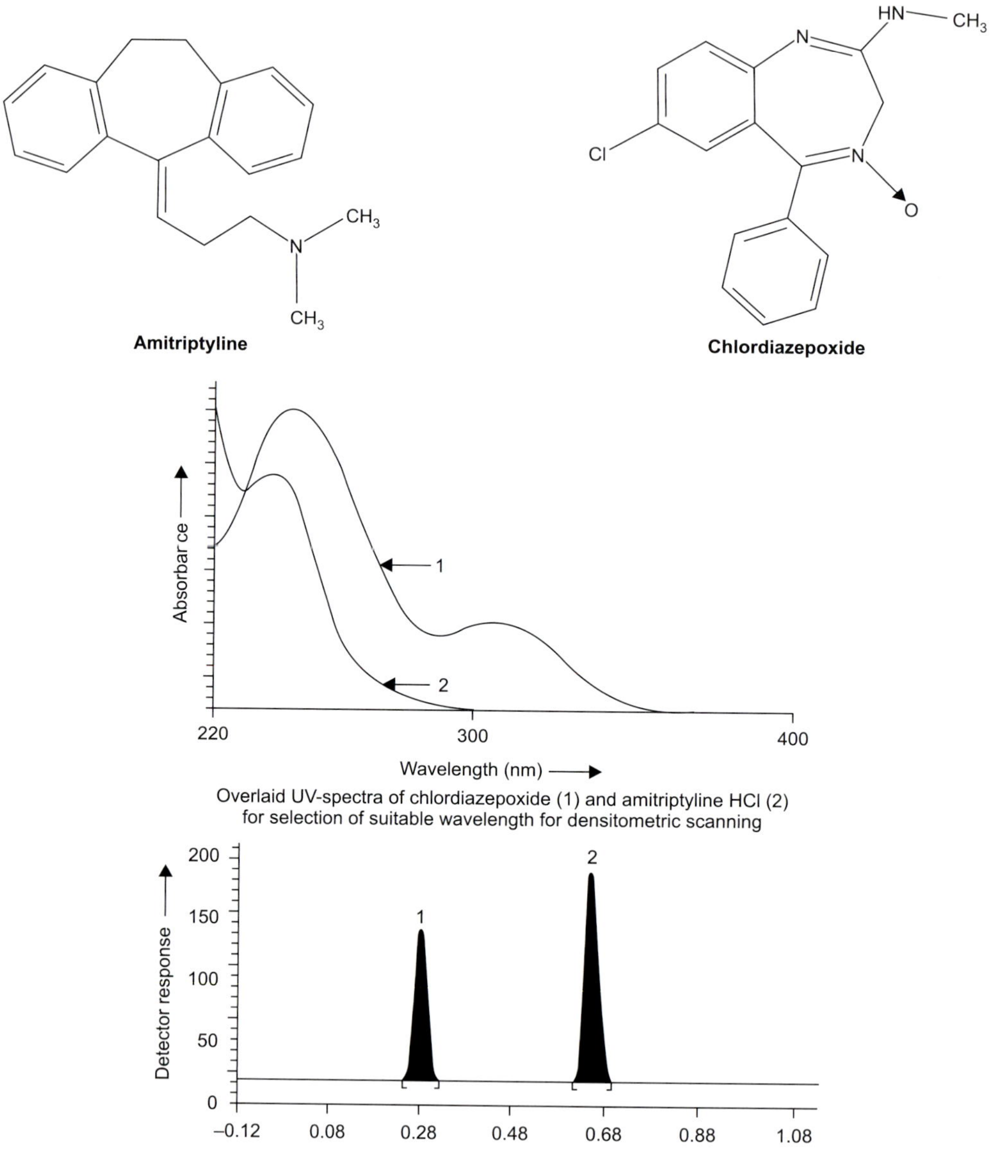

Typical densitogram of the standard containing amitriptyline hydrochloride and chlordiazepoxide. For detailed experimental and chromatographic conditions, refer to Protocol No. 400. Peaks identification: 1. Chlordiazepoxide; 2. Amitriptyline HCl.

PROTOCOL FOR HPTLC ANALYSIS OF PHARMACEUTICAL FORMULATION

Protocol No. 400

Formulation: Amitriptyline hydrochloride, Chlordiazepoxide

Classification: Central Nervous System **Dosage form:** Tablets

Standard preparation: Prepare standard solution of each compound separately in methanol to get 100 μg/ml (amitriptyline HCl) and 40 μg/ml (chlordiazepoxide). Apply different volumes (0.5–6 μl).

Sample preparation: Powdered sample equivalent to 25 mg of amitriptyline HCl and 10 mg of chlordiazepoxide suspended in methanol, sonicated, diluted to 50 ml, filtered and the filtrate suitably diluted with methanol as under standard solution and used for assay.

Chromatographic equipments:

Sample applicator: Camag Linomat–V

Development chamber: Camag twin-trough glass chamber, 10 × 10 cm

Densitometric scanner: Camag TLC Scanner–III

Chromatographic conditions:

1. Stationary phase: Silica gel $60F_{254}$ pre-coated TLC plates, 10 × 10 cm (250 μm) – Merck
2. Mobile phase (MP): Carbon tetrachloride–acetone–triethylamine (6 : 3 : 0.2 v/v)
3. Standard/Sample application:
   Band length: 5 mm Volume applied: 4 μl Spacing: 5 mm
4. Chamber saturation: 30 min (MP)
5. RH (%): 55 ± 5
6. Temperature °C: 25 ± 2
7. Separation technique: Ascending
8. Quantity of mobile phase: 18 ml
9. Migration distance: 80 mm
10. Migration time: 20 min

Densitometric evaluation:

Wavelength: UV–240 nm Scanning mode: Reflectance/Absorbance

HRF: Chlordiazepoxide—29; Amitriptyline HCl—68

Linearity (ng/band): Amitriptyline HCl—50–600; Chlordiazepoxide—20–240

Recovery (%): 100.16–100.80 for both the compounds

References: Sejal Patel and N.J. Patel, *Ind. J. Pharm. Sci.*, **71(4)**, 472–476, 2009.

Comments:

- The method validated for accuracy, precision, linearity, LOD, LOQ, specificity, robustness and ruggedness.
- The sample was simultaneously analysed by first-derivative spectroscopy, HPLC and HPTLC. The results were comparable.

HPTLC : High Performance Thin Layer Chromatography
HPTLC Densitogram

No. 401

• HCl

$CH_2CH_2CH_2 — N(CH_3)_2$

Imipramine hydrochloride

Diazepam

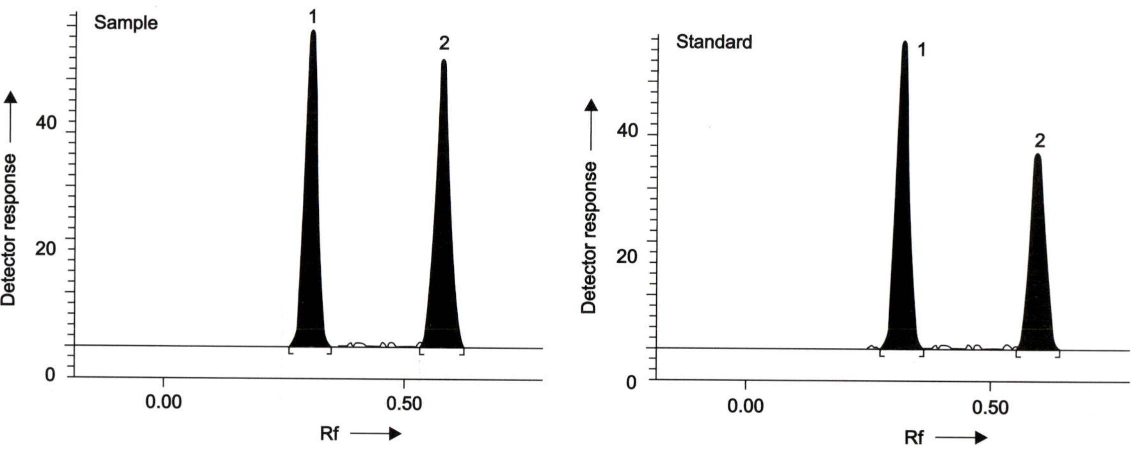

Typical densitogram of the standard and sample containing diazepam and imipramine hydrochloride. For detailed experimental and chromatographic conditions, refer to Protocol No. 401. Peaks identification: 1. Imipramine HCl; 2. Diazepam.

PROTOCOL FOR HPTLC ANALYSIS OF PHARMACEUTICAL FORMULATION

Protocol No. 401

Formulation: Imipramine hydrochloride, Diazepam

Classification: Central Nervous System **Dosage form:** Tablets

Standard preparation: (a) Prepare 1 mg/ml solution of diazepam (D) in methanol. (b) Weigh about 10 mg of imipramine HCl (I), add 0.8 ml of solution (a) and dilute to 10 ml with methanol. Further dilute 0.5 ml to 10 ml with methanol and use for application.

Sample preparation: Weigh powdered sample accurately equivalent to 25 mg of imipramine HCl, add 30 ml of methanol, vortex for 5 min, dilute to 50 ml. Further dilute 1 ml to 10 ml with methanol for application.

Chromatographic equipments:

Sample applicator: Camag Linomat–IV

Development chamber: Camag twin-trough glass chamber, 10 × 10 cm

Densitometric scanner: Camag TLC Scanner–II

Chromatographic conditions:

1. Stationary phase: Silica gel $60F_{254}$ pre-coated TLC plates, 10 × 10 cm (200 μm) – Merck
2. Mobile phase (MP): Toluene–acetone–25% ammonia (7 : 3 : 0.1 v/v)
3. Standard/Sample application:
   Band length: 5 mm Volume applied: 5 μl Spacing: 5 mm
4. Chamber saturation: 10 min (MP)
5. RH (%): 55 ± 5
6. Temperature °C: 22 ± 2
7. Separation technique: Ascending
8. Quantity of mobile phase: 10 ml
9. Migration distance: 50 mm
10. Migration time: 14 min

Densitometric evaluation:

Wavelength: UV–235 nm Scanning mode: Reflectance/Absorbance

HRF: Imipramine HCl—31; Diazepam—58

Linearity (ng/band): Imipramine HCl—50–500; Diazepam—10–100

Recovery (%): 98.05–102.40 for both the compounds

References: —

Comments:

- The method was optimized and analytical work carried out at **Anchrom's HPTLC Application Laboratory**, Mumbai, India.
- Several market samples of similar composition were analysed by the proposed method with reproducible results.

HPTLC : High Performance Thin Layer Chromatography
HPTLC Densitogram

No. 402

• HCl

$CH_2CH_2CH_2 — N(CH_3)_2$

Imipramine hydrochloride

CH_3 N O Cl N

Diazepam

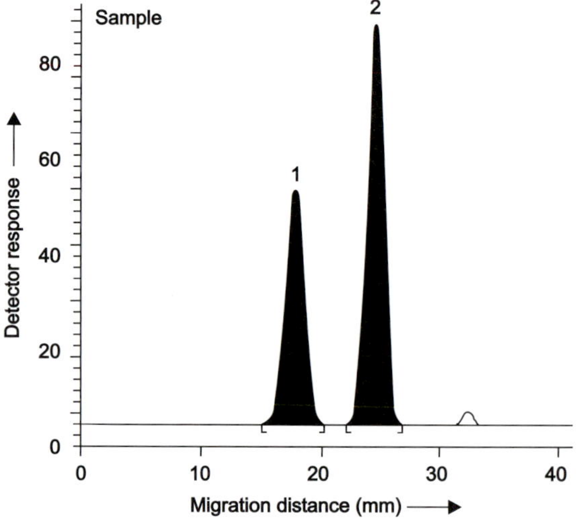

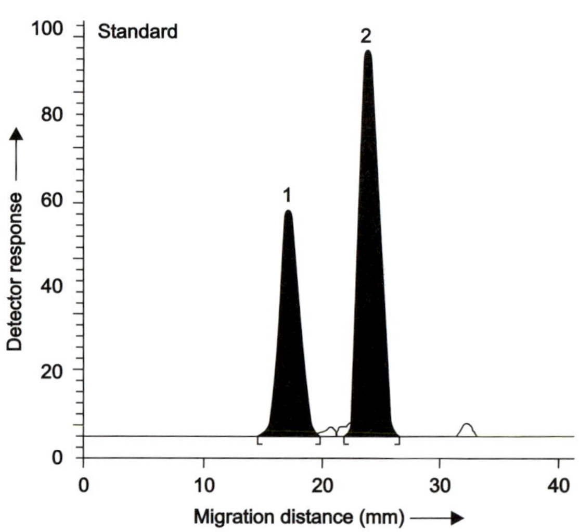

Typical densitogram of the standard and the sample containing diazepam and imipramine hydrochloride. For detailed experimental and chromatographic conditions, refer to Protocol No. 402. Peaks identification: 1. Diazepam; 2. Imipramine HCl.

PROTOCOL FOR HPTLC ANALYSIS OF PHARMACEUTICAL FORMULATION

Protocol No. 402

Formulation: Imipramine hydrochloride, Diazepam
Classification: Central Nervous System **Dosage form:** Tablets
Standard preparation: Prepare 1 mg/ml solution of diazepam (D) in methanol. Take 10 mg of imipramine hydrochloride, add 0.8 ml of solution D, dilute to 10 ml with methanol. Further dilute 0.5 ml of the resulting solution to 10 ml with methanol to use for application.
Sample preparation: Powdered sample equivalent to 25 mg of imipramine hydrochloride suspended in 30 ml of methanol, sonicated for 5 min, diluted to 50 ml, filtered and 1.0 ml of the filtrate diluted to 10 ml and used for chromatographic application.
Chromatographic equipments:
Sample applicator: Camag Linomat–IV
Development chamber: Camag twin-trough glass chamber, 10 × 10 cm
Densitometric scanner: Camag TLC Scanner–II
Chromatographic conditions:

1. Stationary phase: Silica gel 60 RP–18F_{254s} pre-coated HPTLC plates, 5 × 10 cm (200 μm) – Merck
2. Mobile phase (MP): 0.5 M sodium chloride–methanol–acetonitrile–glacial acetic acid (5 : 2 : 3 : 0.1 v/v)
3. Standard/Sample application:
   Band length: 5 mm Volume applied: 5 μl Spacing: 5 mm
4. Chamber saturation: 20 min (MP)
5. RH (%): 55 ± 5
6. Temperature °C: 22 ± 2
7. Separation technique: Ascending
8. Quantity of mobile phase: 10 ml
9. Migration distance: 50 mm
10. Migration time: 20 min

Densitometric evaluation:
Wavelength: UV–235 nm Scanning mode: Reflectance/Absorbance
HRF: Diazepam—30; Imipramine HCl—40
Linearity (ng/band): Imipramine HCl—50–500; Diazepam—10–100
Recovery (%): 97.60–101.50 for both the compounds
References: —
Comments:

- The method was optimized and analytical work carried out at **Anchrom's HPTLC Application Laboratory**, Mumbai, India.
- Reversal of retention order observed in RP–chromatography as compared to NP-chromatography.
- Several market samples of similar composition were analysed by the proposed method with reproducible results.

HPTLC : High Performance Thin Layer Chromatography
HPTLC Densitogram

No. 403

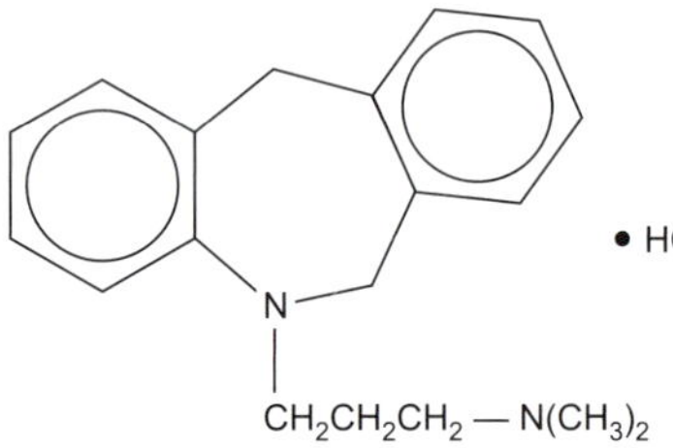

• HCl

$CH_2CH_2CH_2 — N(CH_3)_2$

Imipramine hydrochloride

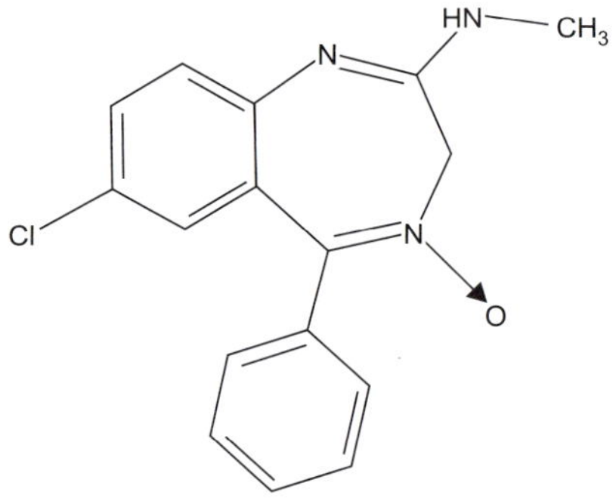

Chlordiazepoxide

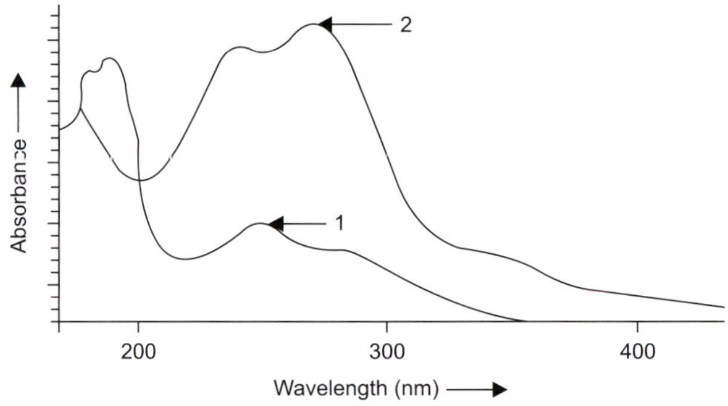

Overlaid UV-spectra of imipramine HCl (1) and chlordiazepoxide (2) for selection of suitable wavelength for densitometric scanning

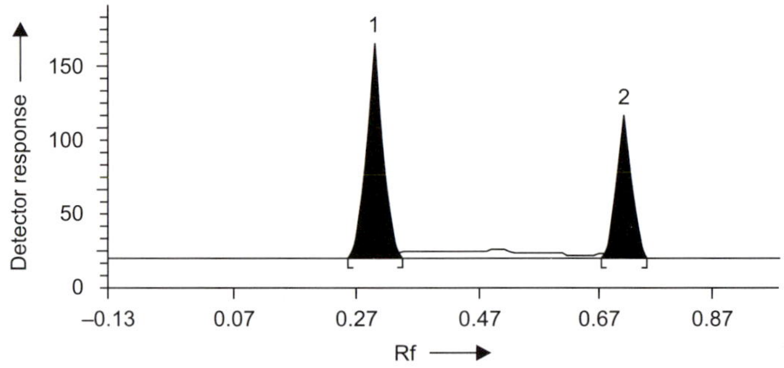

Typical densitogram of the standard containing imipramine HCl and chlordiazepoxide. For detailed experimental and chromatographic conditions, refer to Protocol No. 403. Peaks identification: 1. Imipramine HCl; 2. Chlordiazepoxide.

PROTOCOL FOR HPTLC ANALYSIS OF PHARMACEUTICAL FORMULATION

Protocol No. 403

Formulation: Imipramine hydrochloride, Chlordiazepoxide

Classification: Central Nervous System **Dosage form:** Tablets

Standard preparation: Prepare 1 mg/ml solution of each compound in methanol. Further dilutions made with methanol to get 100 μg/ml (imipramine) and 40 μg/ml (chlordiazepoxide). Apply 0.5–6 μl for linearity studies.

Sample preparation: Powdered sample equivalent to 10 mg of chlordiazepoxide suspended in methanol, sonicated for 10 min, diluted and filtered. The filtrate suitably diluted to get 100 μg/ml (imipramine) and 400 μg/ml (chlordiazepoxide). Apply 4 μl for assay.

Chromatographic equipments:

Sample applicator: Camag Linomat–V

Development chamber: Camag twin-trough glass chamber, 10 × 10 cm

Densitometric scanner: Camag TLC Scanner–III

Chromatographic conditions:

1. Stationary phase: Silica gel 60F_{254} pre-coated HPTLC plates, 10 × 10 cm (200 μm) – Merck
2. Mobile phase (MP): Carbon tetrachloride–acetone–triethylamine (6 : 3 : 0.3 v/v)
3. Standard/Sample application:
   Band length: 5 mm Volume applied: 0.5–6 μl Spacing: 10 mm
4. Chamber saturation: 30 min (MP)
5. RH (%): 55 ± 5
6. Temperature °C: 25 ± 2
7. Separation technique: Ascending
8. Quantity of mobile phase: 18 ml
9. Migration distance: 80 mm
10. Migration time: 25 min

Densitometric evaluation:

Wavelength: UV–240 nm Scanning mode: Reflectance/Absorbance

HRF: Chlordiazepoxide—32; Imipramine—73

Linearity (ng/band): Imipramine HCl—50–600; Chlordiazepoxide—20–240

Recovery (%): 99.51–100.59 for both the compounds

References: Sejal K Patel and N.J. Patel, *J. AOAC*, **91(3)**, 904–910, 2010.

Comments:

- The method validated for accuracy, precision, linearity, LOD, LOQ, specificity, robustness and ruggedness.
- The method was compared with spectrophotometric and RP–HPLC methods with comparable results.

HPTLC : High Performance Thin Layer Chromatography
HPTLC Densitogram

No. 404

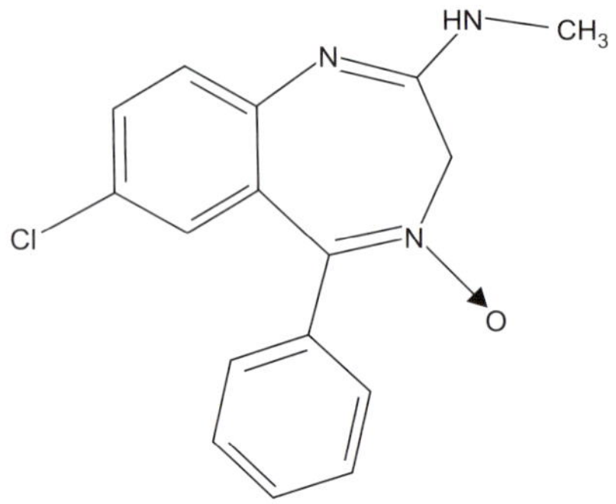

Chlordiazepoxide

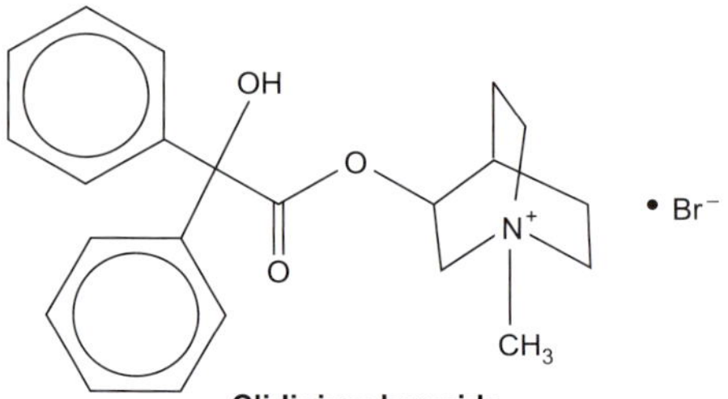

Clidinium bromide

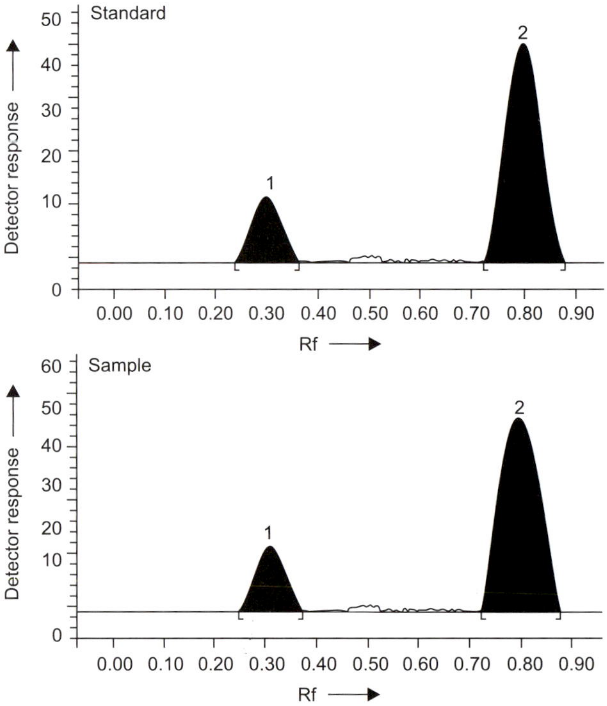

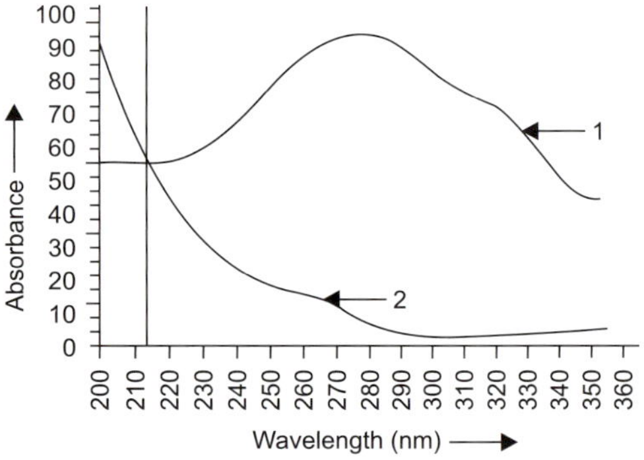

Overlaid UV-spectra of chlordiazepoxide (1) and clidinium bromide (2) for selection of suitable wavelength for densitometric scanning

Typical densitogram of the standard and the sample containing chlordiazepoxide and clidinium bromide. For detailed experimental and chromatographic conditions, refer to Protocol No. 404. Peaks identification: 1. Chlordiazepoxide; 2. Clidinium bromide.

PROTOCOL FOR HPTLC ANALYSIS OF PHARMACEUTICAL FORMULATION

Protocol No. 404

Formulation: Chlordiazepoxide, Clidinium bromide

Classification: Central Nervous System **Dosage form:** Tablets

Standard preparation: Prepare 1 mg/ml solution of chlordiazepoxide and 500 μg/ml of clidinium bromide, both in methanol, and use for analysis.

Sample preparation: Powdered sample equivalent to 5 mg of chlordiazepoxide suspended in 20 ml of methanol, shaken for 15 min, diluted to 25 ml, filtered through Whatman No. 1 filter paper and filtrate used for chromatographic application.

Chromatographic equipments:

Sample applicator: Camag Linomat–IV

Development chamber: Camag twin-trough glass chamber, 10 × 10 cm

Densitometric scanner: Camag TLC Scanner–III

Chromatographic conditions:

1. Stationary phase: Silica gel 60F_{254} pre-coated HPTLC plates, 10 × 10 cm (200 μm) – Merck
2. Mobile phase (MP): Methanol–acetonitrile–water–acetic acid (2 : 6.5 : 1 : 0.5 v/v)
3. Standard/Sample application:
   Spot dia: 6 mm Volume applied: 4 μl Spacing: 10 mm
4. Chamber saturation: 10 min (MP)
5. RH (%): 55 ± 5
6. Temperature °C: 22 ± 2
7. Separation technique: Ascending
8. Quantity of mobile phase: 20 ml
9. Migration distance: 70 mm
10. Migration time: 20 min

Densitometric evaluation:

Wavelength: UV–217 nm Scanning mode: Reflectance/Absorbance

HRF: Clidinium bromide—30; Chlordiazepoxide—83

Linearity (μg/band): Chlordiazepoxide—2.2–12.2; Clidinium bromide—1.2–8.8

Recovery (%): Chlordiazepoxide—98.06–99.31; Clidinium bromide—100.04–102.66

References: S.G. Walode, S.B. Bagade, M.R. Rode and M.R. Tajne, *Asian J. Chem.*, **17(4)**, 2517–2523, 2005.

Comments:

- The method validated for accuracy, precision, linearity, LOD, LOQ, specificity, robustness and ruggedness.
- The method is stability indicating (acid, base, oxidative, thermal, photolytic). The degradation products were separated from main compounds.

HPTLC : High Performance Thin Layer Chromatography
HPTLC Densitogram

No. 405

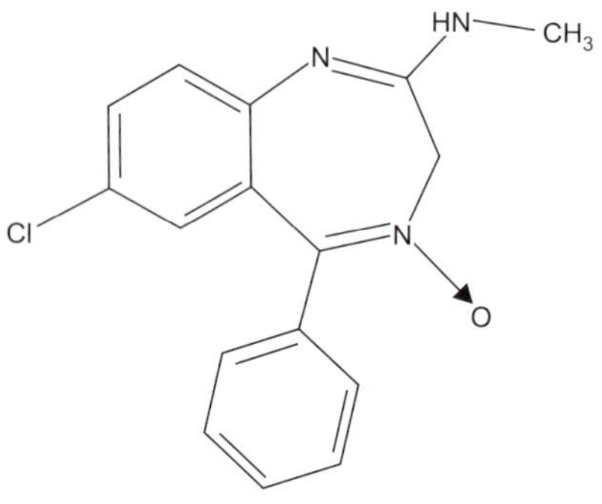

Chlordiazepoxide

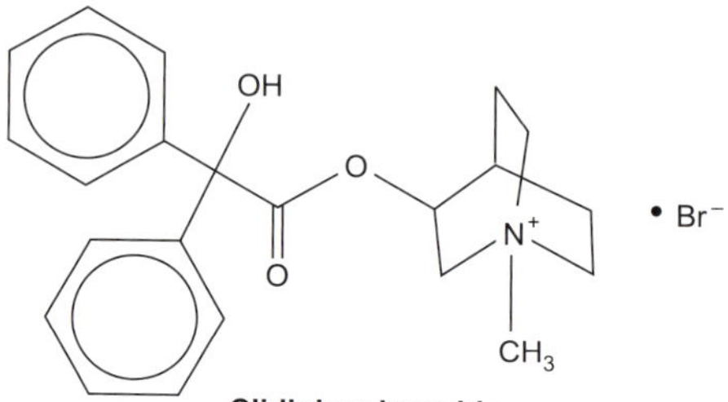

Clidinium bromide

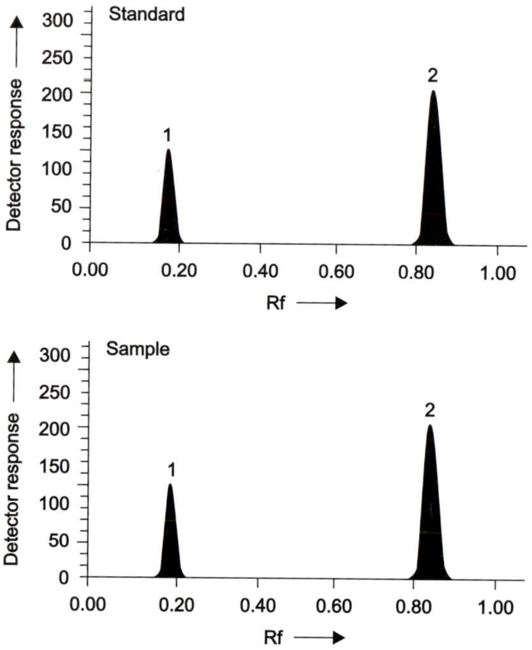

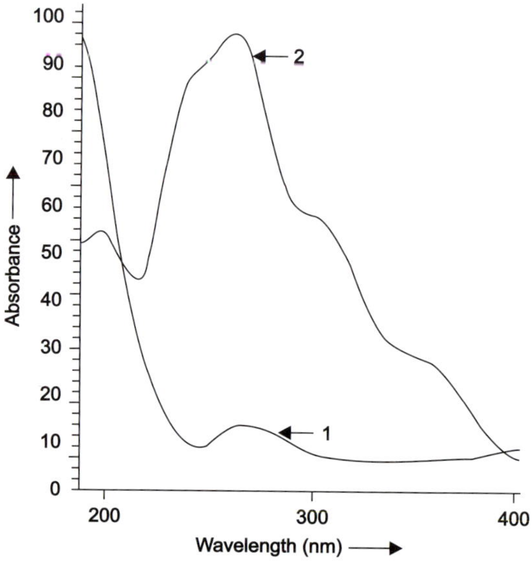

Overlaid UV-spectra of clidinium bromide (1) and chlordiazepoxide (2) for selection of suitable wavelength for densitometric scanning

Typical densitogram of the standard and the sample containing clidinium bromide and chlordiazepoxide. For detailed experimental and chromatographic conditions, refer to Protocol No. 405. Peaks identification: 1. Clidinium bromide; 2. Chlordiazepoxide.

PROTOCOL FOR HPTLC ANALYSIS OF PHARMACEUTICAL FORMULATION

Protocol No. 405

Formulation: Chlordiazepoxide, Clidinium bromide

Classification: Central Nervous System **Dosage form:** Tablets

Standard preparation: Prepare solution of both the compounds in methanol to get 500 μg/ml of chlordiazepoxide and 250 μg/ml of clidinium bromide. Further serial dilutions of each solution are made with methanol for linearity profile. Apply 10 μl of each solution for analysis.

Sample preparation: Suspend powdered sample equivalent to 10 mg of chlordiazepoxide in 15 ml of methanol, sonicate, dilute to 20 ml with methanol, filter and dilute 1 ml of the solution to 10 ml with methanol and use for analysis.

Chromatographic equipments:

Sample applicator: Camag Linomat–V

Development chamber: Camag ADC-2, saturated with Camag saturation pad

Densitometric scanner: Camag TLC Scanner–III

Chromatographic conditions:

1. Stationary phase: Silica gel $60F_{254}$ pre-coated TLC plates glass, 20 × 10 cm (250 μm) – Merck
2. Mobile phase (MP): Acetone–methanol–water–0.2 M HCl (14 : 4 : 1 : 1 v/v)
3. Standard/Sample application:
   Spot dia: 8 mm Volume applied: 10 μl Spacing: 10.6 mm
4. Chamber saturation: 20 min (MP)
5. RH (%): 55 ± 5
6. Temperature °C: 25 ± 1
7. Separation technique: Ascending
8. Quantity of mobile phase: 20 ml
9. Migration distance: 70 mm
10. Migration time: 10 min

Densitometric evaluation:

Wavelength: UV–210 nm Scanning mode: Reflectance/Absorbance

HRF: Clidinium bromide—18; Chlordiazepoxide—85

Linearity (ng/band): Chlordiazepoxide—50–500; Clidinium bromide—25–250

Recovery (%): —

References: —

Comments:

- The method was optimized and analytical work carried out at **Anchrom's HPTLC Application Laboratory**, Mumbai, India.
- Several market samples of similar composition were analysed by the proposed method with reproducible results.

HPTLC : High Performance Thin Layer Chromatography
HPTLC Densitogram

No. 406

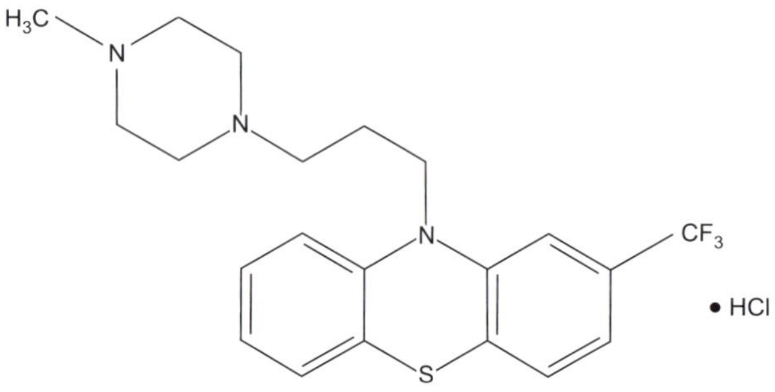

Trifluoperazine hydrochloride

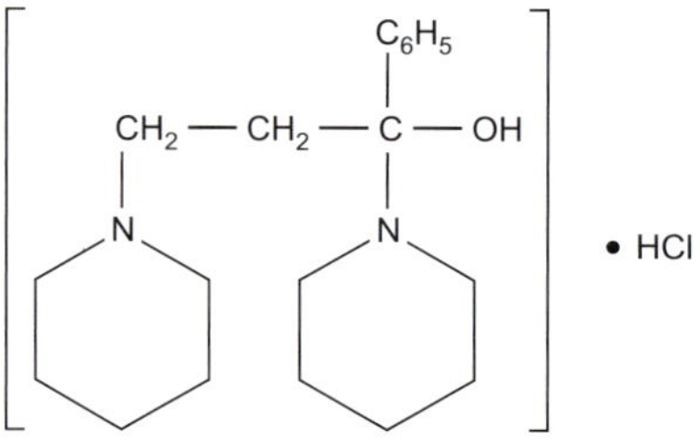

Trihexyphenidyl hydrochloride

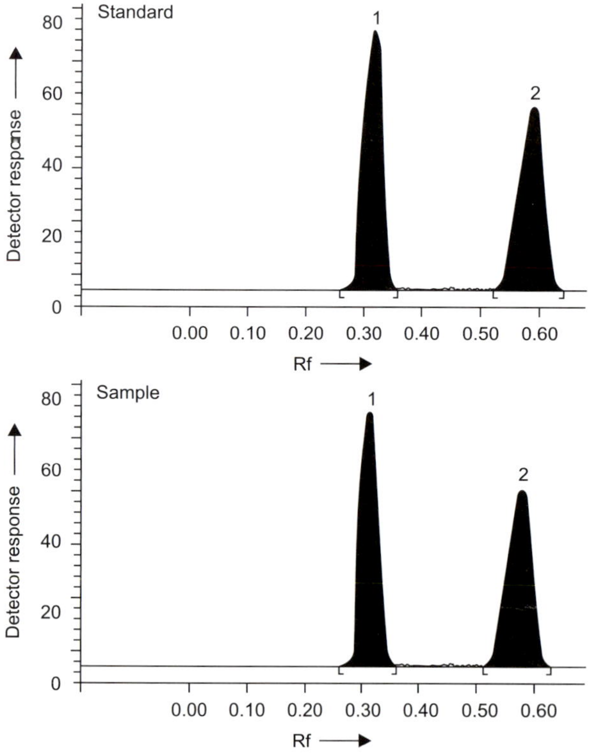

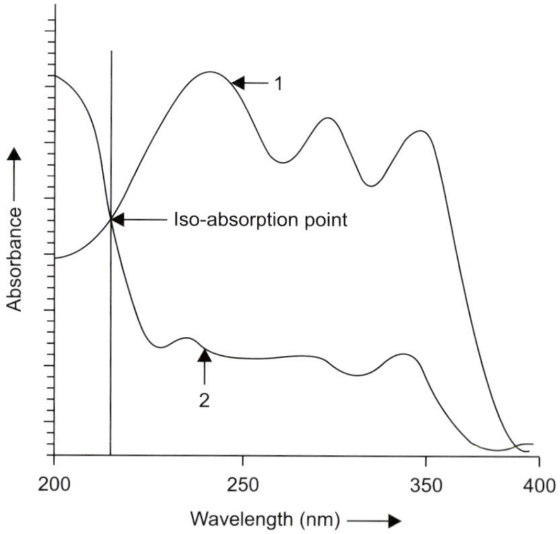

Overlaid UV-spectra of trifluoperazine HCl (1) and trihexyphenidyl HCl (2) for selection of suitable wavelength for densitometric scanning

Typical densitogram of the standard and the sample containing trifluoperazine HCl and trihexyphenidyl HCl. For detailed experimental and chromatographic conditions, refer to Protocol No. 406. Peaks identification: 1. Trifluoperazine HCl; 2. Trihexyphenidyl HCl.

PROTOCOL FOR HPTLC ANALYSIS OF PHARMACEUTICAL FORMULATION

Protocol No. 406

Formulation: Trifluoperazine hydrochloride, Trihexyphenidyl hydrochloride
Classification: Central Nervous System **Dosage form:** Tablets
Standard preparation: Accurately weigh 25 mg of trihexyphenidyl, add 10 mg of trifluoperazine and dissolve in methanol to make 10 ml. Further dilute 0.8 ml to 10 ml with methanol and use for chromatographic evaluation.
Sample preparation: Weigh finely powdered sample equivalent to 10 mg of trifluoperazine HCl, add 5–6 ml of methanol, vortex for 5 min, dilute to 10 ml with methanol, filter. Dilute 0.8 ml to 10 ml with methanol and use for analysis.
Chromatographic equipments:
Sample applicator: Camag Linomat–IV
Development chamber: Camag twin-trough glass chamber, 10 × 10 cm
Densitometric scanner: Camag TLC Scanner–II
Chromatographic conditions:
1. Stationary phase: Silica gel $60F_{254}$ pre-coated HPTLC plates, 10 × 10 cm (200 μm) – Merck
2. Mobile phase (MP): Toluene–acetone–methanol–25% ammonia (8 : 1 : 1 : 0.05 v/v)
3. Standard/Sample application:
Band length: 5 mm Volume applied: 5 μl Spacing: 5 mm
4. Chamber saturation: 10 min (MP)
5. RH (%): 55 ± 5
6. Temperature °C: 22 ± 2
7. Separation technique: Ascending
8. Quantity of mobile phase: 10 ml
9. Migration distance: 50 mm
10. Migration time: 15 min

Densitometric evaluation:
Wavelength: UV–210 nm (iso-absorption point)
Scanning mode: Reflectance/Absorbance
HRF: Trifluoperazine HCl—32; Trihexyphenidyl HCl—59
Linearity (ng/band): Trifluoperazine HCl—250–2000; Trihexyphenidyl HCl—100–1000
Recovery (%): 98.2–98.50 for both the compounds
References: —
Comments:
- The method was optimized and analytical work carried out at **Anchrom's HPTLC Application Laboratory**, Mumbai, India.
- Several market samples of similar composition were analysed by the proposed method with reproducible results.

HPTLC : High Performance Thin Layer Chromatography
HPTLC Densitogram

No. 407

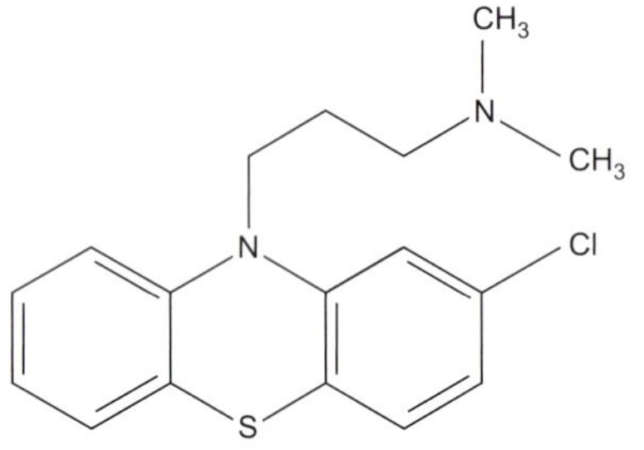

Chlorpromazine

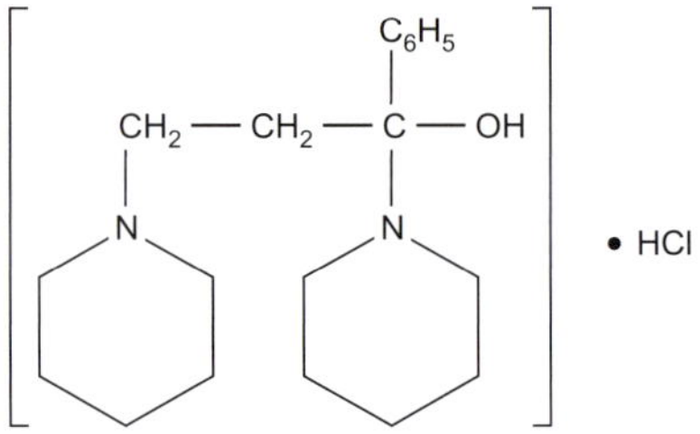

Trihexyphenidyl hydrochloride

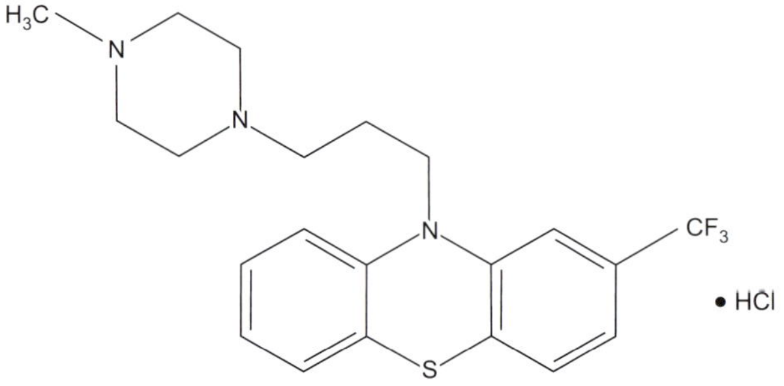

Trifluoperazine hydrochloride

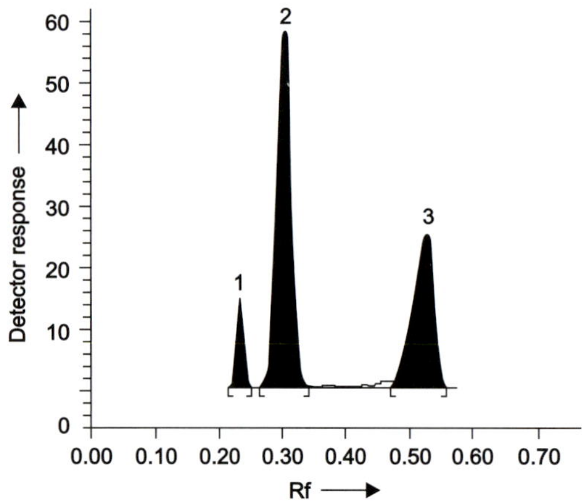

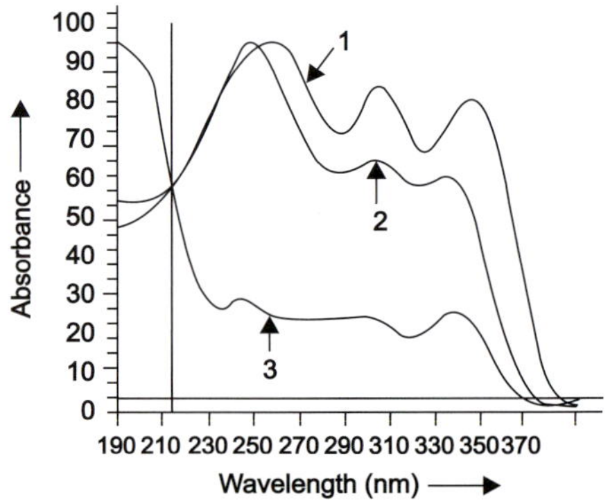

Overlaid UV-spectra of trifluoperazine (1), chlorpromazine (2) and trihexyphenidyl (3) for selection of suitable wavelength for densitometric scanning

Typical densitogram of the standard containing trifluoperazine HCl, chlorpromazine and trihexyphenidyl HCl. For detailed experimental and chromatographic conditions, refer to Protocol No. 407. Peaks identification: 1. Trifluoperazine HCl; 2. Chlorpromazine; 3. Trihexyphenidyl HCl.

PROTOCOL FOR HPTLC ANALYSIS OF PHARMACEUTICAL FORMULATION

Protocol No. 407

Formulation: Trifluoperazine hydrochloride, Trihexyphenidyl hydrochloride, Chlorpromazine hydrochloride

Classification: Central Nervous System **Dosage form:** Tablets

Standard preparation: Prepare stock solution of each compound separately in methanol to get 100 μg/ml of trifluoperazine hydrochloride and 1000 μg/ml each of chlorpromazine hydrochloride and trihexyphenidyl hydrochloride. Further serial dilutions made for linearity studies. Apply 6 μl of each solution for analysis.

Sample preparation: An appropriate quantity of the powdered sample suspended in methanol, sonicated, diluted and filtered. The filtrate was used for analysis by applying 6 μl of the resulting solution.

Chromatographic equipments:

Sample applicator: Camag Linomat–IV

Development chamber: Camag twin-trough glass chamber, 20 × 10 cm

Densitometric scanner: Camag TLC Scanner–III

Chromatographic conditions:

1. Stationary phase: Silica gel 60F_{254} pre-coated HPTLC plates, 20 × 10 cm (200 μm) – Merck, pre-washed with methanol and activated (110°C) for 30 min prior to use
2. Mobile phase (MP): Toluene–methanol–acetone–25% ammonia (7 : 1 : 2 : 0.1 v/v)
3. Standard/Sample application:
   Band length: 6 mm Volume applied: 6 μl Spacing: 6 mm
4. Chamber saturation: 20 min (MP)
5. RH (%): 55 ± 5 6. Temperature °C: 22 ± 2
7. Separation technique: Ascending
8. Quantity of mobile phase: 20 ml
9. Migration distance: 80 mm
10. Migration time: 15 min

Densitometric evaluation:

Wavelength: UV–213 nm Scanning mode: Reflectance/Absorbance

HRF: Trifluoperazine HCl—24; Chlorpromazine HCl—31; Trihexyphenidyl HCl—54

Linearity (μg/band): Trifluoperazine HCl—0.2–1; Chlorpromazine HCl—0.6–12; Trihexyphenidyl HCl—2–10

Recovery (%): 100.43–101.22 for all the three compounds

References: K.R. Mahadik, H. Aggarwal and N. Kaul, *Indian Drugs*, **40(6)**, 340–344, 2003.

Comments: The method validated for accuracy, precision, linearity, LOD, LOQ, specificity, robustness and ruggedness.

HPTLC : High Performance Thin Layer Chromatography
HPTLC Densitogram

No. 408

Amitriptyline

Resperidone

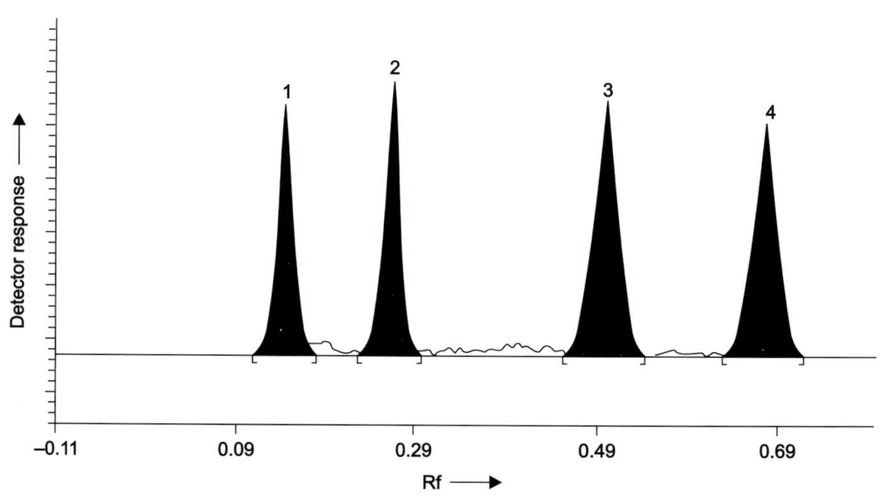

Typical densitogram of the standard containing amitriptyline HCl, trifluoperazine HCl, resperidone and alprazolam. For detailed experimental and chromatographic conditions, refer to Protocol No. 408. Peaks identification: 1. Alprazolam; 2. Resperidone; 3. Trifluoperazine HCl; 4. Amitriptyline HCl.

PROTOCOL FOR HPTLC ANALYSIS OF PHARMACEUTICAL FORMULATION

Protocol No. 408

Formulation: Amitriptyline hydrochloride, Trifluoperazine hydrochloride, Resperidone, Alprazolam

Classification: Central Nervous System **Dosage form:** Tablets

Standard preparation: 1 mg/ml solution of each compound was prepared in methanol. Further serial dilutions made with methanol for linearity studies.

Sample preparation: An appropriate quantity of the powdered sample suspended in methanol, sonicated, diluted, filtered and the filtrate used for chromatographic application and analysis.

Chromatographic equipments:

Sample applicator: Camag Linomat–V

Development chamber: Camag twin-trough glass chamber, 10 × 10 cm

Densitometric scanner: Camag TLC Scanner–III

Chromatographic conditions:

1. Stationary phase: Silica gel $60F_{254}$ pre-coated TLC plates, 10 × 10 cm (250 μm) – Merck
2. Mobile phase (MP): Carbon tetrachloride–acetone–triethylamine (8 : 2 : 3 v/v)
3. Standard/Sample application:
   Band length: 10 mm Volume applied: 0.5–12 μl Spacing: 10 mm
4. Chamber saturation: 25 min (MP)
5. RH (%): 55 ± 5
6. Temperature °C: 25 ± 2
7. Separation technique: Ascending
8. Quantity of mobile phase: 13 ml
9. Migration distance: 80 mm
10. Migration time: 20 min

Densitometric evaluation:

Wavelength: UV–250 nm Scanning mode: Reflectance/Absorbance

HRF: Alprazolam—15; Resperidone—26; Trifluoperazine HCl—50; Amitriptyline HCl—68

Linearity (ng/band): Amitriptyline HCl—50–1200; Trifluoperazine HCl—50–1200; Resperidone—100–2500; Alprazolam—25–600

Recovery (%): 100.65–100.85 for all the four compounds

References: Sejal K. Patel and Natvarlal J. Patel, *Chromatographia*, **69(3–4)**, 393–396, 2009.

Comments: The method validated for accuracy, precision, linearity, LOD, LOQ, specificity, robustness and ruggedness.

HPTLC : High Performance Thin Layer Chromatography
HPTLC Densitogram

No. 409

Propantheline bromide

Haloperidol

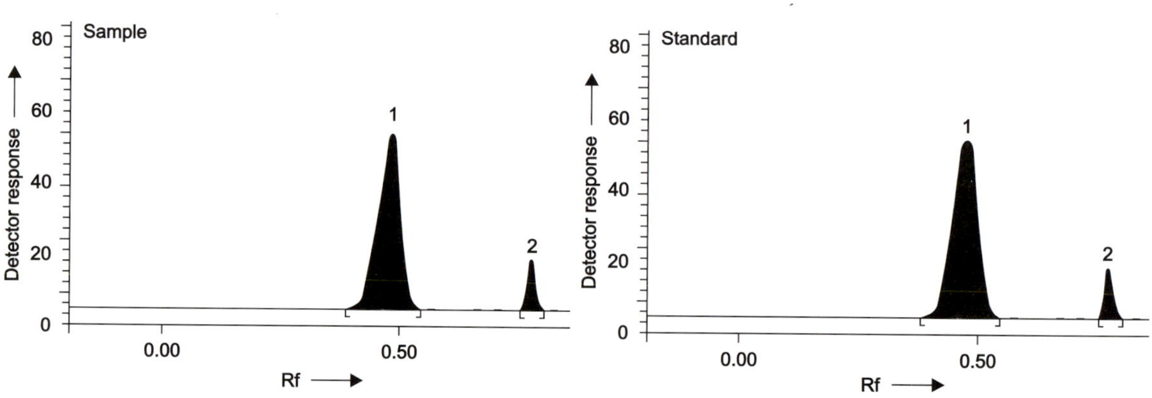

Typical densitogram of the standard and sample containing haloperidol and propantheline bromide. For detailed experimental and chromatographic conditions, refer to Protocol No. 409. Peaks identification: 1. Propantheline bromide; 2. Haloperidol.

PROTOCOL FOR HPTLC ANALYSIS OF PHARMACEUTICAL FORMULATION

Protocol No. 409

Formulation: Haloperidol, Propantheline bromide

Classification: Central Nervous System **Dosage form:** Tablets/Capsules

Standard preparation: (a) Prepare 1 mg/ml solution of haloperidol in methanol. (b) Weigh accurately 15 mg of propantheline bromide, add 0.2 ml of solution (a) and dilute to 10 ml with methanol and use for chromatographic evaluation.

Sample preparation: Weigh sample equivalent to 0.2 mg of haloperidol, add 5–6 ml of methanol, vortex for 5 min, dilute to 10 ml, filter and use for chromatographic analysis.

Chromatographic equipments:

Sample applicator: Camag Linomat–IV

Development chamber: Camag twin-trough glass chamber, 10 × 10 cm

Densitometric scanner: Camag TLC Scanner–II

Chromatographic conditions:

1. Stationary phase: Silica gel 60F_{254} pre-coated HPTLC plates, 7 × 10 cm (200 μm) – Merck
2. Mobile phase (MP): Methanol–acetone–water–glacial acetic acid (6 : 2 : 1 : 0.05 v/v)
3. Standard/Sample application:
   Band length: 5 mm Volume applied: 5 μl Spacing: 5 mm
4. Chamber saturation: 20 min (MP)
5. RH (%): 55 ± 5
6. Temperature °C: 22 ± 2
7. Separation technique: Ascending
8. Quantity of mobile phase: 18 ml
9. Migration distance: 60 mm
10. Migration time: 20 min

Densitometric evaluation:

Wavelength: UV–254 nm Scanning mode: Reflectance/Absorbance

HRF: Propantheline bromide—48; Haloperidol—78

Linearity (ng/band): Propantheline bromide—0.5–10; Haloperidol—50–1000

Recovery (%): 100.75–102.25 for both the compounds

References: —

Comments:

- The method was optimized and analytical work carried out at **Anchrom's HPTLC Application Laboratory**, Mumbai, India.
- Several market samples of similar composition were analysed by the proposed method with reproducible results.

HPTLC : High Performance Thin Layer Chromatography
HPTLC Densitogram

No. 410

C_6H_5
$CH_2 — CH_2 — C — OH$
N N
• HCl

Trihexyphenidyl hydrochloride

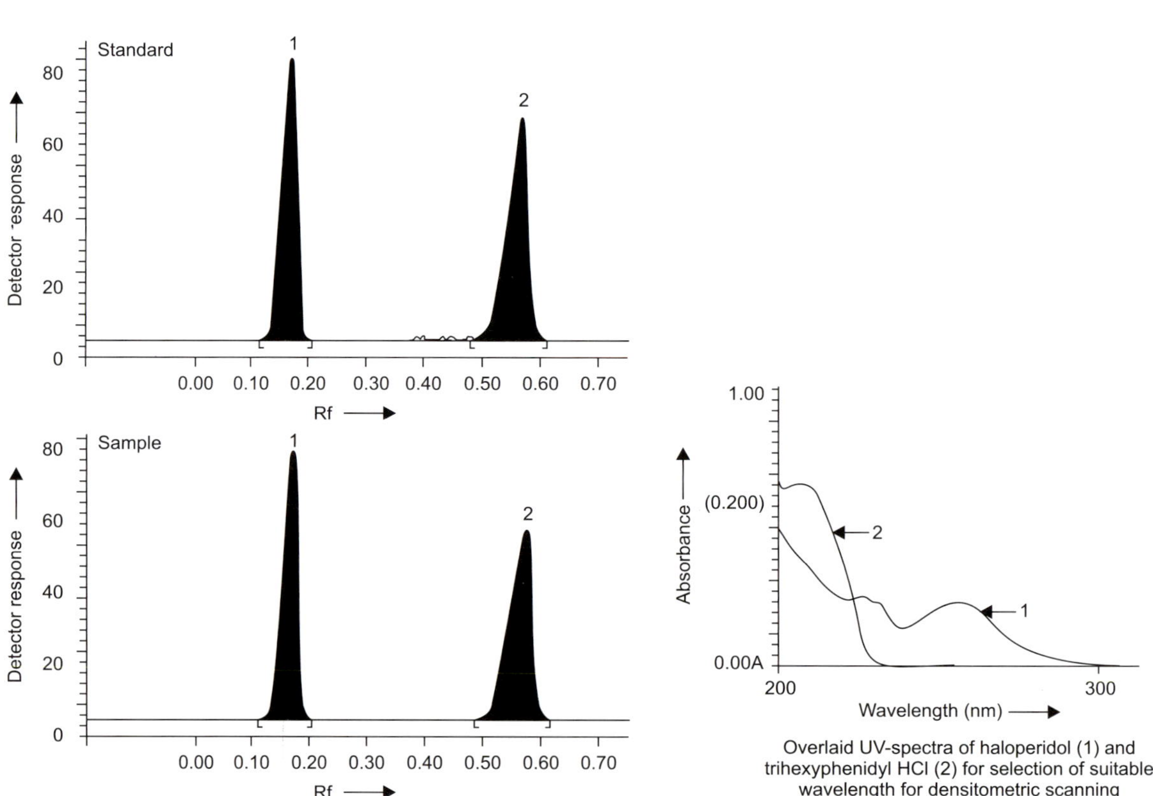

Overlaid UV-spectra of haloperidol (1) and trihexyphenidyl HCl (2) for selection of suitable wavelength for densitometric scanning

Typical densitogram of the standard and the sample containing haloperidol and trihexyphenidyl HCl. For detailed experimental and chromatographic conditions, refer to Protocol No. 410. Peaks identification: 1. Haloperidol; 2. Trihexyphenidyl hydrochloride.

PROTOCOL FOR HPTLC ANALYSIS OF PHARMACEUTICAL FORMULATION

Protocol No. 410

Formulation: Haloperidol, Trihexyphenidyl hydrochloride

Classification: Central Nervous System **Dosage form:** Tablets

Standard preparation: Weigh accurately about 15 mg of haloperidol (H) and 20 mg of trihexyphenidyl HCl (T), dissolve in 10 ml of methanol. Further dilute 0.4 ml to 10 ml with methanol and use for chromatographic analysis.

Sample preparation: Weigh finely powdered sample equivalent to 6 mg of haloperidol, add 50–70 ml methanol, vortex for 5 min, dilute to 100 ml, filter and use for chromatographic analysis.

Chromatographic equipments:

Sample applicator: Camag Linomat–IV

Development chamber: Camag twin-trough glass chamber, 10 × 10 cm

Densitometric scanner: Camag TLC Scanner

Chromatographic conditions:

1. Stationary phase: Silica gel $60F_{254}$ pre-coated HPTLC plates, 7 × 10 cm (200 μm) – Merck
2. Mobile phase (MP): Toluene–acetone–25% ammonia (8 : 2 : 0.05 v/v)
3. Standard/Sample application:
   Band length: 10 mm Volume applied: 10 μl Spacing: 10 mm
4. Chamber saturation: 5 min (MP)
5. RH (%): 55 ± 5
6. Temperature °C: 22 ± 2
7. Separation technique: Ascending
8. Quantity of mobile phase: 10 ml
9. Migration distance: 50 mm
10. Migration time: 15 min

Densitometric evaluation:

Wavelength: UV–210 nm Scanning mode: Reflectance/Absorbance

HRF: Haloperidol—17; Trihexyphenidyl HCl—56

Linearity (ng/band): Haloperidol—50–1000; Trihexyphenidyl HCl—10–1000

Recovery (%): 98.50–99.15 for both the compounds

References: —

Comments:

- The method was optimized and analytical work carried out at **Anchrom's HPTLC Application Laboratory**, Mumbai, India.
- Several market samples of similar composition were analysed by the proposed method with reproducible results.

HPTLC : High Performance Thin Layer Chromatography
HPTLC Densitogram

No. 411

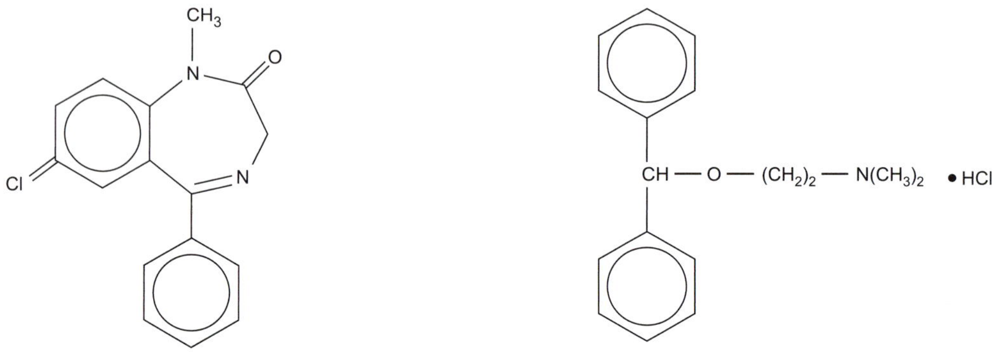

CH3
N
O
Cl
N

Diazepam

CH — O — (CH2)2 — N(CH3)2 • HCl

Diphenhydramine hydrochloride

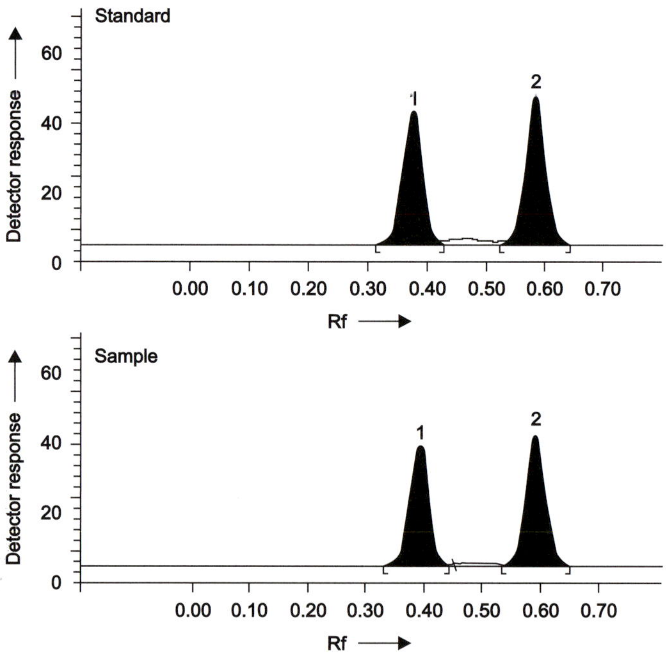

Standard
Detector response
60
40
20
0
1
2
0.00 0.10 0.20 0.30 0.40 0.50 0.60 0.70
Rf

Sample
Detector response
60
40
20
0
1
2
0.00 0.10 0.20 0.30 0.40 0.50 0.60 0.70
Rf

Typical densitogram of the standard and the sample containing diphenhydramine HCl and diazepam. For detailed experimental and chromatographic conditions, refer to Protocol No. 411. Peaks identification: 1. Diphenhydramine HCl; 2. Diazepam.

PROTOCOL FOR HPTLC ANALYSIS OF PHARMACEUTICAL FORMULATION

Protocol No. 411

Formulation: Diphenhydramine hydrochloride, Diazepam

Classification: Central Nervous System **Dosage form:** Tablets

Standard preparation: Prepare (a) 1 mg/ml solution of diphenhydramine HCl in methanol; and (b) 1 mg/ml solution of diazepam, in methanol. Mix 0.5 ml of solution (a) and 0.5 ml of solution (b) and dilute with methanol to 100 ml and use for application.

Sample preparation: Weigh accurately powdered sample equivalent to 0.5 mg of diazepam, add 70 ml of methanol, sonicate for 5 min, dilute to 100 ml, filter and use for application.

Chromatographic equipments:

Sample applicator: Camag Linomat–IV

Development chamber: Camag twin-trough glass chamber, 10 × 10 cm

Densitometric scanner: Camag TLC Scanner–II

Chromatographic conditions:

1. Stationary phase: Silica gel $60F_{254}$ pre-coated HPTLC plates, 7 × 10 cm (200 μm) – Merck
2. Mobile phase (MP): Toluene–acetone–25% ammonia (7 : 3 : 0.1 v/v)
3. Standard/Sample application:
   Band length: 10 mm Volume applied: 5 μl Spacing: 10 mm
4. Chamber saturation: 10 min (MP)
5. RH (%): 55 ± 5
6. Temperature °C: 22 ± 2
7. Separation technique: Ascending
8. Quantity of mobile phase: 10 ml
9. Migration distance: 50 mm
10. Migration time: 14 min

Densitometric evaluation:

Wavelength: UV–230 nm Scanning mode: Reflectance/Absorbance

HRF: Diphenhydramine HCl—38; Diazepam—58

Linearity (ng/band): Diazepam—10–100; Diphenhydramine HCl—100–500

Recovery (%): 98.90–91.2 for both the compounds

References: —

Comments:

- The method was optimized and analytical work carried out at **Anchrom's HPTLC Application Laboratory**, Mumbai, India.
- Several market samples of similar composition were analysed by the proposed method with reproducible results.

HPTLC : High Performance Thin Layer Chromatography
HPTLC Densitogram

No. 412

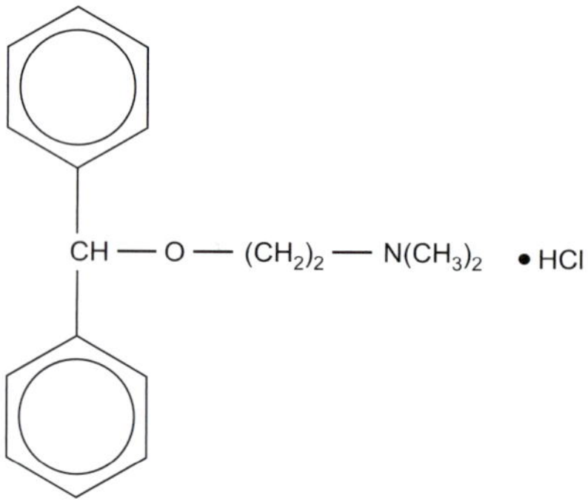

CH — O — $(CH_2)_2$ — $N(CH_3)_2$ • HCl

Diphenhydramine hydrochloride

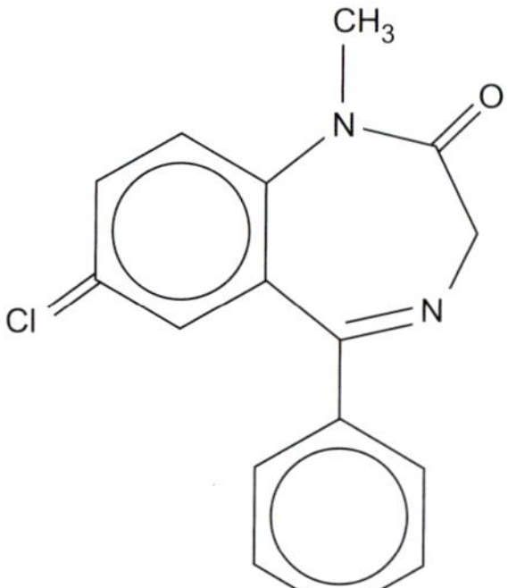

Diazepam

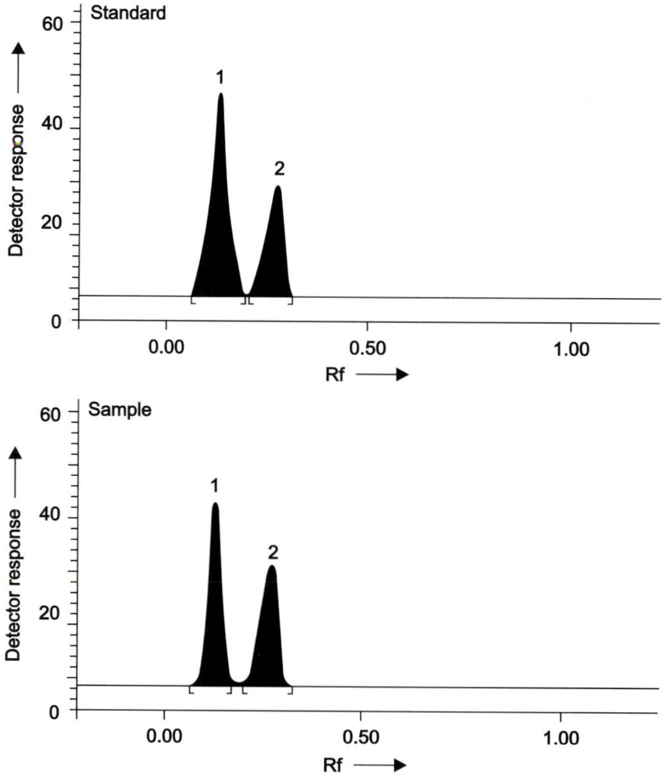

Standard

Sample

Typical densitogram of the standard and the sample containing diazepam and diphenhydramine HCl. For detailed experimental and chromatographic conditions, refer to Protocol No. 412. Peaks identification: 1. Diazepam; 2. Diphenhydramine hydrochloride.

PROTOCOL FOR HPTLC ANALYSIS OF PHARMACEUTICAL FORMULATION

Protocol No. 412

Formulation: Diphenhydramine hydrochloride, Diazepam
Classification: Central Nervous System **Dosage form:** Tablets
Standard preparation: Prepare 1 mg/ml solution of each compound in methanol. Mix 0.5 ml of each solution and dilute to 100 ml with methanol and use for chromatographic analysis.
Sample preparation: Powdered sample equivalent to 0.5 mg of diazepam in suspended in 70 ml of methanol, sonicated for 5 min, diluted to 100 ml, filtered and the filtrate used for application.
Chromatographic equipments:
Sample applicator: Camag Linomat–IV
Development chamber: Camag twin-trough glass chamber, 10 × 10 cm
Densitometric scanner: Camag TLC Scanner–II
Chromatographic conditions:

1. Stationary phase: Silica gel 60 RP–18F_{254s} pre-coated HPTLC plates, 10 × 10 cm (200 μm) – Merck
2. Mobile phase (MP): 0.5 M sod. chloride–methanol–acetonitrile–glacial acetic acid (5 : 2 : 3 : 0.1 v/v)
3. Standard/Sample application:
   Band length: 5 mm Volume applied: 5 μl Spacing: 5 mm
4. Chamber saturation: 20 min (MP)
5. RH (%): 55 ± 5
6. Temperature °C: 22 ± 2
7. Separation technique: Ascending
8. Quantity of mobile phase: 10 ml
9. Migration distance: 50 mm
10. Migration time: 25 min

Densitometric evaluation:
Wavelength: UV–230 nm Scanning mode: Reflectance/Absorbance
HRF: Diazepam—18; Diphenhydramine HCl—27
Linearity (ng/band): Diazepam—10–100; Diphenhydramine HCl—100–500
Recovery (%): 100.25–101.50 for both the compounds
References: —
Comments:

- The method was optimized and analytical work carried out at **Anchrom's HPTLC Application Laboratory**, Mumbai, India.
- Reversal of retention order was observed in RP-chromatography as compared to NP-chromatography.
- Several market samples of similar composition were analysed by the proposed method with reproducible results.

HPTLC : High Performance Thin Layer Chromatography
HPTLC Densitogram

No. 413

CH$_3$ • 2HCl Cl N N

Meclozine hydrochloride

O CH$_3$ H$_3$C N N N O N CH$_3$

Caffeine

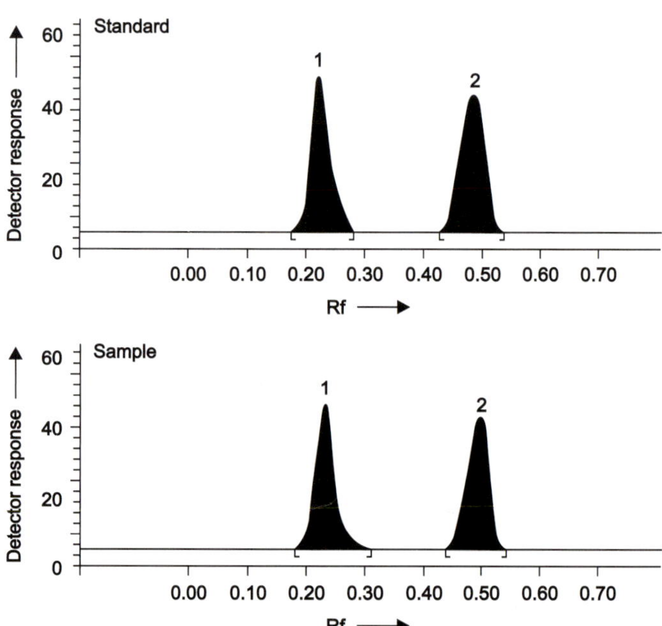

Typical densitogram of the standard and the sample containing caffeine and meclozine hydrochloride. For detailed experimental and chromatographic conditions, refer to Protocol No. 413. Peaks identification: 1. Caffeine citrate; 2. Meclozine HCl.

PROTOCOL FOR HPTLC ANALYSIS OF PHARMACEUTICAL FORMULATION

Protocol No. 413

Formulation: **Meclozine hydrochloride, Caffeine citrate**

Classification: Central Nervous System **Dosage form:** Tablets

Standard preparation: Prepare 100 μg/ml solution of each compound in methanol. Mix 1 ml of solution of meclozine and 0.8 ml of caffeine solution, dilute to 10 ml with methanol and use for chromatographic application.

Sample preparation: Powdered sample equivalent to 25 mg of meclozine hydrochloride suspended in 70 ml of methanol, vortex for 10 min, dilute to 100 ml, filter and dilute 0.4 ml of filtrate to 10 ml with methanol and use for analysis.

Chromatographic equipments:

Sample applicator: Camag Linomat–IV

Development chamber: Camag twin-trough glass chamber, 10 × 10 cm

Densitometric scanner: Camag TLC Scanner–II

Chromatographic conditions:

1. Stationary phase: Silica gel 60F_{254} pre-coated HPTLC plates, 10 × 10 cm (200 μm) – Merck
2. Mobile phase (MP): Toluene–acetone–glacial acetic acid (6 : 1.3 : 0.1 v/v)
3. Standard/Sample application:
   Band length: 10 mm Volume applied: 10 μl Spacing: 10 mm
4. Chamber saturation: 10 min (MP)
5. RH (%): 55 ± 5
6. Temperature °C: 22 ± 2
7. Separation technique: Ascending
8. Quantity of mobile phase: 14 ml
9. Migration distance: 50 mm
10. Migration time: 15 min

Densitometric evaluation:

Wavelength: UV–230 nm or 273 nm Scanning mode: Reflectance/Absorbance

HRF: Caffeine citrate—22; Meclozine HCl—48

Linearity (ng/band): Caffeine citrate—50–150; Meclozine HCl—50–200

Recovery (%): 98.40–99.75 for both the compounds

References: —

Comments:

- The method was optimized and analytical work carried out at **Anchrom's HPTLC Application Laboratory**, Mumbai, India.
- Several market samples of similar composition were analysed by the proposed method with reproducible results.

HPTLC : High Performance Thin Layer Chromatography
HPTLC Densitogram

No. 414

Meclozine hydrochloride

Caffeine

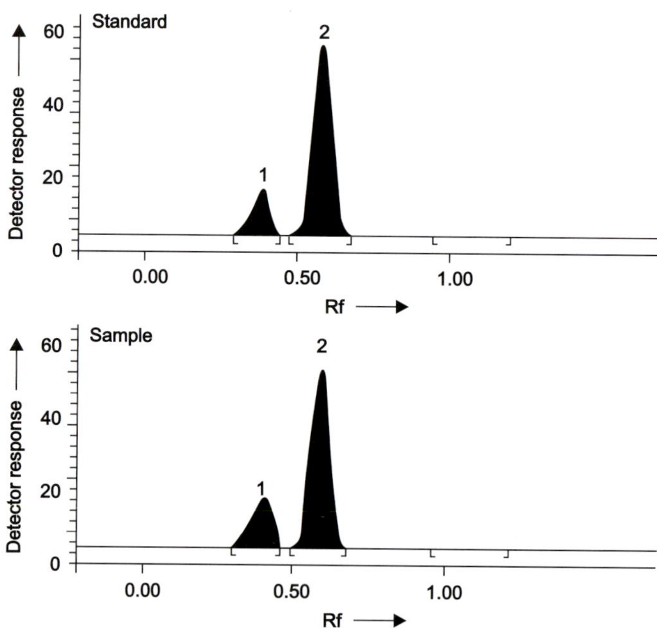

Typical densitogram of the standard and the sample containing caffeine and meclozine hydrochloride. For detailed experimental and chromatographic conditions, refer to Protocol No. 414. Peaks identification: 1. Meclozine HCl; 2. Caffeine citrate.

PROTOCOL FOR HPTLC ANALYSIS OF PHARMACEUTICAL FORMULATION

Protocol No. 414

Formulation: Meclozine hydrochloride, Caffeine citrate

Classification: Central Nervous System **Dosage form:** Tablets

Standard preparation: Prepare (a) 100 μg/ml of meclozine hydrochloride in methanol; and (b) 100 μg/ml of caffeine in methanol. Mix 1 ml of solution (a) and 0.8 ml of solution (b) to produce 10 ml with methanol and use for chromatographic analysis.

Sample preparation: Weigh accurately powdered sample equivalent to 25 mg of meclozine HCl, add 70 ml of methanol, vortex for 10 min, dilute to 10 ml with methanol. Filter and further dilute 0.4 ml to 10 ml with methanol and use for chromatographic analysis.

Chromatographic equipments:

Sample applicator: Camag Linomat–IV
Development chamber: Camag twin-trough glass chamber, 10 × 10 cm
Densitometric scanner: Camag TLC Scanner–II

Chromatographic conditions:

1. Stationary phase: Silica gel 60 RP–18F_{254s} pre-coated HPTLC plates, 10 × 10 cm (200 μm) – Merck
2. Mobile phase (MP): 0.5 M sod. chloride–methanol–acetonitrile–glacial acetic acid (5 : 2 : 3 : 0.1 v/v)
3. Standard/Sample application:
   Band length: 10 mm Volume applied: 10 μl Spacing: 10 mm
4. Chamber saturation: 20 min (MP)
5. RH (%): 55 ± 5
6. Temperature °C: 22 ± 2
7. Separation technique: Ascending
8. Quantity of mobile phase: 10 ml
9. Migration distance: 50 mm
10. Migration time: 25 min

Densitometric evaluation:

Wavelength: UV–230 nm or 273 nm Scanning mode: Reflectance/Absorbance
HRF: Meclozine HCl—30; Caffeine citrate—58
Linearity: 25–250 ng/band for both the compounds
Recovery (%): 97.9–98.75 for both the compounds

References: —

Comments:

- The method was optimized and analytical work carried out at **Anchrom's HPTLC Application Laboratory**, Mumbai, India.
- The plate can be scanned at respective maxima of each compound for better sensitivity; λ_{max} of meclozine hydrochloride—230 nm, and caffeine—273 nm.
- Reversed-phase chromatography resulted in reversal of retention order as compared to normal-phase chromatography.
- Several market samples of similar composition were analysed by the proposed method with reproducible results.

HPTLC : High Performance Thin Layer Chromatography
HPTLC Densitogram

No. 415

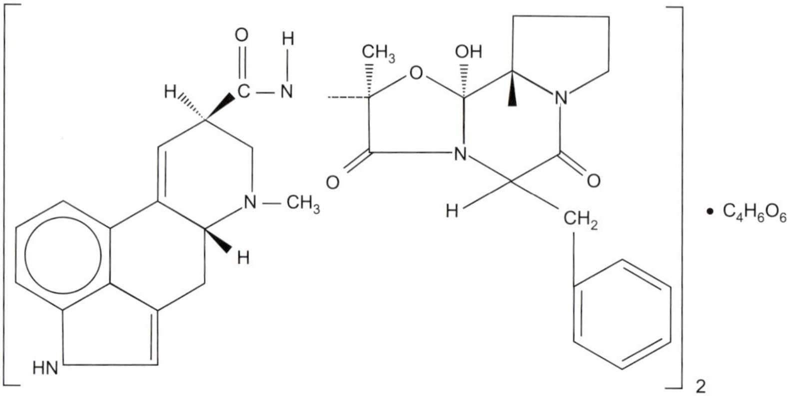

Ergotamine tartrate

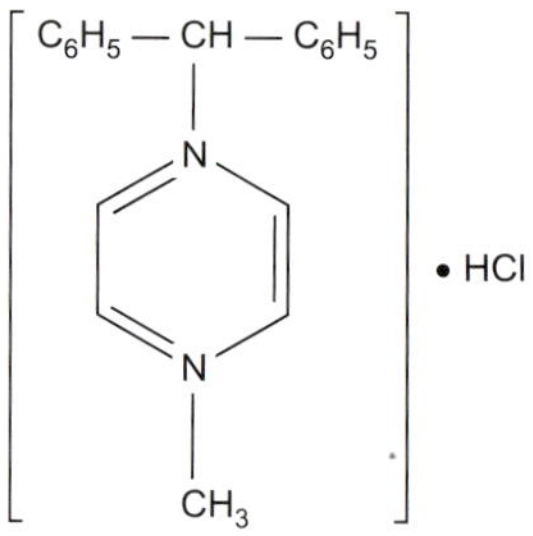

Cyclizine hydrochloride

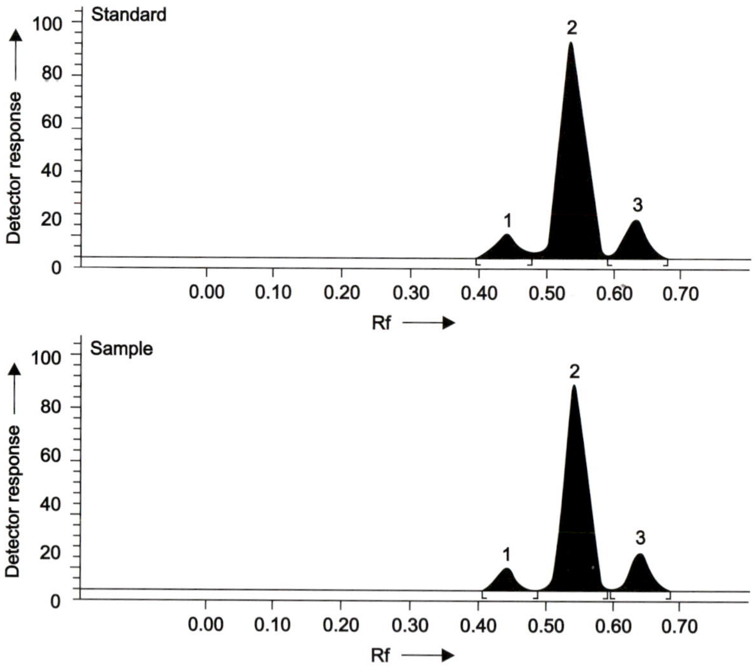

Typical densitogram of the standard and sample containing ergotamine tartrate, cyclizine hydrochloride and caffeine. For detailed experimental and chromatographic conditions, refer to Protocol No. 415. Peaks identification: 1. Ergotamine tartrate; 2. Caffeine; 3. Cyclizine HCl.

PROTOCOL FOR HPTLC ANALYSIS OF PHARMACEUTICAL FORMULATION

Protocol No. 415

Formulation: Ergotamine tartrate, Cyclizine hydrochloride, Caffeine citrate
Classification: Central Nervous System **Dosage form:** Tablets
Standard preparation: Prepare (a) 200 µg/ml of ergotamine tartrate in methanol; and (b) 1 mg/ml of cyclizine HCl in methanol. Weigh 10 mg of caffeine, add to it 1 ml of solution (a) and 5 ml of solution (b) and dilute to 10 ml with methanol and use for chromatographic evaluation.
Sample preparation: Weigh finely powdered sample equivalent to 2 mg of ergotamine tartrate, add about 70 ml of methanol, vortex for 10–15 min, make up the volume to 100 ml with methanol, filter and use for chromatographic analysis.
Chromatographic equipments:
Sample applicator: Camag Linomat–IV
Development chamber: Camag twin-trough glass chamber, 10 × 10 cm
Densitometric scanner: Camag TLC Scanner–II
Chromatographic conditions:

1. Stationary phase: Silica gel $60F_{254}$ pre-coated HPTLC plates, 10 × 10 cm (200 µm) – Merck
2. Mobile phase (MP): Toluene–acetone–25% ammonia (4 : 6 : 0.2 v/v)
3. Standard/Sample application:
   Band length: 5 mm Volume applied: 5 µl Spacing: 5 mm
4. Chamber saturation: 10 min (MP)
5. RH (%): 55 ± 5
6. Temperature °C: 22 ± 2
7. Separation technique: Ascending
8. Quantity of mobile phase: 10 ml
9. Migration distance: 50 mm
10. Migration time: 10 min

Densitometric evaluation:
Wavelength: UV–254 nm or 317 nm Scanning mode: Reflectance/Absorbance
HRF: Ergotamine tartrate—44; Caffeine—54; Cyclizine HCl—65
Linearity (ng/band): Ergotamine tartrate—50–200; Cyclizine HCl—500–3000; Caffeine—100–7500
Recovery (%): 98.44–103.06 for all the three compounds
References: —
Comments:

- The method was optimized and analytical work carried out at **Anchrom's HPTLC Application Laboratory**, Mumbai, India.
- Although the chromatogram has been scanned at 254 nm, the wavelength of 317 nm is the most suitable, being maxima of ergotamine tartrate, the minor component in the formulation.
- Several market samples of similar composition were analysed by the proposed method with reproducible results.

HPTLC : High Performance Thin Layer Chromatography
HPTLC Densitogram

No. 416

Ergotamine tartrate

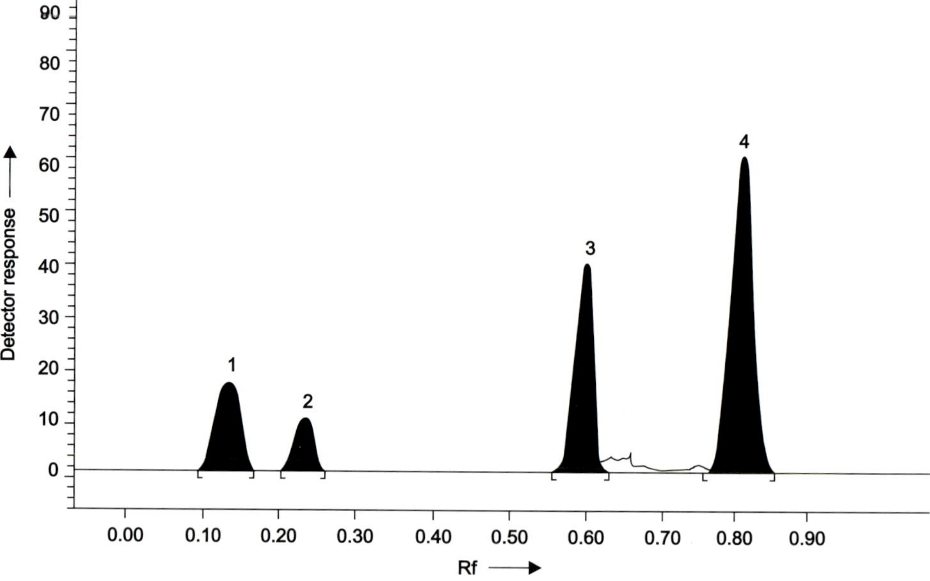

Typical densitogram of the standard containing paracetamol, caffeine citrate, ergotamine tartrate and prochlorperazine maleate. For detailed experimental and chromatographic conditions, refer to Protocol No. 416. Peaks identification: 1. Prochlorperazine maleate; 2. Ergotamine tartrate; 3. Caffeine citrate; 4. Paracetamol.

PROTOCOL FOR HPTLC ANALYSIS OF PHARMACEUTICAL FORMULATION

Protocol No. 416

Formulation: Paracetamol, Caffeine citrate, Ergotamine tartrate, Prochlorperazine maleate

Classification: Central Nervous System **Dosage form:** Tablets

Standard preparation: Prepare 500 μg/ml solution of caffeine and paracetamol and 200 μg/ml solution of ergotamine and prochlorperazine, all in solvent mixture and apply 10 μl of each solution for analysis.

Sample preparation: An appropriate quantity of the powdered sample is dissolved in minimum quantity of ammonia, further dilute with solvent mixture and use for application.

Solvent mixture: Chloroform–methanol (1 : 1 v/v)

Chromatographic equipments:

Sample applicator: Camag Linomat–IV

Development chamber: Normal flat bottom TLC glass chamber, 20 × 15 × 5 cm

Densitometric scanner: Camag TLC Scanner–II

Chromatographic conditions:

1. Stationary phase: Silica gel 60F_{254} pre-coated TLC plates, 20 × 10 cm (250 μm) – Merck
2. Mobile phase (MP): Acetone–n-hexane–chloroform (11 : 11 : 0.04 v/v or toluene–acetone–25% ammonia (4 : 6 : 0.2 v/v)
3. Standard/Sample application:
   Band length: 10 mm Volume applied: 10 μl Spacing: 10 mm
4. Chamber saturation: 20 min (MP)
5. RH (%): 55 ± 5
6. Temperature °C: 22 ± 2
7. Separation technique: Ascending
8. Quantity of mobile phase: 22 ml
9. Migration distance: 120 mm
10. Migration time: 40 min

Densitometric evaluation:

Wavelength: UV-254 nm (Paracetamol and Caffeine), UV-317 nm (Prochlorperazine and Ergotamine)

Scanning mode: Reflectance/Absorbance

HRF: Prochlorperazine maleate—12; Ergotamine tartrate—22; Caffeine citrate—60; Paracetamol—80

Linearity (ng/band): —

Recovery (%): 98.75–100.25 for all the compounds

References: R.B. Patel, M.R. Patel, A.A. Patel and T.N. Bhatt, Abstract No. B-20, 39th IPC, 1987.

Comments:

- Paracetamol and caffeine may be scanned at 254 nm whereas ergotamine and prochlorperazine scanned at 317 nm. It is preferable to scan the entire chromatogram at 317 nm.
- The chromatogram scanned at 317 nm is given in the text.

HPTLC : High Performance Thin Layer Chromatography
HPTLC Densitogram

No. 417

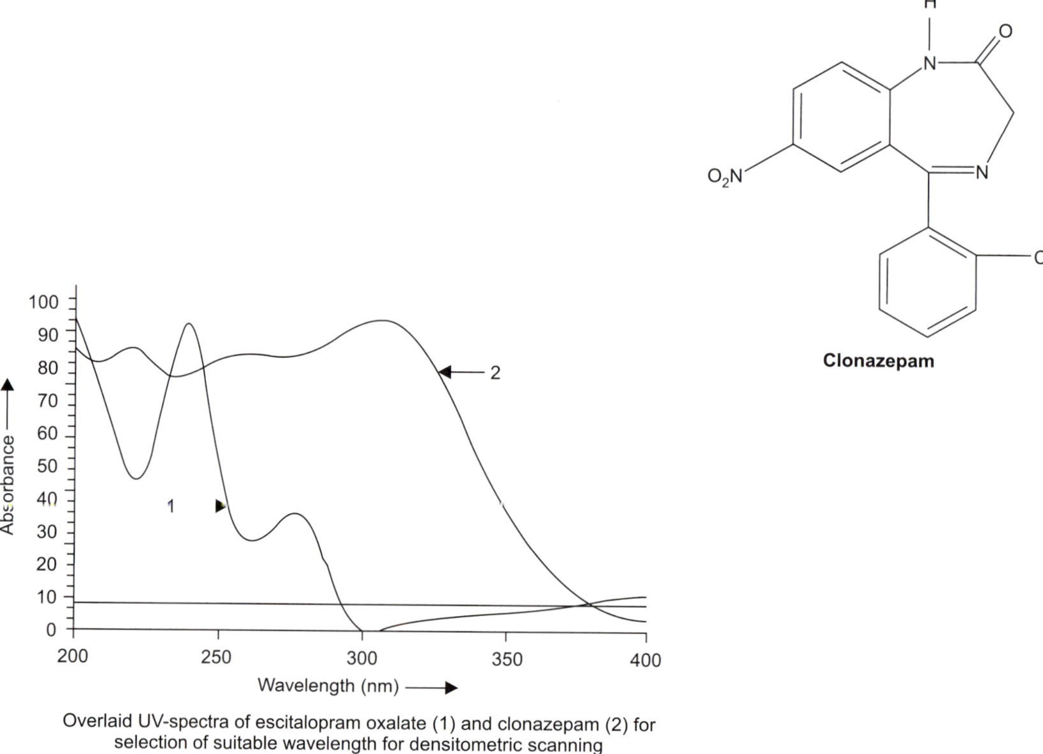

Overlaid UV-spectra of escitalopram oxalate (1) and clonazepam (2) for selection of suitable wavelength for densitometric scanning

Detector response
1
2
–0.13
0.07
0.27
0.47
0.67
0.87
Rf

Typical densitogram of the standard solution containing escitalopram oxalate and clonazepam. For detailed experimental and chromatographic conditions, refer to Protocol No. 417. Peaks identification: 1. Escitalopram oxalate; 2. Clonazepam.

PROTOCOL FOR HPTLC ANALYSIS OF PHARMACEUTICAL FORMULATION

Protocol No. 417

Formulation: **Escitalopram oxalate, Clonazepam**

Classification: Central Nervous System **Dosage form:** Tablets

Standard preparation: Prepare 500 μg/ml solution of escitalopram oxalate and 100 μg/ml solution of clonazepam, both in methanol. Apply 0.5–5 μl of each solution for linearity profile.

Sample preparation: Powdered sample equivalent to 20 mg of escitalopram and 1 mg of clonazepam suspended in 5 ml of methanol, sonicated for 5 min, diluted to 10 ml with methanol, filtered through Whatman No. 41 filter paper and 1 μl of the solution applied for analysis.

Chromatographic equipments:

Sample applicator: Camag Linomat–V

Development chamber: Camag twin-trough glass chamber, 20 × 10 cm

Densitometric scanner: Camag TLC Scanner–III

Chromatographic conditions:

1. Stationary phase: Silica gel 60F_{254} pre-coated TLC plates, 10 × 10 cm (250 μm) – Merck
2. Mobile phase (MP): Toluene–ethyl acetate–triethylamine (7 : 3.5 : 3 v/v)
3. Standard/Sample application:
   Band length: 6 mm Volume applied: 0.5–5 μl Spacing: 5 mm
4. Chamber saturation: 5 min (MP)
5. RH (%): 55 ± 5
6. Temperature °C: 22 ± 2
7. Separation technique: Ascending
8. Quantity of mobile phase: 27 ml
9. Migration distance: 90 mm
10. Migration time: 20 min

Densitometric evaluation:

Wavelength: UV–258 nm Scanning mode: Reflectance/Absorbance

HRF: Escitalopram oxalate—40; Clonazepam—67

Linearity (ng/band): Escitalopram oxalate—250–2500; Clonazepam—50–500

Recovery (%): 99.18–100.07 for both the compounds

References: Nilesh Dhavale, Santhosh Gandhi, Shweta Sabnis and Kailash Bothara, *Chromatographia*, **67(5–6)**, 487–490, 2008.

Comments: The method validated for accuracy, precision, linearity, LOD, LOQ, specificity, robustness and ruggedness.

HPTLC : High Performance Thin Layer Chromatography
HPTLC Densitogram

No. 418

Clonazepam

Escitalopram oxalate

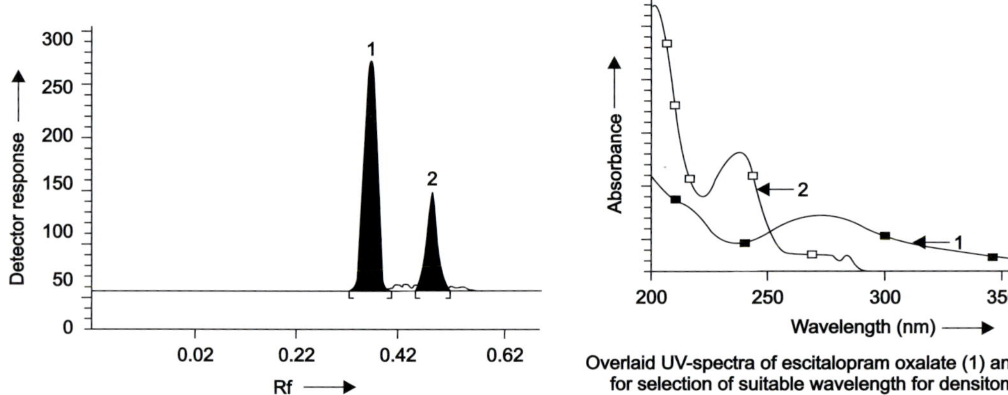

Overlaid UV-spectra of escitalopram oxalate (1) and clonazepam (2) for selection of suitable wavelength for densitometric scanning

Typical densitogram of the standard containing escitalopram oxalate and clonazepam. For detailed experimental and chromatographic conditions, refer to Protocol No. 418. Peaks identification: 1. Escitalopram oxalate; 2. Clonazepam.

PROTOCOL FOR HPTLC ANALYSIS OF PHARMACEUTICAL FORMULATION

Protocol No. 418

Formulation: Escitalopram oxalate, Clonazepam

Classification: Central Nervous System **Dosage form:** Tablets

Standard preparation: Prepare solution of both the drugs in methanol to get 100 μg/ml of escitalopram oxalate and 10 μg/ml of clonazepam. Apply 2–10 μl of each solution for linearity profile.

Sample preparation: An appropriate quantity of the powdered sample suspended in methanol, sonicated for 15 min, diluted, filtered and filtrate suitably diluted with methanol to get 100 μg/ml of escitalopram oxalate and 10 μg/ml of clonazepam for chromatographic evaluation.

Chromatographic equipments:

Sample applicator: Camag Linomat–IV

Development chamber: Normal flat bottom glass chamber, 20 × 15 × 5 cm

Densitometric scanner: Camag TLC Scanner–III

Chromatographic conditions:

1. Stationary phase: Silica gel $60F_{254}$ pre-coated HPTLC plates, 10 × 10 cm (200 μm) – Merck, pre-washed with methanol, dried (115°C) for 30 min before use
2. Mobile phase (MP): Toluene–methanol–triethylamine (3.5 : 1 : 0.1 v/v)
3. Standard/Sample application:
   Band length: 4 mm Volume applied: 2–10 μl Spacing: 4 mm
4. Chamber saturation: 30 min (MP)
5. RH (%): 55 ± 5
6. Temperature °C: 25 ± 2
7. Separation technique: Ascending
8. Quantity of mobile phase: 23 ml
9. Migration distance: 70 mm
10. Migration time: 20 min

Densitometric evaluation:

Wavelength: UV–253 nm Scanning mode: Reflectance/Absorbance

HRF: Escitalopram oxalate—36; Clonazepam—49

Linearity (ng/band): Escitalopram oxalate—100–300; Clonazepam—10–30

Recovery (%): 99.99–100.21 for both the drugs

References: Rajendra Kakde, Dinesh Satone and Nilesh Bawane, *J. Planar Chromatogr.*, **22(6)**, 417–420, 2009.

Comments:

- The method validated for accuracy, precision, linearity, LOD, LOQ, specificity, robustness and ruggedness.
- The method is stability indicating (acid, base, oxidative, thermal, photolytic). The degradation products were separated from main compounds.
- Both the drugs degraded in acidic and basic media but stable under other stress conditions.

HPTLC : High Performance Thin Layer Chromatography
HPTLC Densitogram

No. 419

H₃C, N, N, N, N, Cl

Alprazolam

H, HN — CH₃, H, Cl, Cl

Sertraline

Detector response ⟶

1 2

–0.14 0.06 0.26 0.46 0.66 0.86

Rf ⟶

Typical densitogram of the standard containing alprazolam and sertraline. For detailed experimental and chromatographic conditions, refer to Protocol No. 419. Peaks identification: 1. Sertraline; 2. Alprazolam.

PROTOCOL FOR HPTLC ANALYSIS OF PHARMACEUTICAL FORMULATION

Protocol No. 419

Formulation: Alprazolam, Sertraline

Classification: Central Nervous System **Dosage form:** Tablets

Standard preparation: Prepare 50 μg/ml solution of sertraline and 10 μg/ml solution of alprazolam, both in methanol, and use for chromatographic analysis.

Sample preparation: Powdered sample equivalent to 0.86 mg of alprazolam and 4.17 mg of sertraline suspended in 80 ml of methanol, sonicated for 10 min, diluted to 100 ml with methanol, filtered and the filtrate used for spotting.

Chromatographic equipments:

Sample applicator: Camag Linomat–IV

Development chamber: Camag twin-trough glass chamber, 10 × 10 cm

Densitometric scanner: Camag TLC Scanner–III

Chromatographic conditions:

1. Stationary phase: Silica gel $60F_{254}$ pre-coated HPTLC plates, 10 × 10 cm (200 μm) – Merck, pre-washed with methanol and dried (110°C) for 30 min prior to use
2. Mobile phase (MP): Toluene–ethyl acetate–methanol–acetic acid (9 : 3 : 2 : 0.3 v/v)
3. Standard/Sample application:
   Band length: 5 mm Volume applied: 5 μl Spacing: 5 mm
4. Chamber saturation: —
5. RH (%): 55 ± 5
6. Temperature °C: 25 ± 2
7. Separation technique: Ascending
8. Quantity of mobile phase: 14 ml
9. Migration distance: 70 mm
10. Migration time: 20 min

Densitometric evaluation:

Wavelength: UV–217 nm Scanning mode: Reflectance/Absorbance

HRF: Sertraline—28; Alprazolam—42

Linearity (ng/band): Alprazolam—20–100; Sertraline—100–500

Recovery (%): 98.72–10.24 for both the compounds

References: J.K. Verma and A.V. Joshi, *Indian Drugs*, **42(12)**, 805–807, 2005.

Comments: The method validated for accuracy, precision, linearity, LOD, LOQ, specificity, robustness and ruggedness.

HPTLC : High Performance Thin Layer Chromatography
HPTLC Densitogram

No. 420

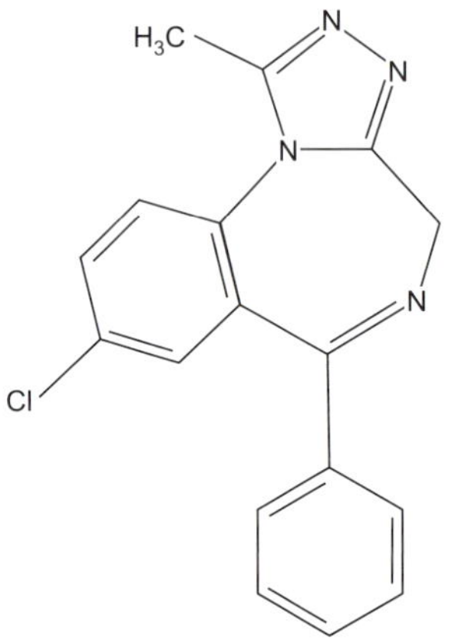

Alprazolam

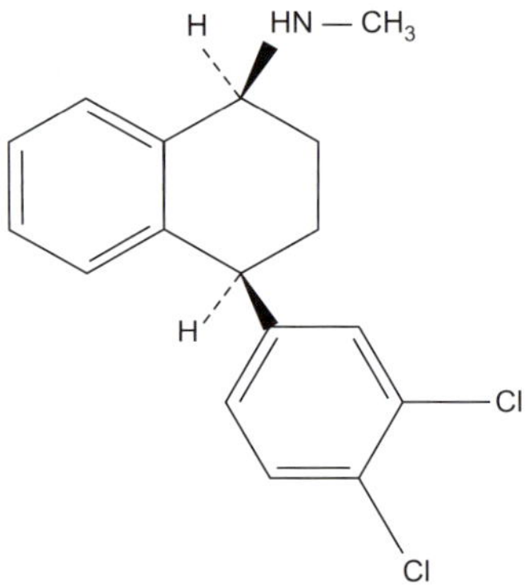

Sertraline

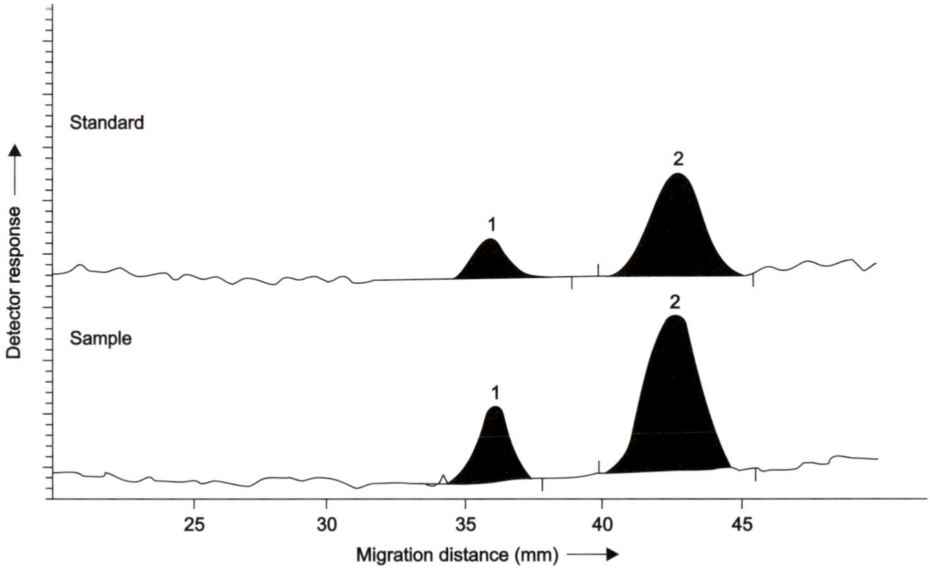

Typical densitogram of the standard and the sample containing alprazolam and sertraline. For detailed experimental and chromatographic conditions, refer to Protocol No. 420. Peaks identification: 1. Alprazolam; 2. Sertraline.

PROTOCOL FOR HPTLC ANALYSIS OF PHARMACEUTICAL FORMULATION

Protocol No. 420

Formulation: Alprazolam, Sertraline

Classification: Central Nervous System **Dosage form:** Tablets

Standard preparation: Prepare 1 mg/ml solution of alprazolam and 5 mg/ml of sertraline, both in methanol. Further serial dilutions made for linearity studies.

Sample preparation: Powdered sample equivalent to 2.5 mg of alprazolam and 12.5 mg of sertraline suspended in 20 ml of methanol, sonicated for 15 min, diluted, filtered and the filtrate suitably diluted for analysis.

Chromatographic equipments:

Sample applicator: Desaga automated sample applicator

Development chamber: Desaga glass chamber, 20 × 20 cm

Densitometric scanner: Desaga CD60 scanner

Chromatographic conditions:

1. Stationary phase: Silica gel 60F_{254} pre-coated TLC plates, 20 × 20 cm (250 μm) – Merck
2. Mobile phase (MP): Carbon tetrachloride–methanol–acetone–25% ammonia (12 : 3 : 5 : 0.1 v/v)
3. Standard/Sample application:
   Band length: 6 mm Volume applied: 3.5 μl Spacing: 2 mm
4. Chamber saturation: 25 min (MP)
5. RH (%): 55 ± 5
6. Temperature °C: 25 ± 2
7. Separation technique: Ascending
8. Quantity of mobile phase: 40 ml
9. Migration distance: 70 mm
10. Migration time: 15 min

Densitometric evaluation:

Wavelength: UV–254 nm Scanning mode: Reflectance/Absorbance

HRF: Alprazolam—52; Sertraline—70

Linearity (ng/band): Alprazolam—200–650; Sertraline—100–325

Recovery (%): Alprazolam—97.7–102.82; Sertraline—96.5–99.9

References: K. Venkateswarlu, R.K. Venisetty, N.R. Yellu, S. Keshetty and M.G. Pai, *J. Chromatogr. Sci.*, **45**, 537–539, 2007.

Comments: The method validated for accuracy, precision, linearity, LOD, LOQ, specificity, robustness and ruggedness.

HPTLC : High Performance Thin Layer Chromatography
HPTLC Densitogram

No. 421

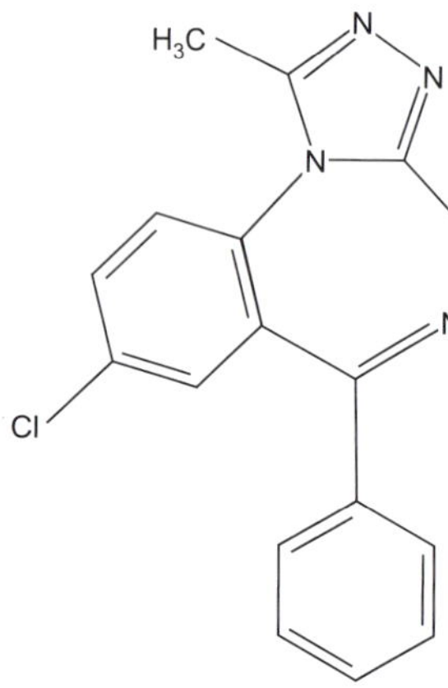

Alprazolam

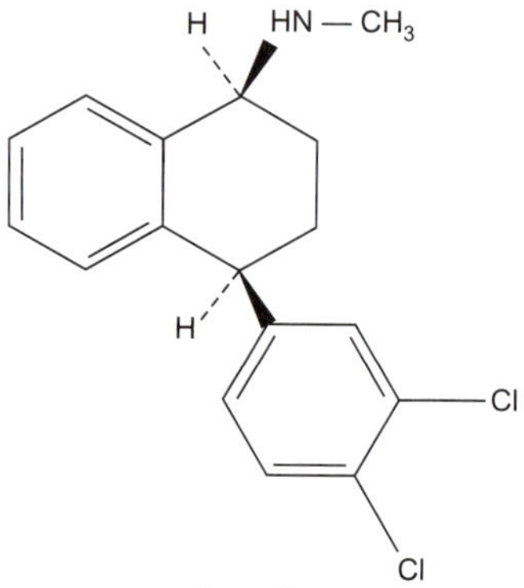

Sertraline

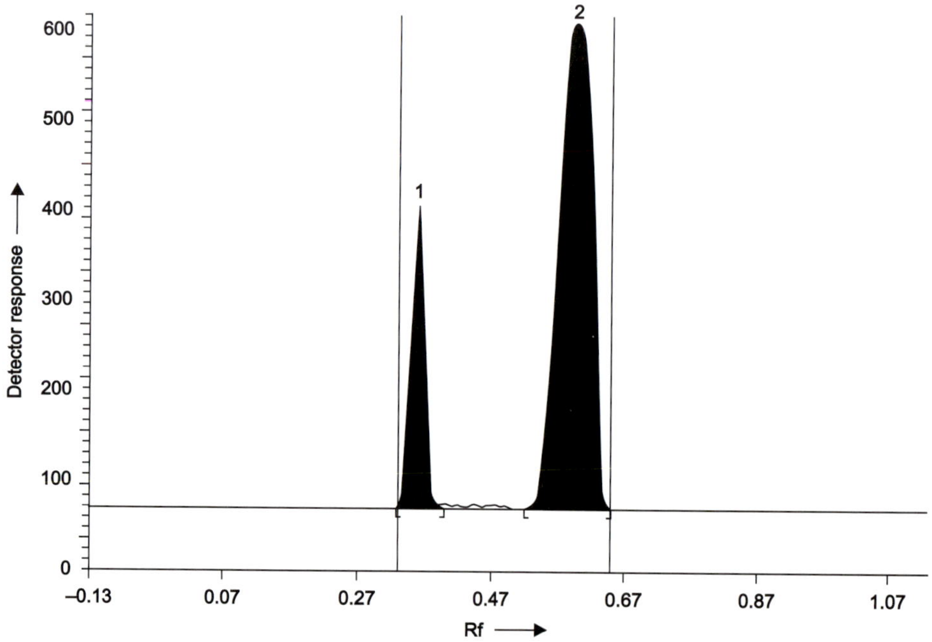

Typical densitogram of the standard containing alprazolam and sertraline. For detailed experimental and chromatographic conditions, refer to Protocol No. 421. Peaks identification: 1. Alprazolam; 2. Sertraline.

PROTOCOL FOR HPTLC ANALYSIS OF PHARMACEUTICAL FORMULATION

Protocol No. 421

Formulation: Alprazolam, Sertraline

Classification: Central Nervous System **Dosage form:** Raw material/Tablets

Standard preparation: Prepare mixed standard solution of both the drugs in methanol to get 5000 μg/ml of sertraline and 100 μg/ml of alprazolam. Further suitably diluted with methanol to get 2 μg/ml (alprazolam) and 100 μg/ml (sertraline). Apply suitable volume to cover the linearity range.

Sample preparation: Powdered sample equivalent to 0.5 mg of alprazolam or 25 mg of sertraline suspended in 30 ml of methanol, sonicated for 15 min, diluted to 50 ml. Filter and dilute 1 ml of the filtrate to 50 ml with methanol and use for chromatographic analysis.

Chromatographic equipments:

Sample applicator: Camag Linomat–V

Development chamber: Camag twin-trough glass chamber, 10 × 10 cm

Densitometric scanner: Camag TLC Scanner–III

Chromatographic conditions:

1. Stationary phase: Silica gel $60F_{254}$ pre-coated HPTLC plates, 10 × 10 cm (200 μm) – Merck
2. Mobile phase (MP): Acetone–toluene–25% ammonia (6 : 3 : 1 v/v)
3. Standard/Sample application:
   Band length: 6 mm Volume applied: 10 μl Spacing: 5 mm
4. Chamber saturation: 30 min (MP)
5. RH (%): 55 ± 5
6. Temperature °C: 22 ± 2
7. Separation technique: Ascending
8. Quantity of mobile phase: 10 ml
9. Migration distance: 80 mm
10. Migration time: 25 min

Densitometric evaluation:

Wavelength: UV–230 nm Scanning mode: Reflectance/Absorbance

HRF: Alprazolam—33; Sertraline—52

Linearity: 400–1400 ng/band for both the drugs

Recovery (%): 99.17–101.47 for both the drugs

References: Rashmin B. Patel, Arpita B. Patel, Mrunali R. Patel, Madhura B. Shankar and Kashyap K. Bhatt, *Analytical Letters*, **42**, 1588–1602, 2009.

Comments: The method validated for accuracy, precision, linearity, LOD, LOQ, specificity, robustness and ruggedness.

HPTLC : High Performance Thin Layer Chromatography
HPTLC Densitogram

No. 422

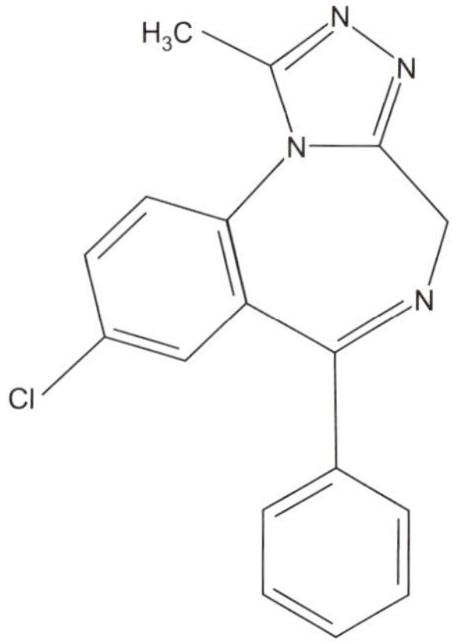

Alprazolam

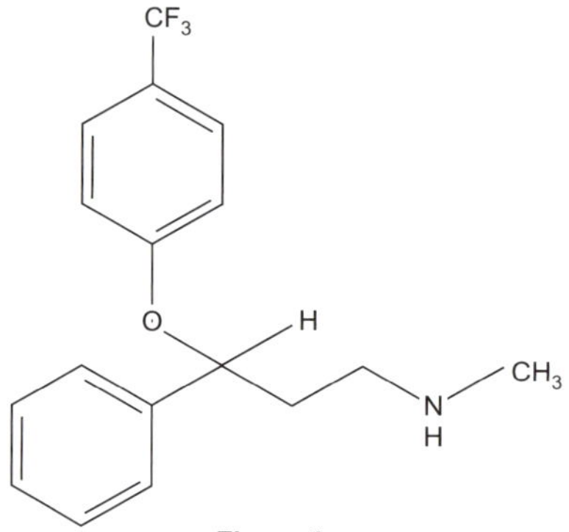

Fluoxetine

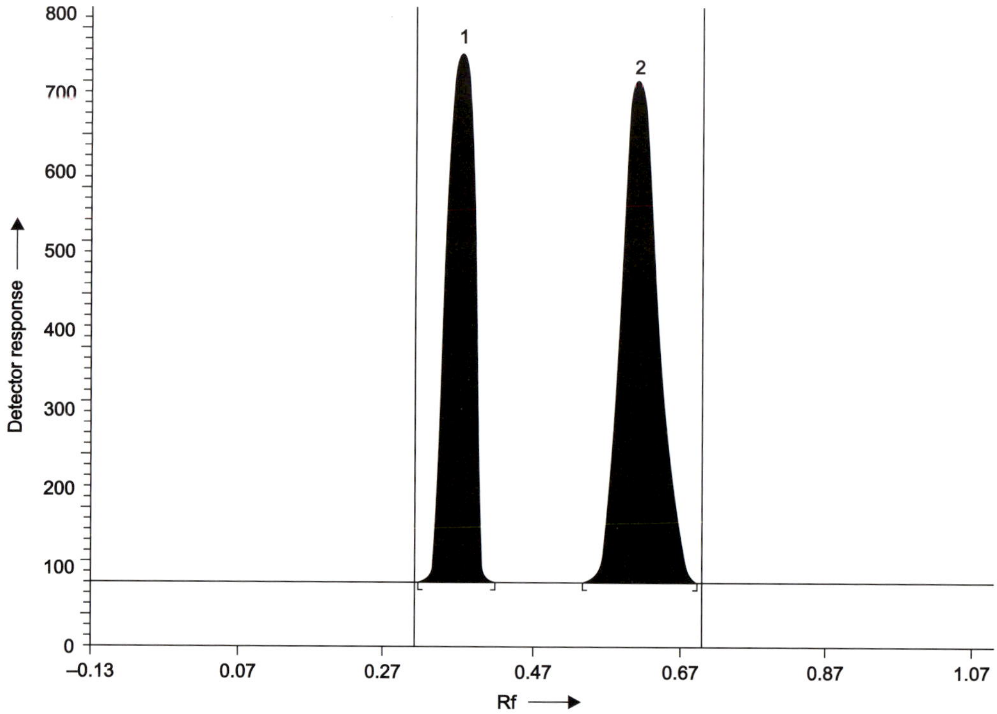

Typical densitogram of the standard containing alprazolam and fluoxetine HCl. For detailed experimental and chromatographic conditions, refer to Protocol No. 422. Peaks identification: 1. Alprazolam; 2. Fluoxetine HCl.

PROTOCOL FOR HPTLC ANALYSIS OF PHARMACEUTICAL FORMULATION

Protocol No. 422

Formulation: Alprazolam, Fluoxetine hydrochloride
Classification: Central Nervous System **Dosage form:** Tablets
Standard preparation: Prepare solution of both the compounds in methanol to get 100 μg/ml (alprazolam) and 8000 μg/ml (fluoxetine). Mix 2 ml of each solution and dilute to 100 ml with methanol, the final concentration being 0.5 μg/ml (alprazolam) and 40 μg/ml (fluoxetine).
Sample preparation: Powdered sample equivalent to 0.25 mg of alprazolam and 20 mg of fluoxetine suspended in 15 ml of methanol, sonicated for 15 min, diluted to 25 ml and used for determination of alprazolam. 0.125 ml of solution diluted to 10 ml and used for determination of fluoxetine.
Chromatographic equipments:
Sample applicator: Camag Linomat–V
Development chamber: Camag twin-trough glass chamber, 10 × 10 cm
Densitometric scanner: Camag TLC Scanner–III
Chromatographic conditions:
1. Stationary phase: Silica gel $60F_{254}$ pre-coated HPTLC plates, 10 × 10 cm (200 μm) – Merck, pre-washed with methanol to dried (110°C) for 5 min prior to use
2. Mobile phase (MP): Acetone–toluene–25% ammonia (6.0 : 3.5 : 0.5 v/v)
3. Standard/Sample application:
   Band length: 6 mm Volume applied: 5 μl Spacing: 5 mm
4. Chamber saturation: 30 min (MP)
5. RH (%): 55 ± 5
6. Temperature °C: 22 ± 2
7. Separation technique: Ascending
8. Quantity of mobile phase: 20 ml
9. Migration distance: 80 mm
10. Migration time: 20 min

Densitometric evaluation:
Wavelength: UV–230 nm Scanning mode: Reflectance/Absorbance
HRF: Alprazolam—39; Fluoxetine HCl—62
Linearity: 400–1400 ng/band for both the drugs
Recovery (%): 99.85–99.95 for both the drugs
References: Rashmin B. Patel, Mrunali R. Patel, Madhura B. Shankar and Kashyap K. Bhatt, *J. AOAC. Int.*, **92(4)**, 1082–87, 2009.
Comments:
- The method validated for accuracy, precision, linearity, LOD, LOQ, specificity, robustness and ruggedness.
- The method was comparable with RP–HPLC.

HPTLC : High Performance Thin Layer Chromatography
HPTLC Densitogram

No. 423

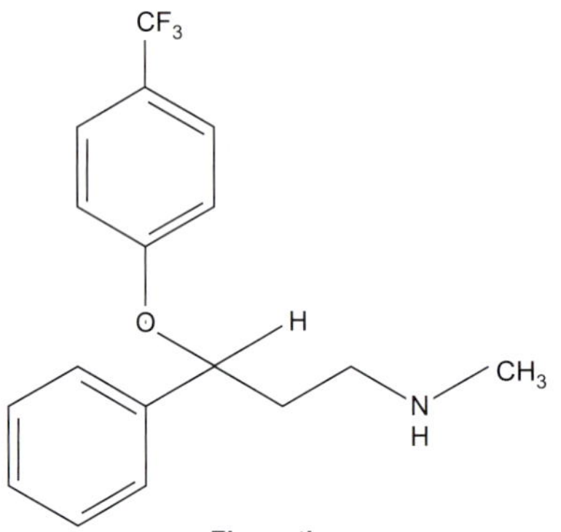

Fluoxetine

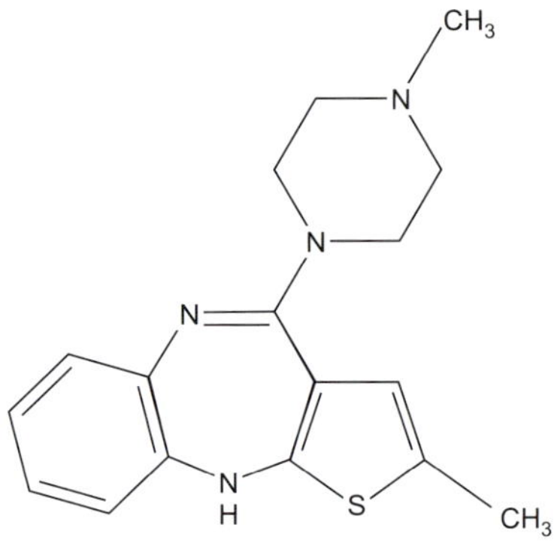

Olanzapine

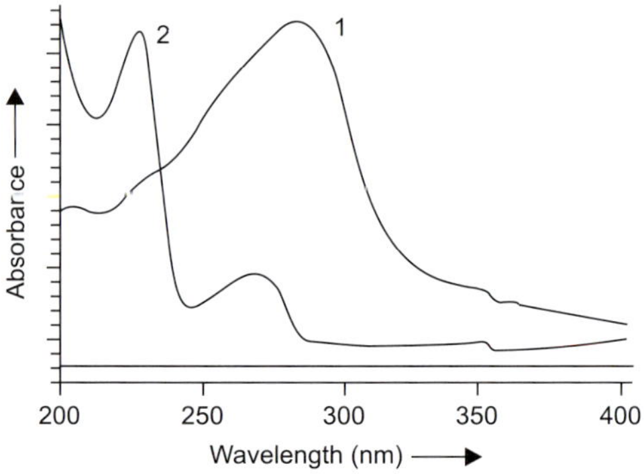

Overlaid UV-spectra of olanzapine (1) and fluoxetine HCl (2) for selection of suitable wavelength for densitometric scanning

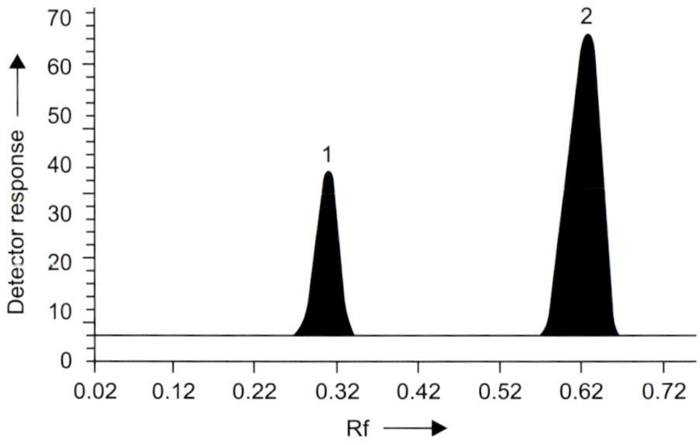

Typical densitogram of the sample containing olanzapine and fluoxetine HCl. For detailed experimental and chromatographic conditions, refer to Protocol No. 423. Peaks identification: 1. Fluoxetine HCl; 2. Olanzapine.

PROTOCOL FOR HPTLC ANALYSIS OF PHARMACEUTICAL FORMULATION

Protocol No. 423

Formulation: Fluoxetine hydrochloride, Olanzapine

Classification: Central Nervous System **Dosage form:** Tablets

Standard preparation: Prepare mixed standard solution of both the compounds in methanol to get 100 μg/ml of olanzapine and 400 μg/ml of fluoxetine. Apply 1–8 μl of the solution for linearity profile.

Sample preparation: An appropriate quantity of powdered sample equivalent to 20 mg of fluoxetine and 5 mg of olanzapine suspended in 40 ml of methanol, sonicated for 15 min, diluted to 50 ml, filtered through 0.2 μm nylon membrane filter and used for application.

Chromatographic equipments:

Sample applicator: Camag Linomat–V

Development chamber: Camag twin-trough glass chamber, 10 × 10 cm

Densitometric scanner: Camag TLC Scanner–III

Chromatographic conditions:

1. Stationary phase: Silica gel $60F_{254}$ pre-coated TLC plates, 10 × 10 cm (250 μm) – Merck
2. Mobile phase (MP): Methanol–toluene (4 : 2 v/v)
3. Standard/Sample application:
   Band length: 6 mm Volume applied: 1–8 μl Spacing: 8 mm
4. Chamber saturation: 30 min (MP)
5. RH (%): 55 ± 5
6. Temperature °C: 22 ± 2
7. Separation technique: Ascending
8. Quantity of mobile phase: 12 ml
9. Migration distance: 70 mm
10. Migration time: 20 min

Densitometric evaluation:

Wavelength: UV-233 nm Scanning mode: Reflectance/Absorbance

HRF: Fluoxetine HCl—31; Olanzapine—63

Linearity (ng/band): Fluoxetine HCl—400–3200; Olanzapine—100–800

Recovery (%): Olanzapine 99.54–99.73; Fluoxetine HCl—100.02–101.35

References: Charmy R. Shah, Nihal J. Shah, B.N. Suhagia and Natvarlal M. Patel, *J. AOAC. Int.*, **90(6)**, 1573–1977, 2007.

Comments:

- The method validated for accuracy, precision, linearity, LOD, LOQ, specificity, robustness and ruggedness.
- The method is stability indicating (acid, base, oxidative, thermal, photolytic). The degradation products were separated from the main compounds.

HPTLC : High Performance Thin Layer Chromatography
HPTLC Densitogram

No. 424

Fluoxetine

Olanzapine

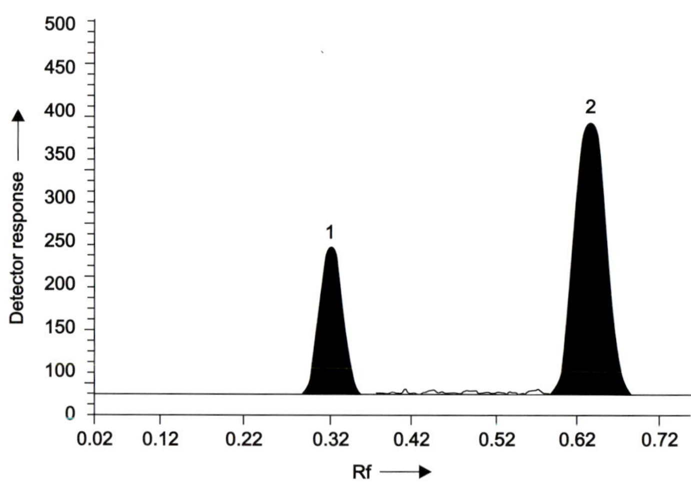

Typical densitogram of the standard containing fluoxetine HCl and olanzapine. For detailed experimental and chromatographic conditions, refer to Protocol No. 424. Peaks identification: 1. Fluoxetine HCl; 2. Olanzapine.

PROTOCOL FOR HPTLC ANALYSIS OF PHARMACEUTICAL FORMULATION

Protocol No. 424

Formulation: Fluoxetine hydrochloride, Olanzapine

Classification: Central Nervous System **Dosage form:** Tablets

Standard preparation: Prepare standard solution of both the compounds in methanol to get 1000 μg/ml of fluoxetine HCl and 100 μg/ml of olanzapine. Apply different volumes for linearity profile.

Sample preparation: Accurately weighed quantity of powder extracted with methanol by sonication, diluted suitably and filtered. Filtrate further diluted with methanol to get 1000 μg/μl of fluoxetine HCl and 100 μg/ml of olanzapine. Final solution used for chromatographic analysis.

Chromatographic equipments:

Sample applicator: Camag Linomat–V

Development chamber: Camag twin-trough glass chamber, 10 × 10 cm

Densitometric scanner: Camag TLC Scanner–III

Chromatographic conditions:

1. Stationary phase: Silica gel $60F_{254}$ pre-coated TLC plates, 10 × 10 cm (250 μm) – Merck, pre-washed with methanol, dried at 50°C (5 min) prior to use
2. Mobile phase (MP): Toluene–methanol (4 : 8 v/v)
3. Standard/Sample application:
   Band length: 10 mm Volume applied: 1–8 μl Spacing: 5 mm
4. Chamber saturation: 30 min (MP)
5. RH (%): 55 ± 5
6. Temperature °C: 22 ± 2
7. Separation technique: Ascending
8. Quantity of mobile phase: 12 ml
9. Migration distance: 72 mm
10. Migration time: 20 min

Densitometric evaluation:

Wavelength: UV–233 nm Scanning mode: Reflectance/Absorbance

HRF: Fluoxetine HCl—31; Olanzapine—65

Linearity (ng/band): Fluoxetine HCl—1000–8000; Olanzapine—100–800

Recovery (%): 99.92–99.96 for both the drugs

References: C.R. Shah, B.N. Suhagia, N.J. Shah, D.R. Patel and N.M. Patel, *Ind. J. Pharm Sci.*, **70(2)**, 251–254, 2008.

Comments:

- The method validated for accuracy, precision, linearity, LOD, LOQ, specificity, robustness and ruggedness.
- The method is stability indicating (acid, base, oxidative, thermal, photolytic). The degradation products were separated from the main compounds.

HPTLC : High Performance Thin Layer Chromatography
HPTLC Densitogram

No. 425

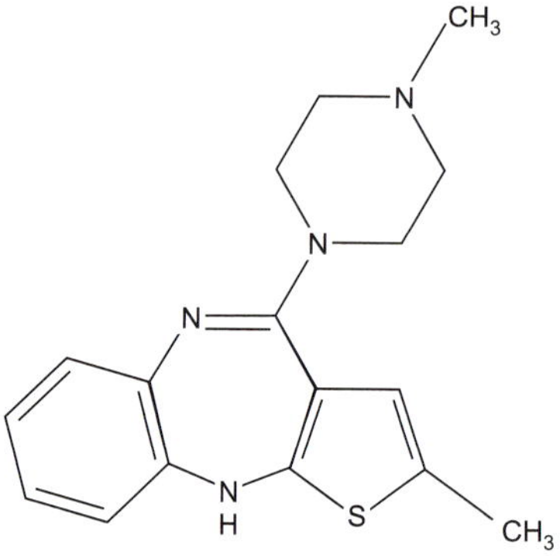

Olanzapine

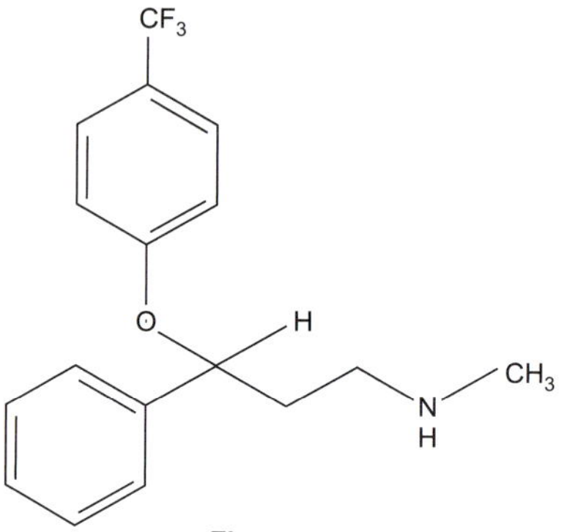

Fluoxetine

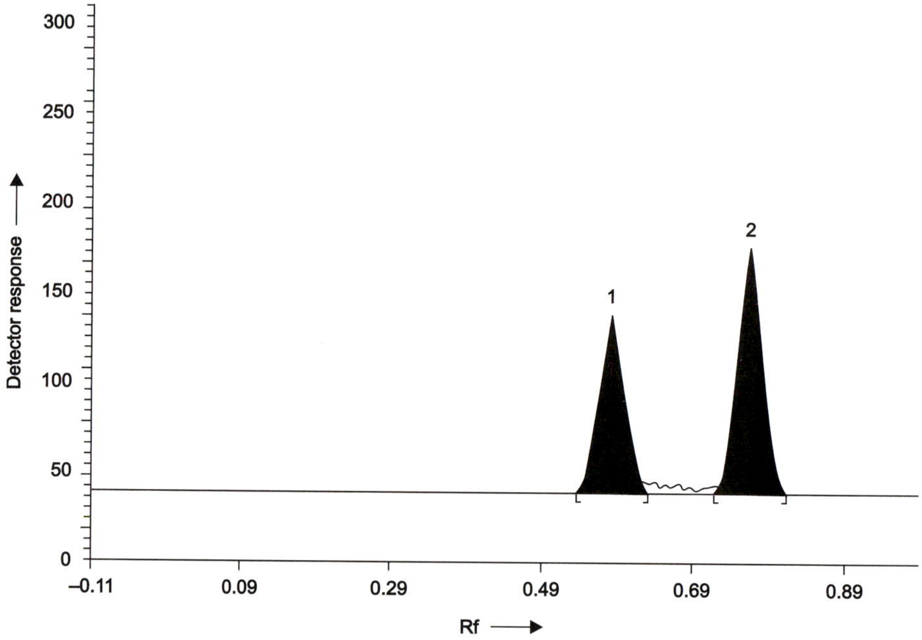

Typical densitogram of the standard containing fluoxetine HCl and olanzapine. For detailed experimental and chromatographic conditions, refer to Protocol No. 425. Peaks identification: 1. Fluoxetine HCl; 2. Olanzapine.

PROTOCOL FOR HPTLC ANALYSIS OF PHARMACEUTICAL FORMULATION

Protocol No. 425

Formulation: Fluoxetine hydrochloride, Olanzapine

Classification: Central Nervous System **Dosage form:** Tablets

Standard preparation: Prepare standard solution of both the compounds in methanol to get 100 μg/ml (fluoxetine HCl) and 50 μg/ml (olanzapine). Apply different volumes (3–10 μl) of each for linearity profile.

Sample preparation: The powdered sample equivalent to 20 mg of fluoxetine HCl or 10 mg of olanzapine suspended in 40 ml of methanol, sonicated, diluted to 50 ml, filtered and suitably diluted with methanol to get 500 μg/ml (fluoxetine HCl) and 250 μg/ml (olanzapine). Further dilutions made as under standard solution for assay.

Chromatographic equipments:

Sample applicator: Camag Linomat–V

Development chamber: Camag twin-trough glass chamber, 10 × 10 cm

Densitometric scanner: Camag TLC Scanner–III

Chromatographic conditions:

1. Stationary phase: Silica gel 60F_{254} pre-coated TLC plates, 10 × 10 cm (250 μm) – Merck
2. Mobile phase (MP): Acetone–methanol–triethylamine (5 : 3 : 0.5 v/v)
3. Standard/Sample application:
   Band length: 5 mm Volume applied: 8 μl Spacing: 5 mm
4. Chamber saturation: 20 min (MP)
5. RH (%): 55 ± 5
6. Temperature °C: 25 ± 2
7. Separation technique: Ascending
8. Quantity of mobile phase: 16 ml
9. Migration distance: 80 mm
10. Migration time: 30 min

Densitometric evaluation:

Wavelength: UV–235 nm Scanning mode: Reflectance/Absorbance

HRF: Fluoxetine HCl—58; Olanzapine—77

Linearity (ng/band): Fluoxetine HCl—300–1000; Olanzapine—150–500

Recovery (%): 99.38–100.95 for both the compounds

References: Sejal Patel and N.J. Patel, *Ind. J. Pharm. Sci.*, **71(4)**, 477–480, 2009.

Comments:

- The method validated for accuracy, precision, linearity, LOD, LOQ, specificity, robustness and ruggedness.
- The results were co-related with RP-HPLC method carried out simultaneously.

HPTLC : High Performance Thin Layer Chromatography
HPTLC Densitogram

No. 426

Fluoxetine

Citalopram hydrobromide

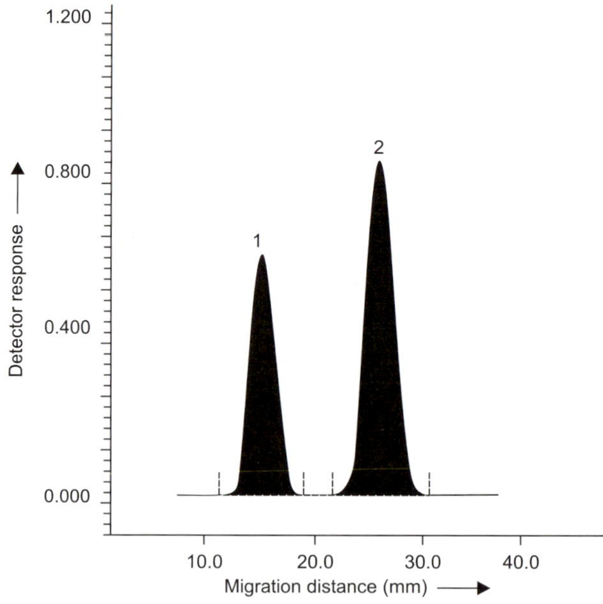

Typical densitogram of the standard containing fluoxetine hydrochloride and citalopram hydrobromide. For detailed experimental and chromatographic conditions, refer to Protocol No. 426. Peaks identification: 1. Fluoxetine HCl; 2. Citalopram HBr.

PROTOCOL FOR HPTLC ANALYSIS OF PHARMACEUTICAL FORMULATION

Protocol No. 426

Formulation: Fluoxetine hydrochloride, Citalopram hydrobromide

Classification: Central Nervous System **Dosage form:** Tablets

Standard preparation: Prepare 1 mg/ml solution of each drug in methanol and stored at 4°C. Prepare serial dilutions with methanol to get 100–1000 μg/ml. Apply 5 μl of each solution for linearity profile.

Sample preparation: Powdered sample equivalent to 20 mg of fluoxetine hydrochloride suspended in 20 ml of methanol, sonicated for 10 min, diluted to 25 ml with methanol, filtered and further dilutions made with methanol for analysis.

Chromatographic equipments:

Sample applicator: Camag Linomat–II

Development chamber: Flat bottom glass chamber (20 × 15 × 5 cm)

Densitometric scanner: Shimadzu CS–930 dual wavelength TLC scanner

Chromatographic conditions:

1. Stationary phase: RP-18F_{254s} pre-coated TLC plates, 10 × 10 cm (250 μm) – Merck
2. Mobile phase (MP): Methanol–0.05 M phosphate buffer pH 5–triethylamine (68 : 27 : 5 v/v)
3. Standard/Sample application:
   Band length: 5 mm Volume applied: 5 μl Spacing: 10 mm
4. Chamber saturation: 15 min (MP)
5. RH (%): —
6. Temperature °C: Ambient
7. Separation technique: Ascending
8. Quantity of mobile phase: 50 ml
9. Migration distance: 80 mm
10. Migration time: —

Densitometric evaluation:

Wavelength: UV–230 nm Scanning mode: Reflectance/Absorbance

HRF: Fluoxetine HCl—12; Citalopram HBr—28

Linearity: 500–5000 ng/band for both the drugs

Recovery (%): 99.10–101.70 for both the drugs

References: Tatána Gondová and Ibrahim A. Amar, *J. Planar Chromatogr.*, **24(1)**, 40–43, 2011.

Comments: The method validated for accuracy, precision, linearity, LOD, LOQ, specificity, robustness and ruggedness.

HPTLC : High Performance Thin Layer Chromatography
HPTLC Densitogram

No. 427

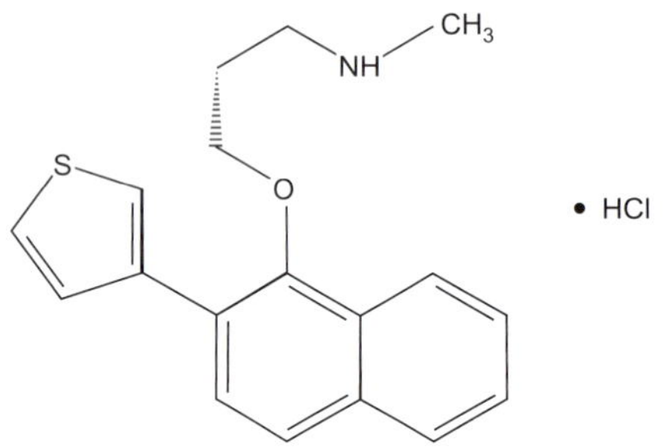

• HCl

Duloxetine hydrochloride

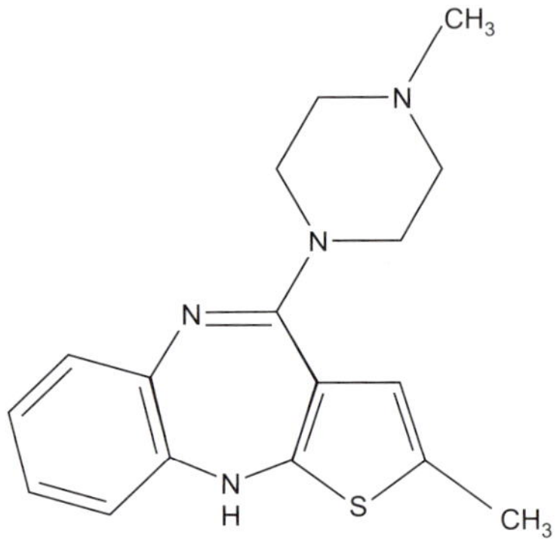

Olanzapine

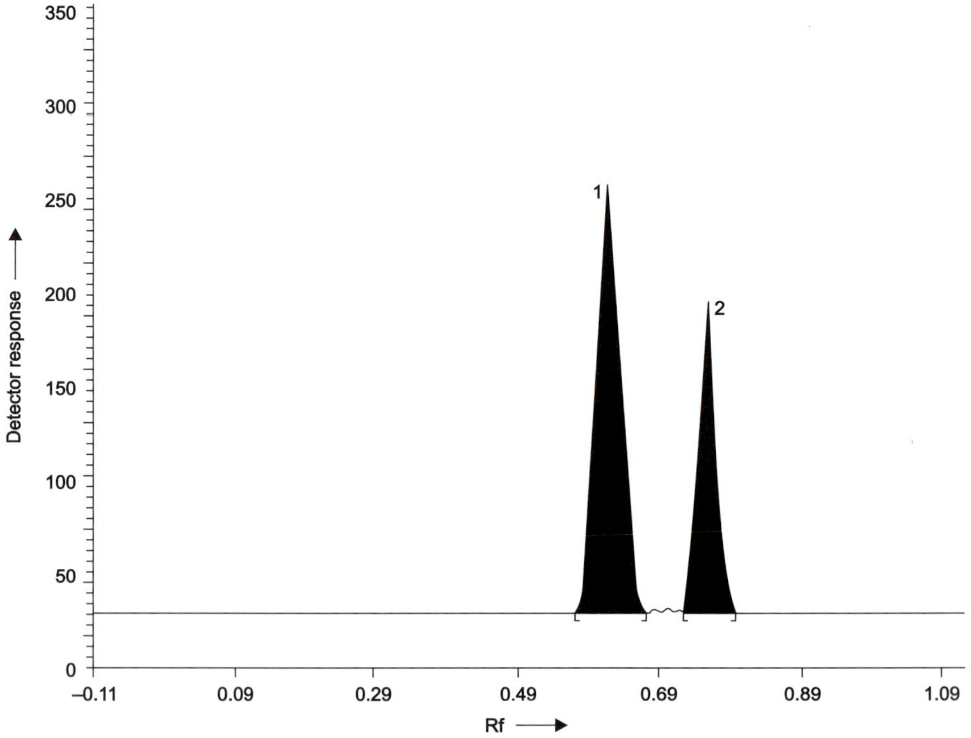

Detector response ⟶

350
300
250
200
150
100
50
0

–0.11 0.09 0.29 0.49 0.69 0.89 1.09

Rf ⟶

1
2

Typical densitogram of the standard containing duloxetine HCl and olanzapine. For detailed experimental and chromatographic conditions, refer to Protocol No. 427. Peaks identification: 1. Duloxetine HCl; 2. Olanzapine.

PROTOCOL FOR HPTLC ANALYSIS OF PHARMACEUTICAL FORMULATION

Protocol No. 427

Formulation: Duloxetine hydrochloride, Olanzapine
Classification: Central Nervous System **Dosage form:** Analyte mixture
Standard preparation: Prepare 1 mg/ml solution of each compound in methanol. Further dilutions made to get 60 μg/ml. Apply varying volumes (1–8 μl) for linearity profile.
Sample preparation: Powdered sample equivalent to 20 mg of duloxetine hydrochloride and 10 mg of olanzapine suspended in 40 ml of methanol, sonicated, diluted, filtered and filtrate suitably diluted for assay. Apply 4 μl of the solution for analysis.
Chromatographic equipments:
Sample applicator: Camag Linomat–V
Development chamber: Camag twin-trough glass chamber, 10 × 10 cm
Densitometric scanner: Camag TLC Scanner–III
Chromatographic conditions:

1. Stationary phase: Silica gel F_{254} pre-coated HPTLC plates, 10 × 10 cm (200 μm) – Merck
2. Mobile phase (MP): Acetone–methanol–triethylamine (5 : 3 : 0.5 v/v)
3. Standard/Sample application:
   Band length: 6 mm Volume applied: 4 μl Spacing: 8 mm
4. Chamber saturation: 20 min (MP)
5. RH (%): 55 ± 5
6. Temperature °C: 25 ± 2
7. Separation technique: Ascending
8. Quantity of mobile phase: 16 ml
9. Migration distance: 80 mm
10. Migration time: 20 min

Densitometric evaluation:
Wavelength: UV–240 nm Scanning mode: Reflectance/Absorbance
HRF: Duloxetine HCl—62; Olanzapine—75
Linearity (ng/band): Olanzapine—50–400; Duloxetine HCl—100–800
Recovery (%): Duloxetine HCl—99.75–100.85; Olanzapine—99.25–99.35
References: Sejal K. Patel, Natvarlal J. Patel, Paresh U. Patel, Dipti B. Patel, Arun M. Prajapati and Satish A. Patel, *J. Planar. Chromatogr.*, **22(2)**, 121–126, 2009.
Comments:

- The method validated for accuracy, precision, linearity, LOD, LOQ, specificity, robustness and ruggedness.
- The method is stability indicating (acid, base, oxidative, thermal, photolytic). The degradation products were separated from main compounds.

HPTLC : High Performance Thin Layer Chromatography
HPTLC Densitogram

No. 428

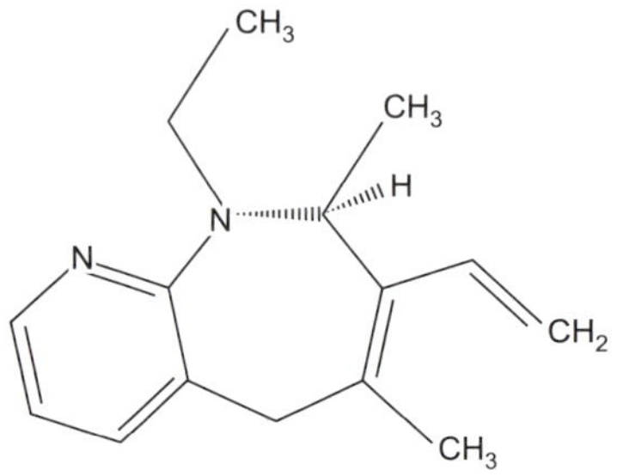

CH3 CH3 H N N CH2 CH3

Mirtazapine

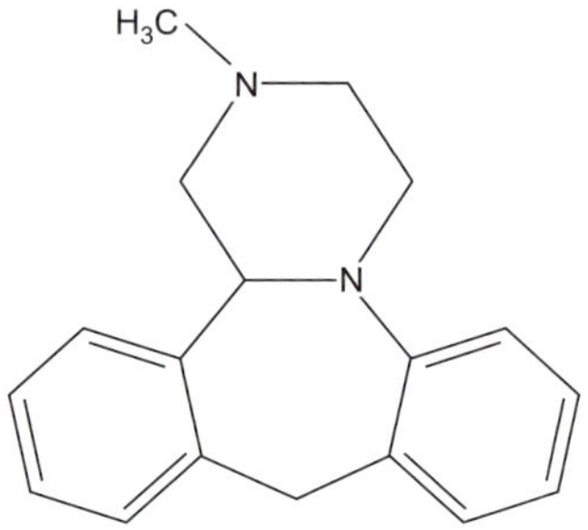

H3C N N

Mianserine

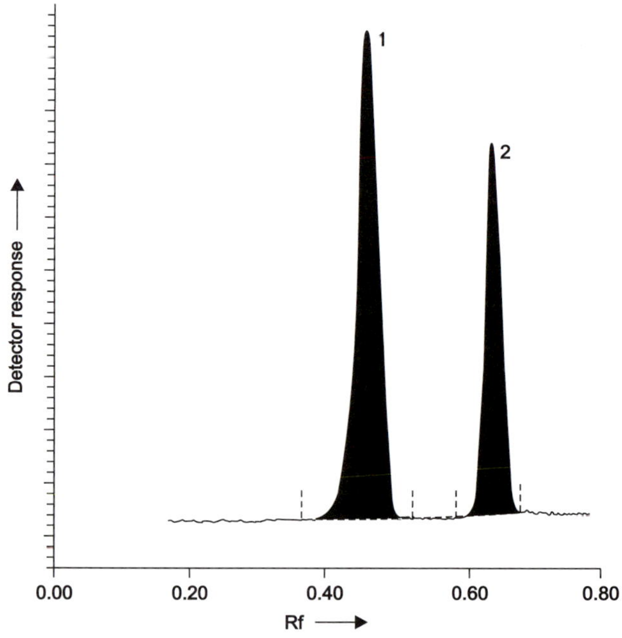

1 2

Detector response →

0.00 0.20 0.40 0.60 0.80

Rf →

Typical densitogram of the standard containing mirtazapine and mianserine. For detailed experimental and chromatographic conditions, refer to Protocol No. 428. Peaks identification: 1. Mirtazapine; 2. Mianserine.

PROTOCOL FOR HPTLC ANALYSIS OF PHARMACEUTICAL FORMULATION

Protocol No. 428

Formulation: Mirtazapine, Mianserine

Classification: Central Nervous System **Dosage form:** Tablets

Standard preparation: Prepare standard solution of each compound in methanol to get 100–400 μg/ml (mirtazapine) and 100–800 μg/ml (mianserine). Apply 5 μl of each of above solutions for linearity studies.

Sample preparation: Powdered sample equivalent to 30 mg of one of the components suspended in methanol, sonicated for 20 min, filtered and filtrate diluted suitably with methanol to get concentration within linearity range. Apply 5 μl for assay.

Chromatographic equipments:

Sample applicator: Camag 5 μl syringe

Development chamber: Flat-bottom glass chamber, 20 × 15 × 5 cm

Densitometric scanner: Shimadzu CS–930 dual wavelength scanner

Chromatographic conditions:

1. Stationary phase: Silica gel 60F_{254} pre-coated HPTLC plates, 10 × 10 cm (250 μm) – Merck
2. Mobile phase (MP): n-hexane–isopropanol–25% ammonia (7 : 2.5 : 0.5 v/v)
3. Standard/Sample application:
   Band length: 5 mm Volume applied: 5 μl Spacing: 5 mm
4. Chamber saturation: 20 min (MP)
5. RH (%): 60 ± 5
6. Temperature °C: 25 ± 1
7. Separation technique: Ascending
8. Quantity of mobile phase: 20 ml
9. Migration distance: 80 mm
10. Migration time: 15 min

Densitometric evaluation:

Wavelength: UV–280 nm Scanning mode: Reflectance/Absorbance

HRF: Mirtazapine—43; Mianserine—62

Linearity (ng/band): Mirtazapine—50–250; Mianserine—500–5000

Recovery (%): 98.86–101.71 for both the compounds

References: Tatana Gondova and Iveta Petrikova, *J. AOAC Int.*, **93(3)**, 778–782, 2010.

Comments: The method validated for accuracy, precision, linearity, LOD, LOQ, specificity, robustness and ruggedness.

HPTLC : High Performance Thin Layer Chromatography
HPTLC Densitogram

No. 429

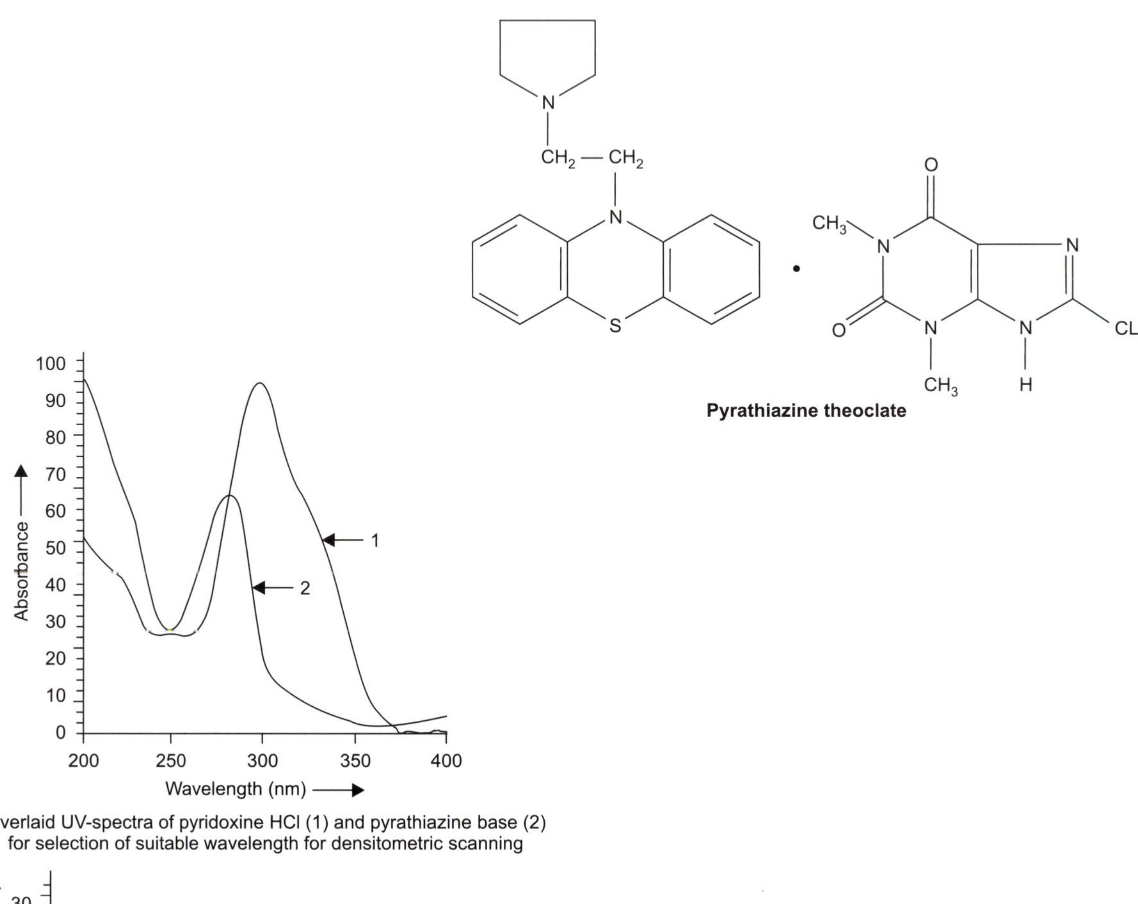

Overlaid UV-spectra of pyridoxine HCl (1) and pyrathiazine base (2) for selection of suitable wavelength for densitometric scanning

Typical densitogram of the standard containing pyridoxine HCl, pyrathiazine, theoclate. For detailed experimental and chromatographic conditions, refer to Protocol No. 429. Peaks identification: 1. Pyridoxine HCl; 2. Pyrathiazine; 3. Theoclate.

PROTOCOL FOR HPTLC ANALYSIS OF PHARMACEUTICAL FORMULATION

Protocol No. 429

Formulation: Pyridoxine hydrochloride, Pyrathiazine theoclate

Classification: Central Nervous System **Dosage form:** Tablets

Standard preparation: Prepare 5 mg/ml solution of both the compounds in ethanol (96%). Further serial dilutions made to get 750–2750 μg/ml solution. Apply 2 μl of each solution for linearity profile.

Sample preparation: Powdered sample equivalent to 16 mg of pyrathiazine theoclate and 15 mg of pyridoxine HCl suspended in 5 ml of ethanol, sonicated for 10 min, diluted to 10 ml, filter and apply 2 μl for assay.

Chromatographic equipments:

Sample applicator: Camag Nanomat–III

Development chamber: Camag twin-trough glass chamber, 20 × 10 cm

Densitometric scanner: Camag TLC Scanner–III

Chromatographic conditions:

1. Stationary phase: Silica gel F_{254} pre-coated TLC plates, 10 × 20 cm (250 μm) – Merck
2. Mobile phase (MP): Dichloromethane–methanol–acetone–acetic acid (19.5 : 6.0 : 3.0 : 1.5 v/v)
3. Standard/Sample application:
   Band length: 2 mm Volume applied: 2 μl Spacing: 10 mm
4. Chamber saturation: 60 min (MP)
5. RH (%): 55 ± 5
6. Temperature °C: 24 ± 2
7. Separation technique: Ascending
8. Quantity of mobile phase: 30 ml
9. Migration distance: 80 mm
10. Migration time: 20 min

Densitometric evaluation:

Wavelength: UV–254 nm Scanning mode: Reflectance/Absorbance

HRF: Pyridoxine HCl—39; Pyrathiazine (base)—59; Theoclate—95

Linearity (ng/band): 750–2750 μg/ml for both the compounds

Recovery (%): 100.92–11.54 for both the compounds

References: Dian Widiretnani, Sari Indah Wahyuni, Farina Kartinasari and Gunawan Indrayanto, *J. Liq. Chromatogr. and Related Tech.*, **32**, 154–165, 2009.

Comments:

- The method validated for accuracy, precision, linearity, LOD, LOQ, specificity, robustness and ruggedness.
- The method is suitable for dissolution profile (phosphate buffer, pH 6.8; 900 ml; 75 rpm; 60 min).

HPTLC : High Performance Thin Layer Chromatography
HPTLC Densitogram

No. 430

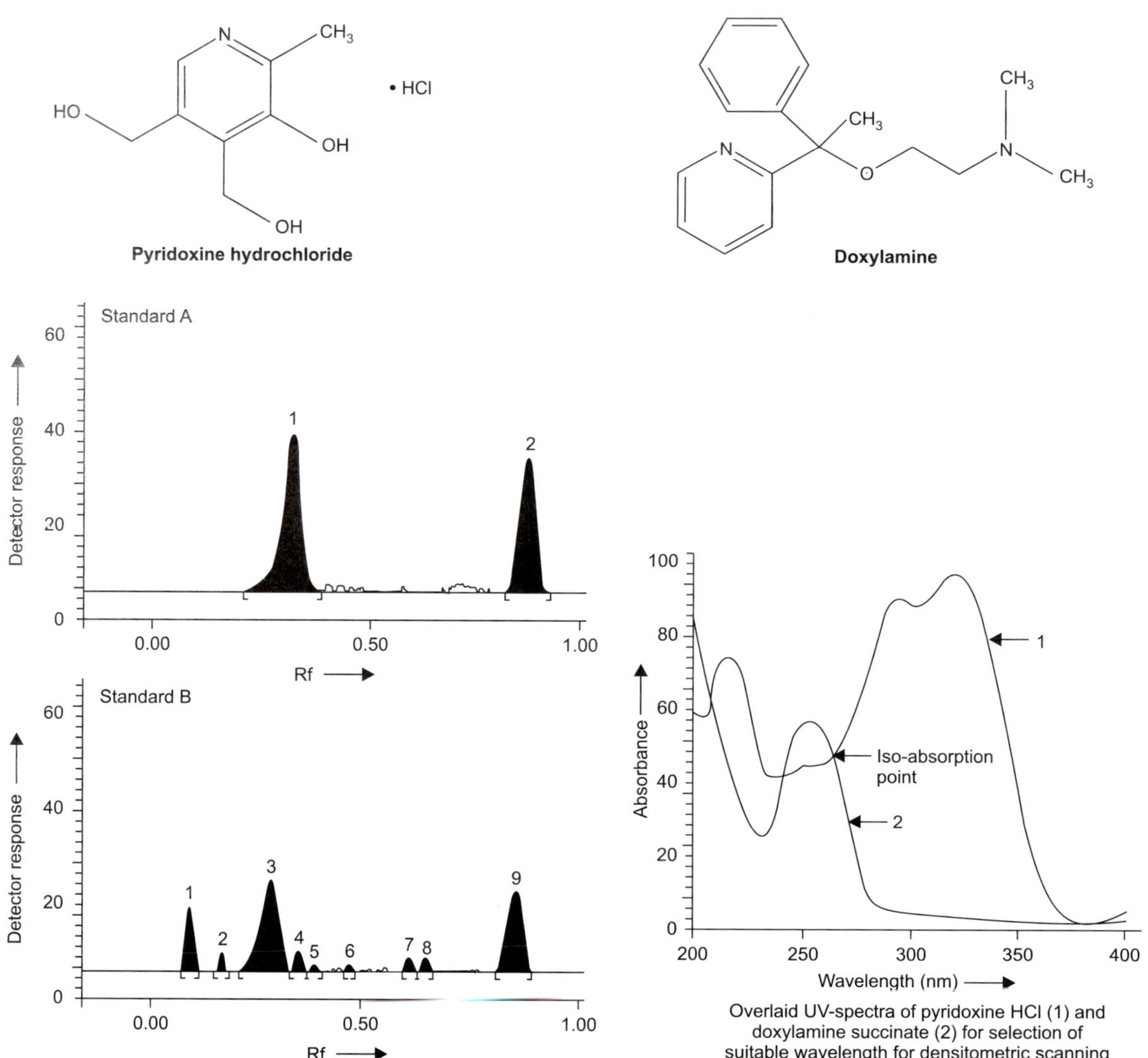

Overlaid UV-spectra of pyridoxine HCl (1) and doxylamine succinate (2) for selection of suitable wavelength for densitometric scanning

A. Typical densitogram of the standard containing pyridoxine HCl and doxylamine succinate. For detailed experimental and chromatographic conditions, refer to Protocol No. 430. Peaks identification: 1. Pyridoxine HCl; 2. Doxylamine succinate.

B. Densitogram of the sample showing degradation profile under oxidative stress condition. Peaks 3 and 9 correspond to pyridoxine and doxylamine.

PROTOCOL FOR HPTLC ANALYSIS OF PHARMACEUTICAL FORMULATION

Protocol No. 430

Formulation: Pyridoxine hydrochloride, Doxylamine succinate

Classification: Central Nervous System **Dosage form:** Tablets

Standard preparation: Prepare 500 μg/ml solution of each compound in methanol. Dilute 5 ml to 10 ml with methanol and use for chromatographic application for linearity profile.

Sample preparation: Powdered sample equivalent to 25 mg of pyridoxine or doxylamine suspended in 20 ml of methanol, sonicated for 10 min, dilute to 25 ml, filter through Whatman No. 42 filter paper, dilute 5 ml of filtrate to 10 ml with methanol and use for analysis.

Chromatographic equipments:

Sample applicator: Camag Linomat–IV

Development chamber: Camag twin-trough glass chamber, 10 × 10 cm

Densitometric scanner: Camag TLC Scanner–III

Chromatographic conditions:

1. Stationary phase: Silica gel 60F_{254} pre-coated HPTLC plates, 10 × 10 cm (200 μm) – Merck
2. Mobile phase (MP): Acetone–chloroform–methanol–25% ammonia (7 : 1.5 : 0.3 : 1.2 v/v)
3. Standard/Sample application:
   Band length: 6 mm Volume applied: 5 μl Spacing: 10 mm
4. Chamber saturation: 20 min (MP)
5. RH (%): 55 ± 5
6. Temperature °C: 22 ± 2
7. Separation technique: Ascending
8. Quantity of mobile phase: 20 ml
9. Migration distance: 60 mm
10. Migration time: 15 min

Densitometric evaluation:

Wavelength: UV–269 nm (iso-absorption point)

Scanning mode: Reflectance/Absorbance

HRF: See densitogram–A

Linearity: 0.5–2 μg/band for both the compounds

Recovery (%): 100.1–101.18 for both the compounds

References: A.P. Argekar and J.G. Sawant, *J. Liq. Chromatogr. and Related Technol.*, **22(13)**, 2051–260, 1996.

Comments:

- The method validated for accuracy, precision, linearity, LOD, LOQ, specificity, robustness and ruggedness.
- The method is stability indicating (acid, base, oxidative, thermal, photolytic). The degradation products were separated from main compounds.
- However, there was significant degradation when exposed to oxidative (30% H_2O_2) stress. All the degradation peaks were well separated from principal peaks.

HPTLC : High Performance Thin Layer Chromatography
HPTLC Densitogram

No. 431

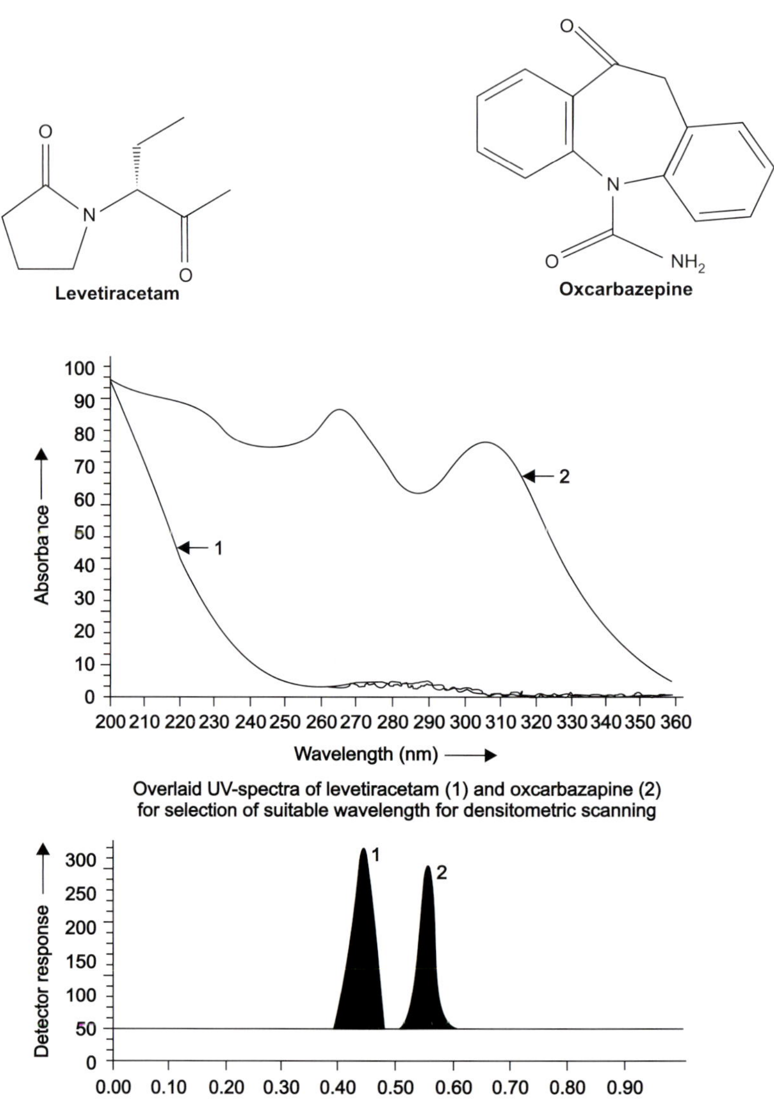

Overlaid UV-spectra of levetiracetam (1) and oxcarbazapine (2) for selection of suitable wavelength for densitometric scanning

Typical densitogram of the sample containing oxcarbazepine and levetiracetam. For detailed experimental and chromatographic conditions, refer to Protocol No. 431. Peaks identification: 1. Levetiracetam; 2. Oxcarbazepine.

PROTOCOL FOR HPTLC ANALYSIS OF PHARMACEUTICAL FORMULATION

Protocol No. 431

Formulation: Oxcarbazepine, Levetiracetam
Classification: Central Nervous System **Dosage form:** Tablets
Standard preparation: Prepare 5 mg/ml solution of each compound in methanol. Further serial dilutions suitably made for linearity studies or apply varying volumes of standard solution (5–10 μl) to study linearity profile.
Sample preparation: Powdered sample equivalent to 25 mg of levetiracetam and 100 mg of oxcarbazepine suspended in methanol, sonicated for 30 min, diluted, filtered and filtrate suitably diluted for assay.
Chromatographic equipments:
Sample applicator: Camag Linomat–IV
Development chamber: Camag twin-trough glass chamber, 20 × 10 cm
Densitometric scanner: Camag TLC Scanner–III
Chromatographic conditions:
1. Stationary phase: Silica gel $60F_{254}$ pre-coated TLC plates, 20 × 10 cm (250 μm) – Merck
2. Mobile phase (MP): Toluene–acetone–methanol (6 : 2 : 2 v/v)
3. Standard/Sample application:
   Band length: 4 mm Volume applied: 1 μl Spacing: 4 mm
4. Chamber saturation: 20 min (MP)
5. RH (%): 60 ± 5
6. Temperature °C: 25 ± 2
7. Separation technique: Ascending
8. Quantity of mobile phase: 20 ml
9. Migration distance: 80 mm
10. Migration time: 20 min

Densitometric evaluation:
Wavelength: UV–200 nm (Levetiracetam); 261 nm (Oxcarbazepine)
Scanning mode: Reflectance/Absorbance
HRF: Levetiracetam—45; Oxcarbazepine—55
Linearity (ng/band): Levetiracetam—5–10; Oxcarbazepine—100–600
Recovery (%): 99.05–99.30 for both the compounds
References: T.S. Reddy and P. Sita Devi, *J. Planar. Chromatogr.*, **20(6)**, 451–457, 2007.
Comments:
- The method validated for accuracy, precision, linearity, LOD, LOQ, specificity, robustness and ruggedness.
- The sample was unstable when exposed to photochemical stress (direct sunlight – 24 h).

HPTLC : High Performance Thin Layer Chromatography
HPTLC Densitogram

No. 432

Phenytoin sodium

Carbamazepine

Phenobarbitone

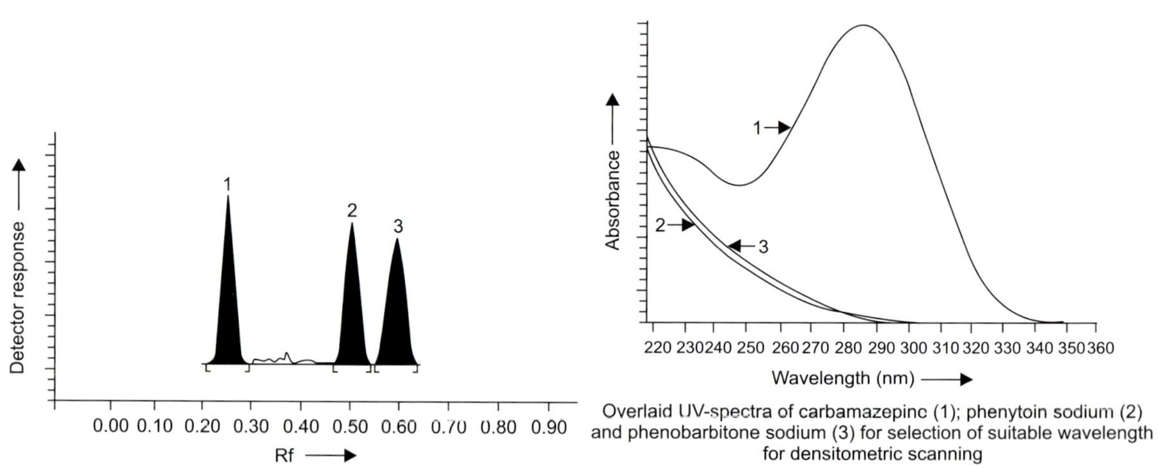

Overlaid UV-spectra of carbamazepine (1); phenytoin sodium (2) and phenobarbitone sodium (3) for selection of suitable wavelength for densitometric scanning

Typical densitogram of the standard containing phenobarbitone sodium, phenytoin sodium and carbamazepine. For detailed experimental and chromatographic conditions, refer to Protocol No. 432. Peaks identification: 1. Carbamazepine; 2. Phenytoin sodium; 3. Phenobarbitone sodium.

PROTOCOL FOR HPTLC ANALYSIS OF PHARMACEUTICAL FORMULATION

Protocol No. 432

Formulation: Phenobarbitone sodium, Phenytoin sodium, Carbamazepine
Classification: Central Nervous System **Dosage form:** Tablets
Standard preparation: Dissolve appropriate quantity of pure compounds in methanol to get 100 μg/ml solution. Apply 5–10 μl of each solution for linearity profile.
Sample preparation: Powdered sample equivalent to 50 mg of phenobarbitone sodium, 100 mg of phenytoin sodium and 200 mg of carbamazepine suspended in 80 ml of methanol, sonicated, diluted to 100 ml, filtered through Whatman No. 1 filter. 10 ml of the filtrate diluted to 100 ml with methanol to get 50 μg/ml (phenobarbitone sodium), 100 μg/ml (phenytoin sodium) and 200 μg/ml (carbamazepine). Apply 10 μl for assay.
Chromatographic equipments:
Sample applicator: Camag Linomat–IV
Development chamber: Camag twin-trough glass chamber, 10 × 10 cm
Densitometric scanner: Camag TLC Scanner–III
Chromatographic conditions:
1. Stationary phase: Silica gel $60F_{254}$ pre-coated TLC plates, 10 × 10 cm (250 μm) – Merck
2. Mobile phase (MP): Acetone–toluene (10 : 4 v/v) or (4 : 10 v/v)
3. Standard/Sample application:
   Band length: 10 mm Volume applied: 5–10 μl Spacing: 10 mm
4. Chamber saturation: —
5. RH (%): 55 ± 5
6. Temperature °C: 22 ± 2
7. Separation technique: Ascending
8. Quantity of mobile phase: 14 ml
9. Migration distance: 80 mm
10. Migration time: 20 min

Densitometric evaluation:
Wavelength: UV–217 Scanning mode: Reflectance/Absorbance
HRF: Carbamazepine—25; Phenytoin sodium—50; Phenobarbitone sodium—59
Linearity (ng/band): Phenobarbitone and Phenytoin—500–1000; Carbamazepine—500–1100
Recovery (%): 99.80–100.4 for all the three compounds.
References: K.M. Patil and S.L. Bodhankar, *Ind. J. Pharm. Sci.*, **67(3)**, 351–355, 2005.
Comments:
- The method validated for accuracy, precision, linearity, LOD, LOQ, specificity, robustness and ruggedness.
- The authors have published HPTLC method for analysis of above antiepileptic drugs in biological sample (*Indian Drugs*, **42(10)**, 665–670, 2005). There is some discrepancy in composition of mobile phase in two publications i.e. toluene–acetone (10 : 4) or (4 : 10), all Rf values are similar in both MP.

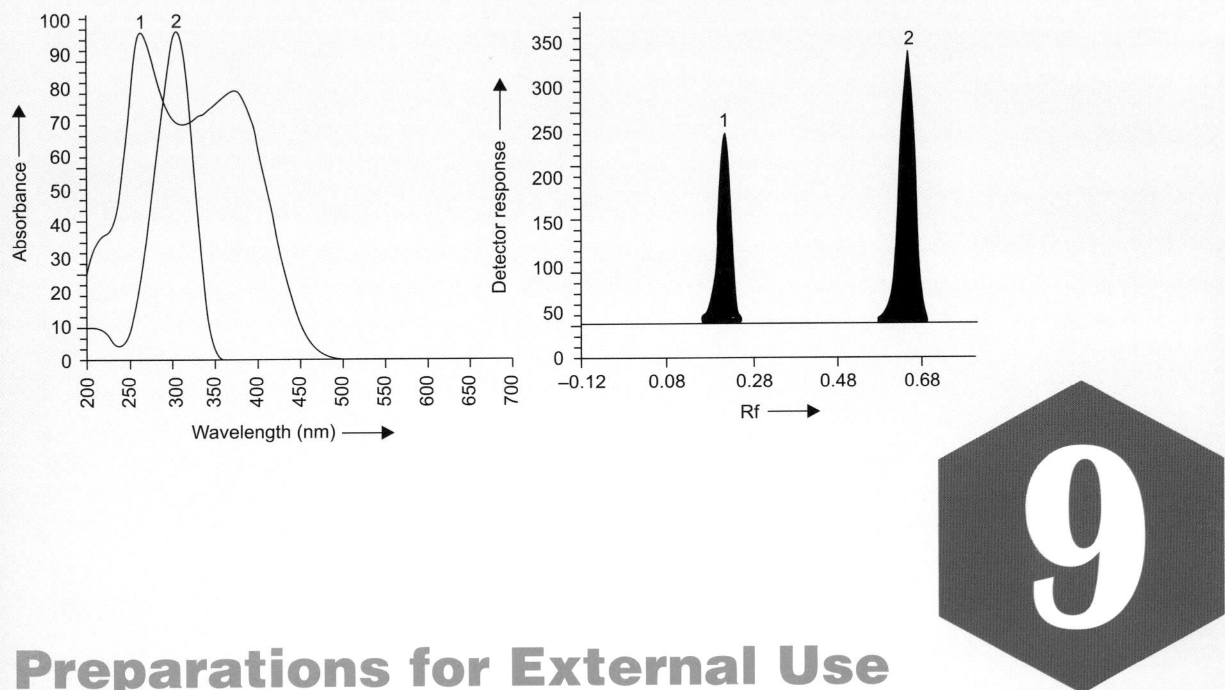

9

Preparations for External Use

- Topical antifungals
- Anti-infectives
- Keratolytics and cleansers
- Topical steroidal preparations
- Rubefacients
- Eye, ear and nasal preparations

Protocols and Densitograms from 433 to 459

Do not think expensive equipments will make up for the lack of talent or experience.

HPTLC : High Performance Thin Layer Chromatography
HPTLC Densitogram

No. 433

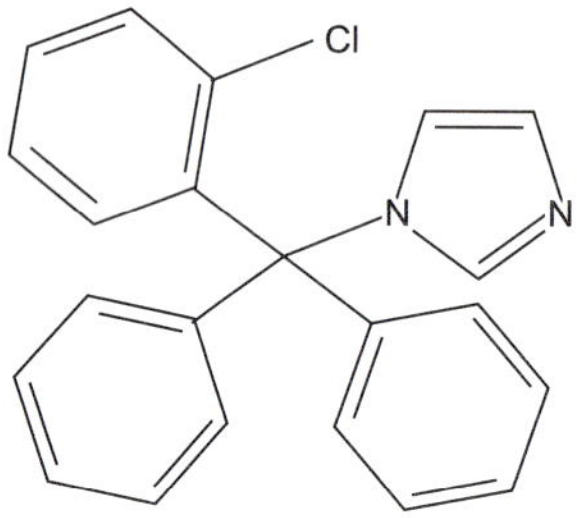

Clotrimazole

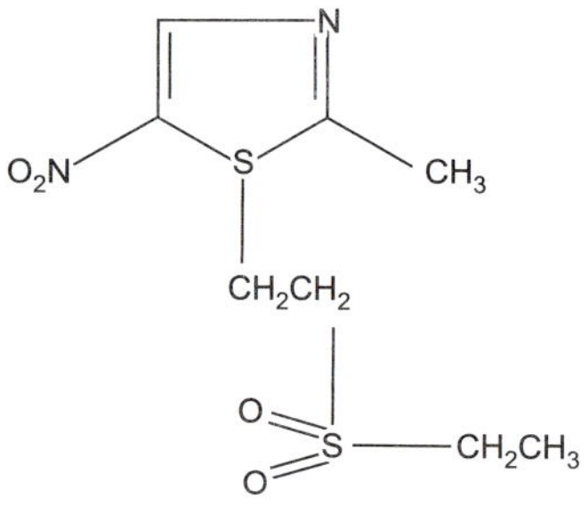

Tinidazole

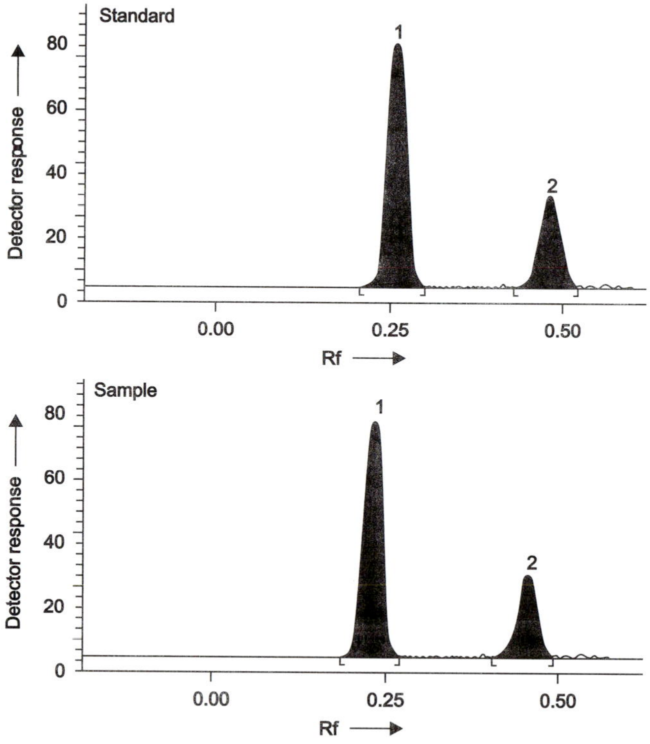

Standard

Sample

Typical densitogram of the sample and standard containing tinidazole and clotrimazole. For detailed experimental and chromatographic conditions, refer to Protocol No. 433. Peaks identification: 1. Tinidazole; 2. Clotrimazole.

PROTOCOL FOR HPTLC ANALYSIS OF PHARMACEUTICAL FORMULATION

Protocol No. 433

Formulation: Tinidazole, Clotrimazole

Classification: External **Dosage form:** Cream, Vaginal tablets

Standard preparation: Prepare 1 mg/ml each of tinidazole (T) and clotrimazole (C) in methanol. Mix 0.5 ml of solution (T) and 0.2 ml of solution (C) and dilute to 10 ml with methanol.

Sample preparation: The sample suspended in methanol, shaken for 10 min, filtered and diluted to get 200 μg/ml of clotrimazole and 500 μg/ml for tinidazole. Apply 10 μl for chromatographic separation and analysis.

Chromatographic equipments:

Sample applicator: Camag Linomat–IV

Development chamber: Camag twin-trough glass chamber, 10 × 10 cm

Densitometric scanner: Camag TLC Scanner–II

Chromatographic conditions:

1. Stationary phase: Silica gel $60F_{254}$ pre-coated HPTLC plates, 10 × 10 cm (200 μm) – Merck
2. Mobile phase (MP): Toluene–acetone–25% ammonia (7 : 3 : 0.1 v/v)
3. Standard/Sample application:
   Band length: 5 mm Volume applied: 5 μl Spacing: 10 mm
4. Chamber saturation: 30 mm (MP)
5. RH (%): 55 ± 5
6. Temperature °C: 22 ± 2
7. Separation technique: Ascending
8. Quantity of mobile phase: 10 ml
9. Migration distance: 50 mm
10. Migration time: 14 min

Densitometric evaluation:

Wavelength: UV–210 or 254 nm Scanning mode: Reflectance/Absorbance

HRF: Tinidazole—25; Clotrimazole—49

Linearity (ng/band): Tinidazole—100–500; Clotrimazole—50–250

Recovery (%): 98.27–99.66 for both the compounds

References: —

Comments:

- The method was optimized and analytical work carried out at **Anchrom's HPTLC Application Laboratory**, Mumbai, India.
- For extraction from cream, suspend the sample in methanol, keep the samples in methanol in refrigerator overnight, decant and use for application.
- Scanning at UV–210 nm is more suitable as both the compounds have significant absorbance.
- Several market samples of similar composition were analysed by the proposed method with reproducible results.

HPTLC : High Performance Thin Layer Chromatography
HPTLC Densitogram

No. 434

Clotrimazole

Tinidazole

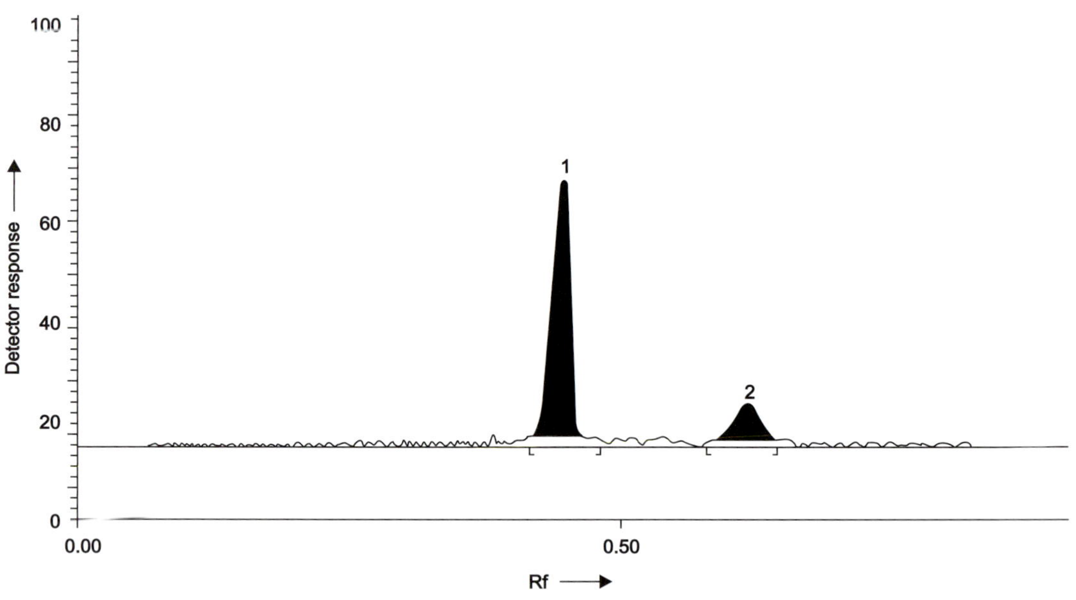

Typical densitogram of the sample containing clotrimazole and tinidazole. For detailed experimental and chromatographic conditions, refer to Protocol No. 434. Peaks identification: 1. Clotrimazole; 2. Tinidazole.

PROTOCOL FOR HPTLC ANALYSIS OF PHARMACEUTICAL FORMULATION

Protocol No. 434

Formulation: Tinidazole, Clotrimazole

Classification: External **Dosage form:** Tablets

Standard preparation: Prepare 5 mg/ml solution of clotrimazole and 10 mg/ml solution of tinidazole, both in methanol. Further diluted suitably with methanol for linearity profile. Apply 10 μl of each solution.

Sample preparation: The sample suspended in methanol, shaken for 10 min, filtered and diluted to get 200 μg/ml of clotrimazole and 500 μg/ml for tinidazole. Apply 10 μl for chromatographic separation and analysis.

Chromatographic equipments:

Sample applicator: Camag Linomat–IV

Development chamber: Camag twin-trough glass chamber, 20 × 10 cm

Densitometric scanner: Camag TLC Scanner–II

Chromatographic conditions:

1. Stationary phase: Silica gel 60F_{254} pre-coated HPTLC plates, 10 × 10 cm (200 μm) – Merck
2. Mobile phase (MP): Toluene–acetone–methanol–glacial acetic acid (6 : 3 : 1 : 0.3 v/v)
3. Standard/Sample application:
   Band length: 7 mm Volume applied: 10 μl Spacing: 10 mm
4. Chamber saturation: 10 mm (MP)
5. RH (%): 55 ± 5
6. Temperature °C: 22 ± 2
7. Separation technique: Ascending
8. Quantity of mobile phase: 20 ml
9. Migration distance: 80 mm
10. Migration time: 30 min

Densitometric evaluation:

Wavelength: UV–254 nm Scanning mode: Reflectance/Absorbance

HRF: Clotrimazole—44; Tinidazole—61

Linearity (ng/band): Clotrimazole—1000–3000; Tinidazole—3000–8000

Recovery (%): 99.98–100.27 for both the compounds

References: Vikas V. Vaidya, Sasikumar N. Menon, Ganesh R. Singh, Maharudra B. Kekare, and Milind P. Choukekar, *J. Planar Chromatogr.*, **20(2)**, 145–147, 2007.

Comments: The method validated for accuracy, precision, linearity, LOD, LOQ, specificity, robustness and ruggedness.

HPTLC : High Performance Thin Layer Chromatography
HPTLC Densitogram

No. 435

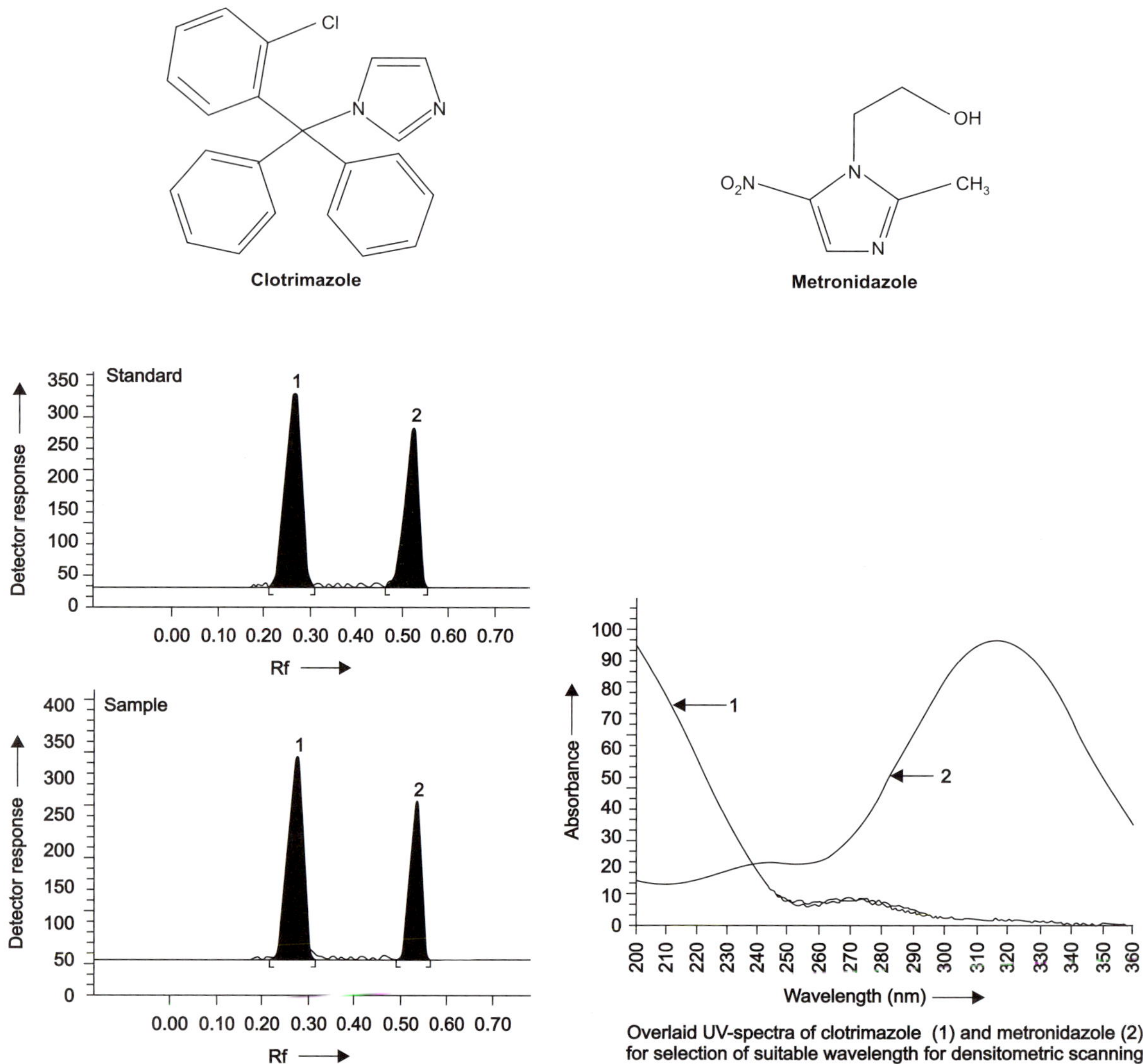

Overlaid UV-spectra of clotrimazole (1) and metronidazole (2) for selection of suitable wavelength for densitometric scanning

Typical densitogram of the sample and standard containing clotrimazole and metronidazole. For detailed experimental and chromatographic conditions, refer to Protocol No. 435. Peaks identification: 1. Metronidazole; 2. Clotrimazole.

PROTOCOL FOR HPTLC ANALYSIS OF PHARMACEUTICAL FORMULATION

Protocol No. 435

Formulation: Metronidazole, Clotrimazole
Classification: External **Dosage form:** Tablets, Cream
Standard preparation: Prepare 2 mg/ml solution of each compound in methanol. Carry out further dilutions to get 500 μg/ml (metronidazole) and 100 μg/ml (clotrimazole). Apply appropriate quantity for linearity profile.
Sample preparation: Weigh powdered sample or cream, suspend in methanol, sonicate, dilute, centrifuge and use the supernatant for chromatographic evaluation.
Chromatographic equipments:
Sample applicator: Camag Linomat–IV
Development chamber: Camag twin-trough glass chamber, 10 × 10 cm
Densitometric scanner: Camag TLC Scanner–II
Chromatographic conditions:

1. Stationary phase: Silica gel $60F_{254}$ pre-coated HPTLC plates, 10 × 10 cm (200 μm) – Merck, pre-washed with methanol, activated (110°C) for 10 min prior to use
2. Mobile phase (MP): Toluene–ethyl acetate–methanol–acetic acid (5.5 : 2 : 0.6 : 0.1 v/v)
3. Standard/Sample application:
   Band length: 4 mm Volume applied: 1–10 μl Spacing: 4 mm
4. Chamber saturation: 10 mm (MP)
5. RH (%): 60 ± 5
6. Temperature °C: 25 ± 2
7. Separation technique: Ascending
8. Quantity of mobile phase: 16 ml
9. Migration distance: 70 mm
10. Migration time: 25 min

Densitometric evaluation:
Wavelength: UV–220 nm Scanning mode: Reflectance/Absorbance
HRF: Metronidazole—28; Clotrimazole—53
Linearity (ng/band): Metronidazole—2000–4000; Clotrimazole—400–800
Recovery (%): 99.02–100.18 for both the compounds
References: Dhananjay B. Meshram, Shashikant B. Bagade and Mahukar R. Tajne, *J. Planar Chromatogr.*, **21(4)**, 277–282, 2008.
Comments:

- The method validated for accuracy, precision, linearity, LOD, LOQ, specificity, robustness and ruggedness.
- The method is stability indicating (acid, base, oxidative, thermal, photolytic). The degradation products were separated from main compounds.

HPTLC : High Performance Thin Layer Chromatography
HPTLC Densitogram

No. 436

Metronidazole

Miconazole nitrate

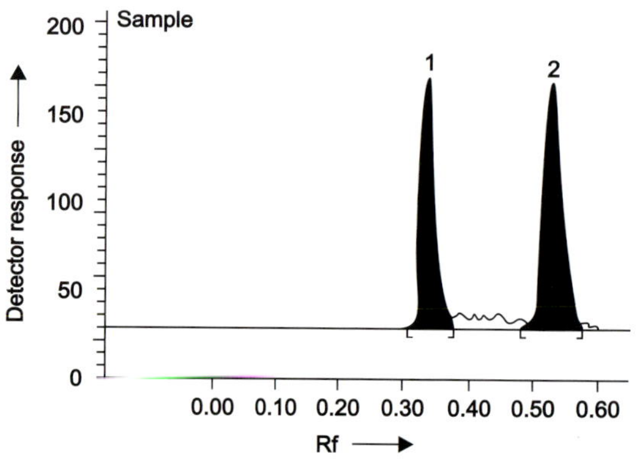

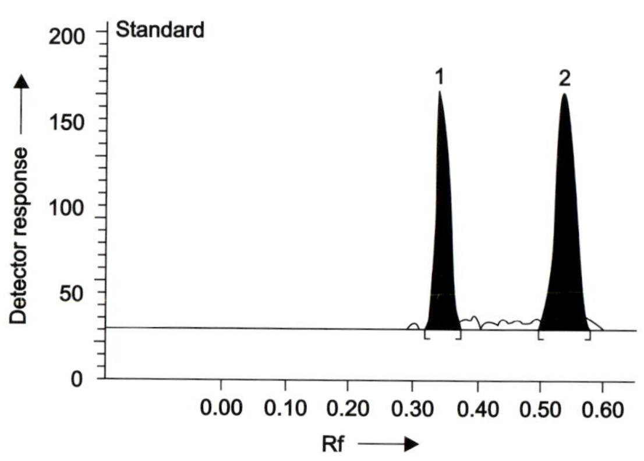

Typical densitogram of the standard and sample containing metronidazole and miconazole nitrate. For detailed experimental and chromatographic conditions, refer to Protocol No. 436. Peaks identification: 1. Metronidazole; 2. Miconazole nitrate.

PROTOCOL FOR HPTLC ANALYSIS OF PHARMACEUTICAL FORMULATION

Protocol No. 436

Formulation: Metronidazole, Miconazole nitrate

Classification: External **Dosage form:** Gel

Standard preparation: Prepare solution of both the compounds in methanol to get 1 mg/ml of metronidazole and 2 mg/ml of miconazole nitrate. Carry out further dilutions to get 100 μg/ml of metronidazole and 200 μg/ml of miconazole nitrate. Apply 1–10 μl of each solution for linearity profile.

Sample preparation: Sample equivalent to 1 mg of metronidazole suspended in 8 ml of methanol, shake for 25 min, dilute to 10 ml with methanol, centrifuge and use the supernatant for chromatographic analysis.

Chromatographic equipments:

Sample applicator: Camag Linomat–IV

Development chamber: Camag twin-trough glass chamber, 10 × 10 cm

Densitometric scanner: Camag TLC Scanner–III

Chromatographic conditions:

1. Stationary phase: Silica gel 60F_{254} pre-coated HPTLC plates, 10 × 10 cm (200 μm) – Merck
2. Mobile phase (MP): Toluene–chloroform–methanol (3 : 2 : 0.6 v/v)
3. Standard/Sample application:
   Band length: 4 mm Volume applied: 5 μl Spacing: 10 mm
4. Chamber saturation: 10 min (MP)
5. RH (%): 60 ± 5
6. Temperature °C: 25 ± 2
7. Separation technique: Ascending
8. Quantity of mobile phase: 11 ml
9. Migration distance: 70 mm
10. Migration time: 15 min

Densitometric evaluation:

Wavelength: UV–240 nm Scanning mode: Reflectance/Absorbance

HRF: Metronidazole—34; Miconazole nitrate—55

Linearity (ng/band): Metronidazole—300–700; Miconazole nitrate—600–1400

Recovery (%): 98.92–100.13 for both the compounds

References: Dhananjay B. Meshram, Shashikant B. Bagade and Madhukar R. Tajne, *Pak. J. Pharm. Sci.*, **22(3)**, 323–328, 2009.

Comments:

- The method validated for accuracy, precision, linearity, LOD, LOQ, specificity, robustness and ruggedness.
- The method is stability indicating (acid, base, oxidative, thermal, photolytic). The degradation products were separated from main compounds.

HPTLC : High Performance Thin Layer Chromatography
HPTLC Densitogram

No. 437

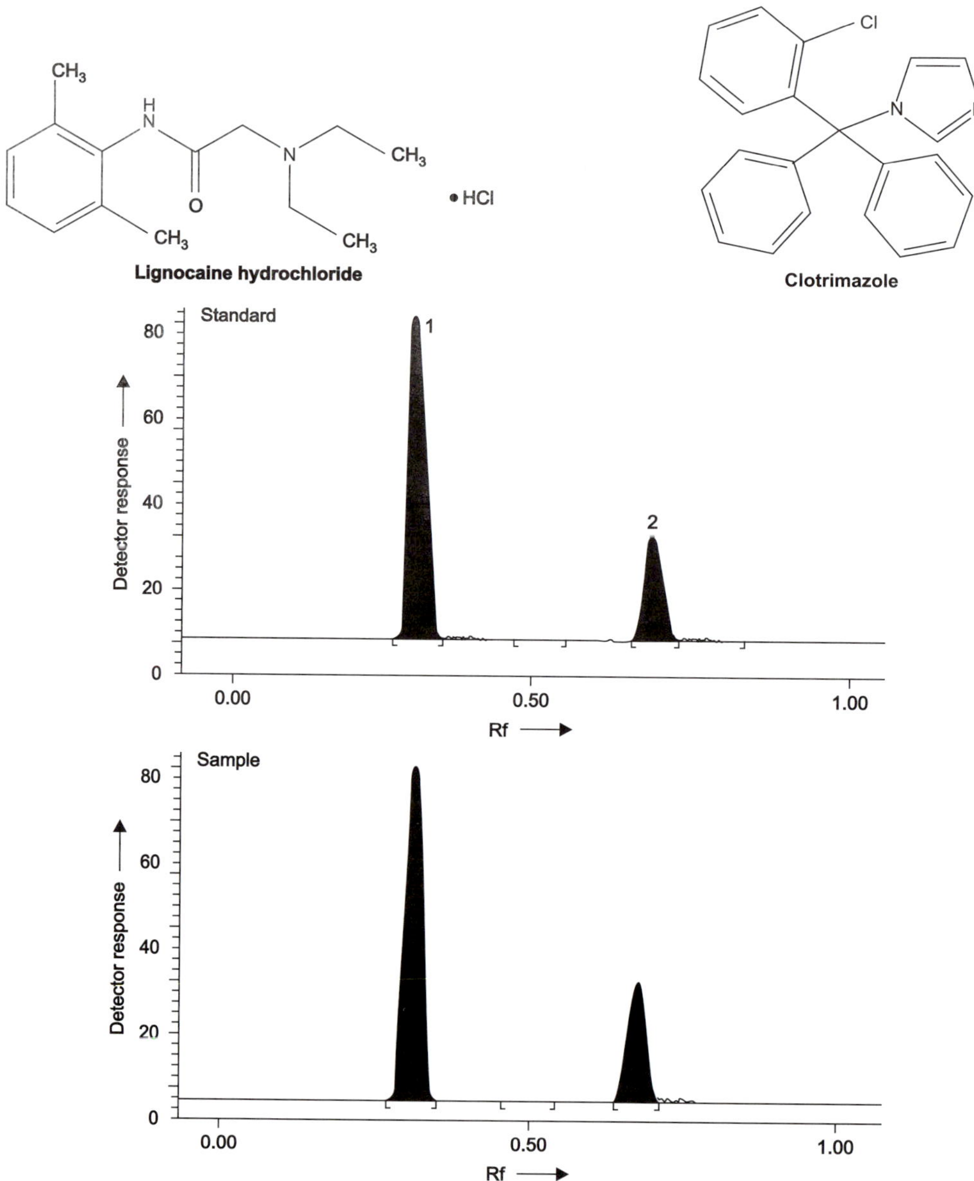

Typical densitogram of the sample and standard containing lidocaine hydrochloride and clotrimazole. For detailed experimental and chromatographic conditions, refer to Protocol No. 437. Peaks identification: 1. Lidocaine HCl; 2. Clotrimazole.

PROTOCOL FOR HPTLC ANALYSIS OF PHARMACEUTICAL FORMULATION

Protocol No. 437

Formulation: **Lidocaine hydrochloride (Lignocaine hydrochloride), Clotrimazole**

Classification: External **Dosage form:** Cream

Standard preparation: Prepare 2 mg/ml solution of each compound in methanol. Further dilutions made to get 100 μg/ml of each. Apply varying volumes of each solution for linearity studies and carry out the chromatographic analysis.

Sample preparation: Weigh appropriate quantity of the sample, suspend in methanol, sonicate, dilute, centrifuge and use the supernatant solution for chromatographic analysis.

Chromatographic equipments:

Sample applicator: Camag Linomat–V

Development chamber: Camag twin-trough glass chamber, 10 × 10 cm

Densitometric scanner: Camag TLC Scanner–III

Chromatographic conditions:

1. Stationary phase: Silica gel $60F_{254}$ pre-coated TLC plates, 10 × 10 cm, (250 μm) – Merck
2. Mobile phase (MP): Toluene–ethyl acetate–methanol–glacial acetic acid (4.5 : 3 : 2 : 0.1 v/v)
3. Standard/Sample application:
   Band length: 6 mm Volume applied: 5 μl Spacing: 6 mm
4. Chamber saturation: 30 min (MP)
5. RH (%): 55 ± 5
6. Temperature °C: 22 ± 2
7. Separation technique: Ascending
8. Quantity of mobile phase: 10 ml
9. Migration distance: 80 mm
10. Migration time: 20 min

Densitometric evaluation:

Wavelength: UV–235 nm Scanning mode: Reflectance/Absorbance

HRF: Lidocaine HCl—28; Clotrimazole—70

Linearity (ng/band): Lidocaine HCl—200–1200; Clotrimazole—100–600

Recovery (%): Lidocaine HCl—99.65; Clotrimazole—99.0

References: R.H. Gharge, G.S. Wankhede, R.R. Kulkarni and K.S. Jain, Abstract No. F-243, 62nd IPC, 2010.

Comments:

- The method validated for different parameters as per ICH guidelines.
- Densitogram as obtained in our laboratory under above chromatographic conditions is included.

HPTLC : High Performance Thin Layer Chromatography
HPTLC Densitogram

No. 438

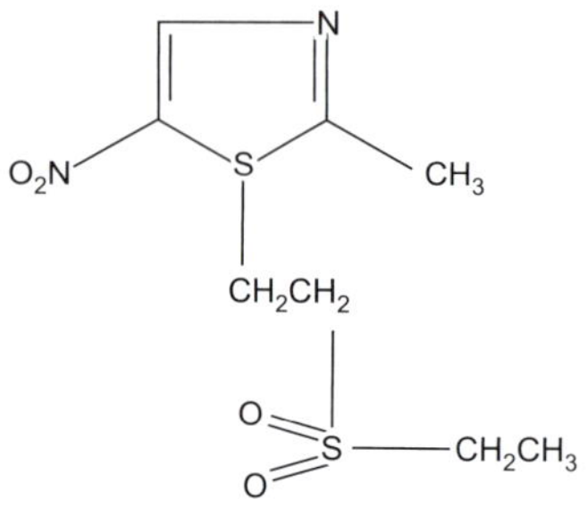

Tinidazole

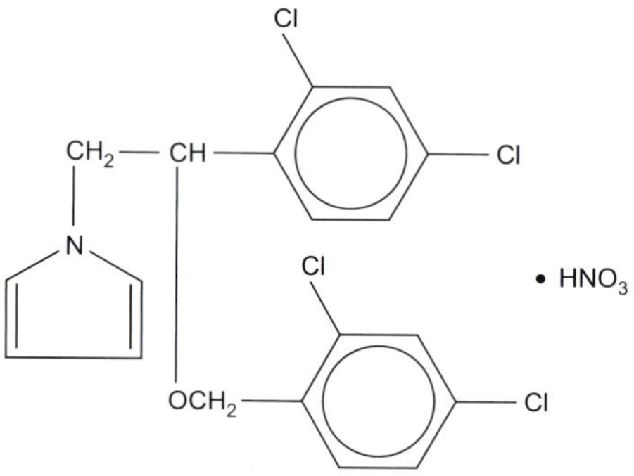

Miconazole nitrate

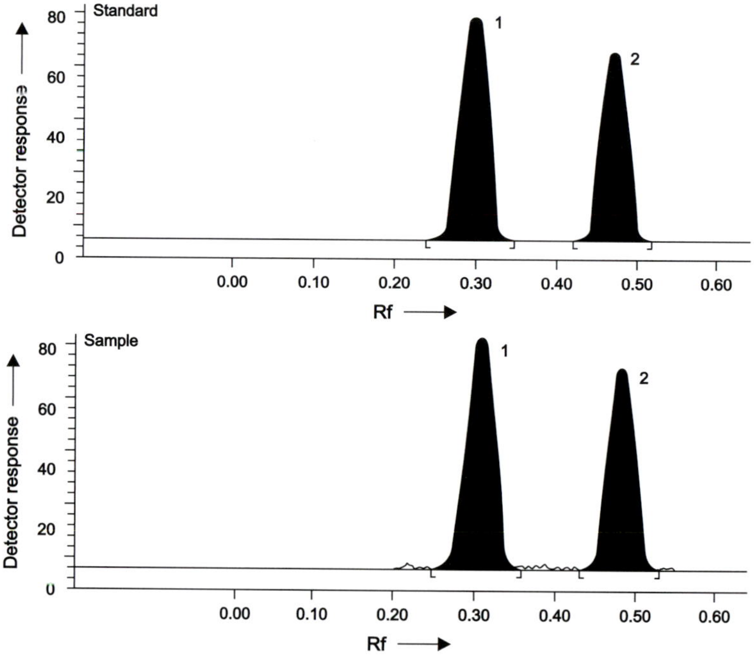

Typical densitogram of the sample and standard containing tinidazole and miconazole nitrate. For detailed experimental and chromatographic conditions, refer to Protocol No. 438. Peaks identification: 1. Tinidazole; 2. Miconazole nitrate.

PROTOCOL FOR HPTLC ANALYSIS OF PHARMACEUTICAL FORMULATION

Protocol No. 438

Formulation: Miconazole nitrate, Tinidazole

Classification: External **Dosage form:** Cream, Vaginal tablets

Standard preparation: Prepare 2.5 mg/ml solution of tinidazole (T) in methanol (1), 1 mg/ml solution of miconazole nitrate (M) in methanol (2). Mix 2 ml of solution (1) and 1 ml of solution (2). Dilute to 10 ml with methanol.

Sample preparation: Weigh sample equivalent to 500 mg of tinidazole, add 70 ml of methanol, vortex for 10 min, dilute to 100 ml with methanol, filter and dilute 1 ml of filtrate to 10 ml and use for application.

Chromatographic equipments:

Sample applicator: Camag Linomat–IV
Development chamber: Camag twin-trough glass chamber, 10 × 10 cm
Densitometric scanner: Camag TLC Scanner–II

Chromatographic conditions:

1. Stationary phase: Silica gel $60F_{254}$ pre-coated HPTLC plates, 7 × 10 cm (200 µm) – Merck
2. Mobile phase (MP): Toluene–acetone–25% ammonia (7 : 3 : 0.1 v/v)
3. Standard/Sample application:
   Band length: 5 mm Volume applied: 5 µl Spacing: 5 mm
4. Chamber saturation: 30 mm (MP)
5. RH (%): 55 ± 5
6. Temperature °C: 22 ± 2
7. Separation technique: Ascending
8. Quantity of mobile phase: 10 ml
9. Migration distance: 50 mm
10. Migration time: 14 min

Densitometric evaluation:

Wavelength: UV–220 or 272 nm Scanning mode: Reflectance/Absorbance
HRF: Tinidazole—30; Miconazole nitrate—47
Linearity (ng/band): Tinidazole—100–250; Miconazole—100–500
Recovery (%): 100.40–100.90 for both the compounds

References: —

Comments:

- The method was optimized and analytical work carried out at **Anchrom's HPTLC Application Laboratory**, Mumbai, India.
- For extraction from cream, leave the sample in refrigerator overnight, then decant and use for application.
- Several market samples of similar composition were analysed by the proposed method with reproducible results.

HPTLC : High Performance Thin Layer Chromatography
HPTLC Densitogram

No. 439

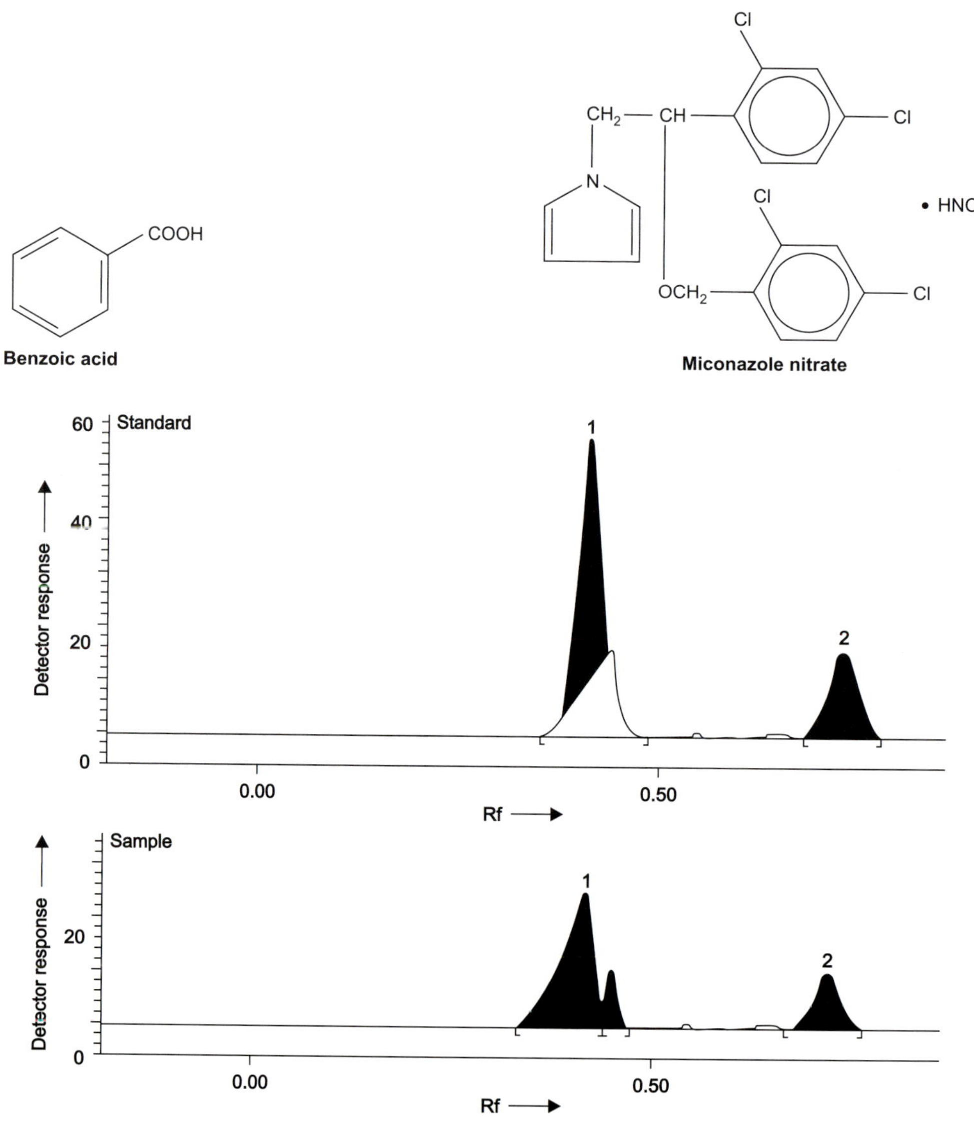

Typical densitogram of the sample and standard containing miconazole nitrate and benzoic acid. For detailed experimental and chromatographic conditions, refer to Protocol No. 439. Peaks identification: 1. Benzoic acid; 2. Miconazole nitrate.

PROTOCOL FOR HPTLC ANALYSIS OF PHARMACEUTICAL FORMULATION

Protocol No. 439

Formulation: Miconazole nitrate, Benzoic acid

Classification: External **Dosage form:** Solution, Paint, Cream

Standard preparation: Prepare 1 mg/ml solution of each compound in methanol. Further dilutions made with methanol for chromatographic analysis.

Sample preparation: An accurately weighed quantity of the sample suspended in methanol, sonicated, diluted and filtered. The filtrate used for application.

Chromatographic equipments:

Sample applicator: Camag Linomat–IV

Development chamber: Normal flat bottom glass chamber, 20 × 20 cm

Densitometric scanner: Camag TLC Scanner–II

Chromatographic conditions:

1. Stationary phase: Silica gel $60F_{254}$ pre-coated TLC plates, 10 × 10 cm (250 μm) – Merck
2. Mobile phase (MP): n-hexane–chloroform–methanol–diethylamine (4.2 : 2.1 : 1.3 : 0.5 v/v)
3. Standard/Sample application:
   Band length: 10 mm Volume applied: 10 μl Spacing: 10 mm
4. Chamber saturation: 30 min (MP)
5. RH (%): 55 ± 5
6. Temperature °C: 22 ± 2
7. Separation technique: Ascending
8. Quantity of mobile phase: 16 ml
9. Migration distance: 50 mm
10. Migration time: 15 min

Densitometric evaluation:

Wavelength: UV–220 nm Scanning mode: Reflectance/Absorbance

HRF: Benzoic acid—45; Miconazole nitrate—70

Linearity (ng/band): Benzoid acid—200–700; Miconazole nitrate—100–500

Recovery (%): 99.25–100.75 for both the compounds

References: Z.H. Qian, W. Yan, Y. Phe, G. Lu, *Chinese J. Hospital Pharma.*, **11**, 435–37, 1991.

Comments: The method checked as per protocol described by the author and found reproducible.

HPTLC : High Performance Thin Layer Chromatography
HPTLC Densitogram

No. 440

COOH
OH

Salicylic acid

OH O OH

Dithranol

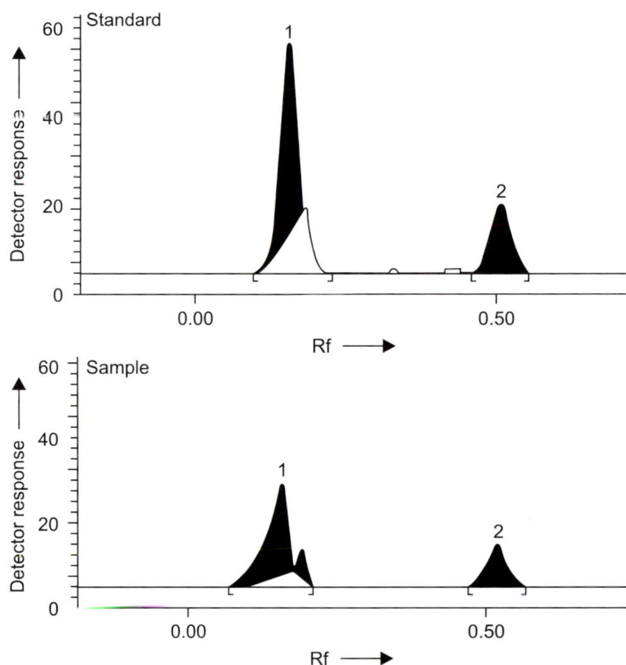

Typical densitogram of the sample and standard containing salicylic acid and dithranol. For detailed experimental and chromatographic conditions, refer to Protocol No. 440. Peaks identification: 1. Salicylic acid; 2. Dithranol.

PROTOCOL FOR HPTLC ANALYSIS OF PHARMACEUTICAL FORMULATION

Protocol No. 440

Formulation: Salicylic acid, Dithranol

Classification: External **Dosage form:** Cream, Ointment

Standard preparation: Prepare 2 mg/ml solution of salicylic acid in methanol (1). 100 mcg/ml solution of dithranol in methanol (2). Mix 2.5 ml each of solution (1) and (2) and dilute to 10 ml with methanol.

Sample preparation: Weigh sample accurately equivalent to 2.5 mg of dithranol, extract with methanol, dilute to 100 ml with methanol, chill, filter and use for analysis.

Chromatographic equipments:

Sample applicator: Camag Linomat–IV

Development chamber: Camag twin-trough glass chamber, 10 × 10 cm

Densitometric scanner: Camag TLC Scanner–II

Chromatographic conditions:

1. Stationary phase: Silica gel 60F_{254} pre-coated HPTLC plates, 10 × 10 cm (200 μm) – Merck
2. Mobile phase (MP): n-hexane–ethyl acetate–glacial acetic acid (9.5 : 0.5 : 0.1 v/v)
3. Standard/Sample application:
   Band length: 5 mm Volume applied: 5 μl Spacing: 5 mm
4. Chamber saturation: 20 min (MP)
5. RH (%): 55 ± 5
6. Temperature °C: 22 ± 2
7. Separation technique: Ascending
8. Quantity of mobile phase: 10 ml
9. Migration distance: 50 mm
10. Migration time: 18 min

Densitometric evaluation:

Wavelength: UV–338 nm Scanning mode: Reflectance/Absorbance

HRF: Salicylic acid—15; Dithranol—52

Linearity (ng/band): Salicylic acid—500–1250; Dithranol—50–200

Recovery (%): 97.75–99.25 for both the compounds

References: —

Comments:

- The method was optimized and analytical work carried out at **Anchrom's HPTLC Application Laboratory**, Mumbai, India.
- The sample was suspended in methanol, stored in refrigerator overnight, decanted and clear supernatant used for application.
- Several market samples of similar composition were analysed by the proposed method with reproducible results.

HPTLC : High Performance Thin Layer Chromatography
HPTLC Densitogram

No. 441

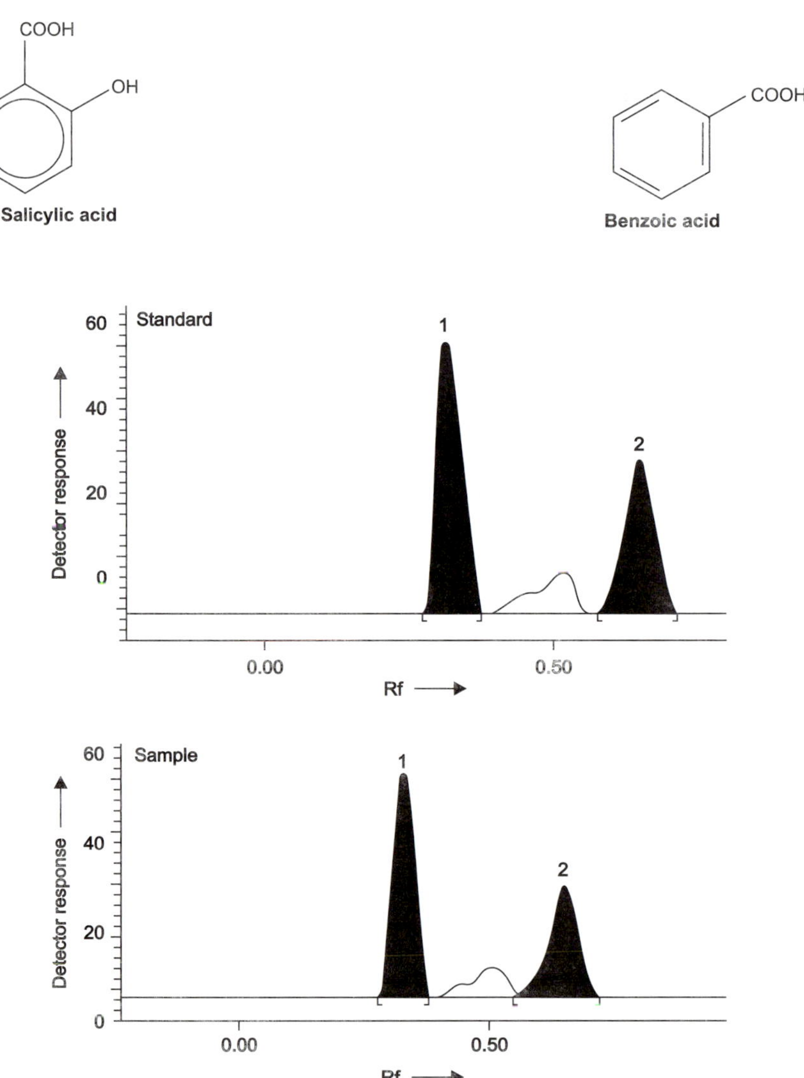

Typical densitogram of the sample and standard containing salicylic acid and benzoid acid. For detailed experimental and chromatographic conditions, refer to Protocol No. 441. Peaks identification: 1. Salicylic acid; 2. Benzoic acid.

PROTOCOL FOR HPTLC ANALYSIS OF PHARMACEUTICAL FORMULATION

Protocol No. 441

Formulation: Salicylic acid, Benzoic acid

Classification: External **Dosage form:** Lotion, Ointment

Standard preparation: Prepare 1 mg/ml solution of each compound in methanol. Further dilutions made with methanol for chromatographic analysis.

Sample preparation: An accurately weighed quantity of the sample suspended in methanol, sonicated, diluted and filtered. The filtrate used for application.

Chromatographic equipments:

Sample applicator: Camag Linomat–IV

Development chamber: Camag flat bottom glass chamber, 20 × 20 cm

Densitometric scanner: Camag TLC Scanner–II

Chromatographic conditions:

1. Stationary phase: Silica gel $60F_{254}$ pre-coated HPTLC plates, 10 × 10 cm (200 μm) – Merck
2. Mobile phase (MP): Ethyl acetate–acetone (9 : 2 v/v) or pet. ether–glacial acetic acid (9 : 1 v/v)
3. Standard/Sample application:
   Band length: 5 mm Volume applied: 3 μl Spacing: 5 mm
4. Chamber saturation: 20 min (MP)
5. RH (%): 55 ± 5
6. Temperature °C: 22 ± 2
7. Separation technique: Ascending
8. Quantity of mobile phase: 10 ml
9. Migration distance: 50 mm
10. Migration time: 15 min

Densitometric evaluation:

Wavelength: UV–295 nm (SA), 223 nm (BA), 267 nm (BA and SA)

Scanning mode: Reflectance/Absorbance

HRF: Salicylic acid—40; Benzoic acid—60

Linearity (ng/band): Salicylic acid—50–250; Benzoic acid—100–500

Recovery (%): 99.10–100.50 for both the compounds

References: (i) Li. Z.G., Shi. T.G., Song. G.P. through *Analytical Abstract*, July, 1993. (ii) Li. Zengguang, *Chinese. J. of Chromatography*, **10**, 313, 1992.

Comments: The chromatogram can be scanned at 223 nm and 295 nm for benzoic acid and salicylic acid respectively, being their absorption maxima, however, wavelength of 267 nm was chosen being the iso-absorption point.

HPTLC : High Performance Thin Layer Chromatography
HPTLC Densitogram

No. 442

O_2N–C_6H_4–CH(H)–CH(NHCOCHCl$_2$)–CH_2OH

Chloramphenicol

H_2N–C_6H_4–$COOC_2H_5$

Benzocaine

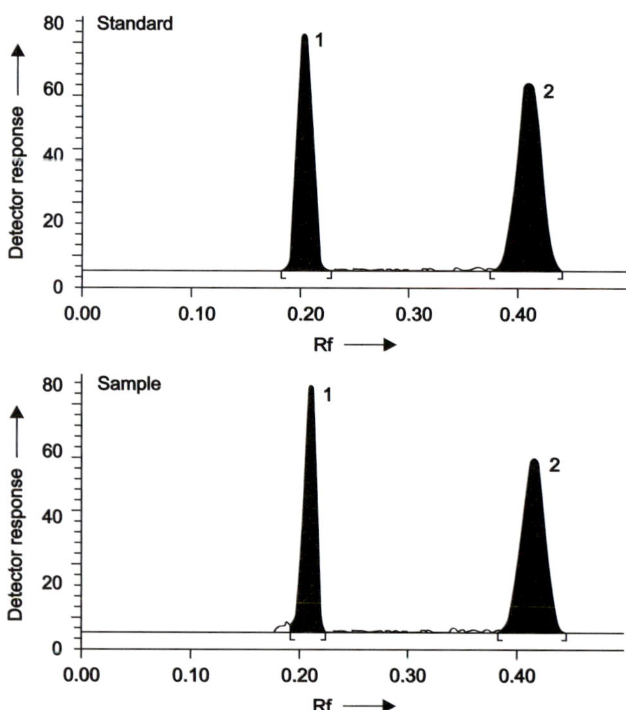

Typical densitogram of the sample and the standard containing chloramphenicol and benzocaine. For detailed experimental and chromatographic conditions, refer to Protocol No. 442. Peaks identification: 1. Chloramphenicol; 2. Benzocaine.

PROTOCOL FOR HPTLC ANALYSIS OF PHARMACEUTICAL FORMULATION

Protocol No. 442

Formulation: Benzocaine, Chloramphenicol

Classification: External **Dosage form:** Ear drops

Standard preparation: Weigh accurately 50 mg of chloramphenicol and 10 mg of benzocaine, dissolve in methanol to produce 10 ml. Further dilute 0.5 ml to 10 ml with methanol and use for application.

Sample preparation: Dilute 1 ml of the sample to 10 ml with methanol. Dilute 0.5 ml of the resulting solution to 10 ml with methanol for chromatographic analysis.

Chromatographic equipments:

Sample applicator: Camag Linomat–IV

Development chamber: Camag twin-trough glass chamber, 10 × 10 cm

Densitometric scanner: Camag TLC Scanner–II

Chromatographic conditions:

1. Stationary phase: Silica gel 60F_{254} pre-coated HPTLC plates, 10 × 10 cm (200 μm) – Merck
2. Mobile phase (MP): Toluene–acetate (7.5 : 2.5 v/v)
3. Standard/Sample application:
   Band length: 5 mm Volume applied: 5 μl Spacing: 5 mm
4. Chamber saturation: 10 min (MP)
5. RH (%): 55 ± 5
6. Temperature °C: 22 ± 2
7. Separation technique: Ascending
8. Quantity of mobile phase: 10 ml
9. Migration distance: 50 mm
10. Migration time: 15 min

Densitometric evaluation:

Wavelength: UV–255 nm Scanning mode: Reflectance/Absorbance

HRF: Chloramphenicol—22; Benzocaine—42

Linearity (ng/band): Benzocaine—50–500; Chloramphenicol—100–200

Recovery (%): 98.60–101.0 for both the compounds

References: —

Comments:

- The method was optimized and analytical work carried out at **Anchrom's HPTLC Application Laboratory**, Mumbai, India.
- Several market samples of similar composition were analysed by the proposed method with reproducible results.

HPTLC : High Performance Thin Layer Chromatography
HPTLC Densitogram

No. 443

Chloramphenicol

Benzocaine

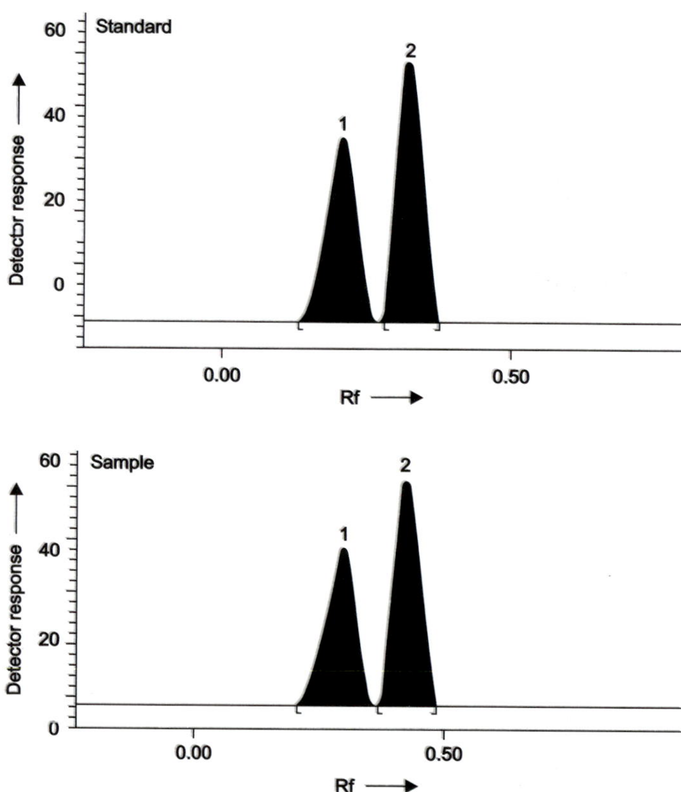

Typical densitogram of the sample and standard containing chloramphenicol and benzocaine. For detailed experimental and chromatographic conditions, refer to Protocol No. 443. Peaks identification: 1. Benzocaine; 2. Chloramphenicol.

PROTOCOL FOR HPTLC ANALYSIS OF PHARMACEUTICAL FORMULATION

Protocol No. 443

Formulation: Benzocaine, Chloramphenicol

Classification: External **Dosage form:** Ear drops

Standard preparation: Weigh accurately 50 mg of chloramphenicol and 10 mg of benzocaine, dissolve in methanol to produce 10 ml. Further dilute 0.5 ml to 10 ml with methanol and use for application.

Sample preparation: Dilute 1 ml of ear drops to 10 ml with methanol. Further dilute 0.5 ml to 10 ml with methanol and use for chromatographic application.

Chromatographic equipments:

Sample applicator: Camag Linomat–IV

Development chamber: Camag twin-trough glass chamber, 10 × 10 cm

Densitometric scanner: Camag TLC Scanner–II

Chromatographic conditions:

1. Stationary phase: Silica gel 60 RP-18F_{254s} pre-coated HPTLC plates, 7 × 10 cm (200 μm) – Merck
2. Mobile phase (MP): 0.5 M sodium chloride–methanol–glacial acetic acid (12 : 8 : 0.01 v/v)
3. Standard/Sample application:
   Band length: 5 mm Volume applied: 5 μl Spacing: 5 mm
4. Chamber saturation: 30 min (MP)
5. RH (%): 55 ± 5
6. Temperature °C: 22 ± 2
7. Separation technique: Ascending
8. Quantity of mobile phase: 20 ml
9. Migration distance: 50 mm
10. Migration time: 40 min

Densitometric evaluation:

Wavelength: UV–285 nm Scanning mode: Reflectance/Absorbance

HRF: Benzocaine—35; Chloramphenicol—45

Linearity (ng/band): Benzocaine—50–500; Chloramphenicol—100–2000

Recovery (%): 98.25–98.75 for both the compounds

References: —

Comments:

- The method was optimized and analytical work carried out at **Anchrom's HPTLC Application Laboratory**, Mumbai, India.
- Reversal of retention order observed in RP-chromatography as compared to NP-chromatography.
- Several market samples of similar composition were analysed by the proposed method with reproducible results.

HPTLC : High Performance Thin Layer Chromatography
HPTLC Densitogram

No. 444

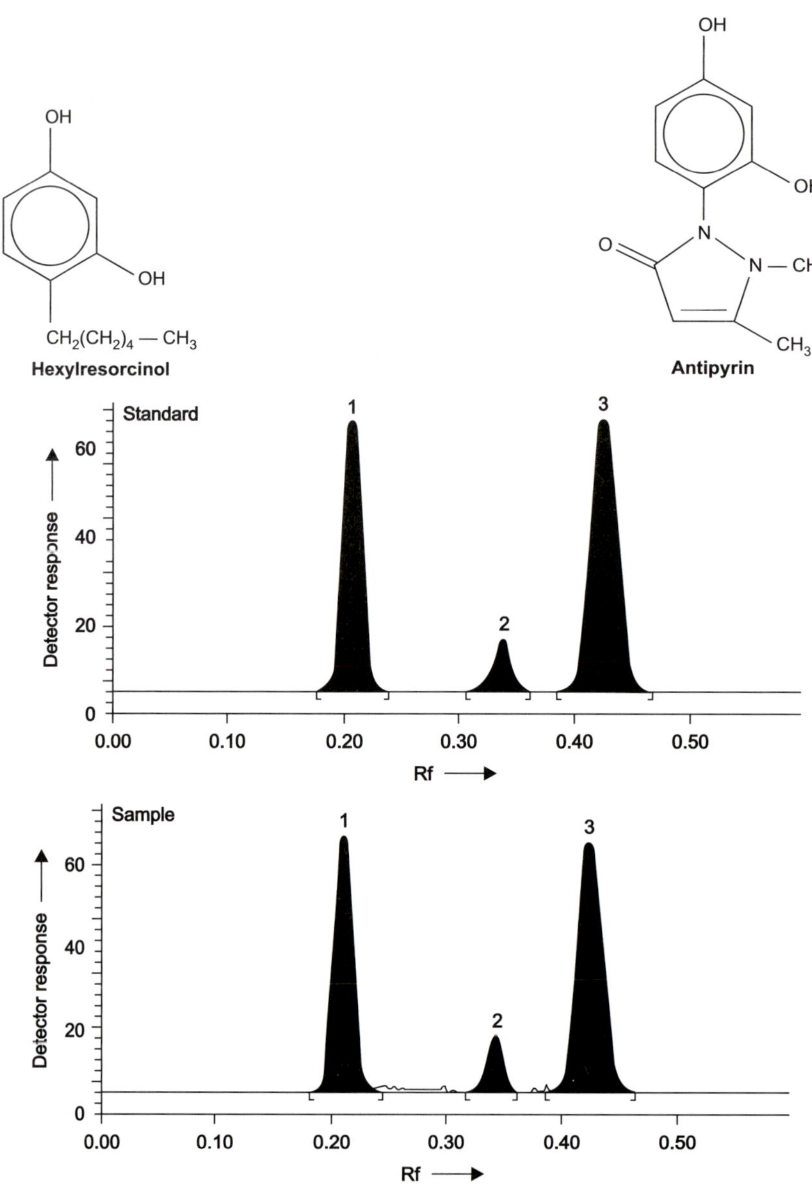

Typical densitogram of the sample and standard containing benzocaine, antipyrin and hexylresorcinol. For detailed experimental and chromatographic conditions, refer to Protocol No. 444. Peaks identification: 1. Antipyrin; 2. Hexylresorcinol; 3. Benzocaine.

PROTOCOL FOR HPTLC ANALYSIS OF PHARMACEUTICAL FORMULATION

Protocol No. 444

Formulation: Benzocaine, Antipyrin, Hexylresorcinol

Classification: External **Dosage form:** Ear drops

Standard preparation: Weigh accurately about 10 mg of hexylresorcinol (H) and dissolve in methanol to get 1 mg/ml solution (1). Weigh 50 mg of antipyrin (A), 12.5 mg of benzocaine (B), add 5–6 ml methanol and 1 ml of solution (1), dilute to 10 ml. Further dilute 0.4 ml to 10 ml with methanol.

Sample preparation: Dilute 1 ml of ear drops to 10 ml with methanol. Further dilute 0.5 ml to 10 ml with methanol and use for chromatographic application.

Chromatographic equipments:

Sample applicator: Camag Linomat–IV
Development chamber: Camag twin-trough glass chamber, 10 × 10 cm
Densitometric scanner: Camag TLC Scanner–II

Chromatographic conditions:

1. Stationary phase: Silica gel $60F_{254}$ pre-coated HPTLC plates, 7 × 10 cm (200 μm) – Merck
2. Mobile phase (MP): Toluene–acetone (7 : 3 v/v)
3. Standard/Sample application:
   Band length: 5 mm Volume applied: 5 μl Spacing: 10 mm
4. Chamber saturation: 20 min (MP)
5. RH (%): 55 ± 5
6. Temperature °C: 22 ± 2
7. Separation technique: Ascending
8. Quantity of mobile phase: 10 ml
9. Migration distance: 70 mm
10. Migration time: 20 min

Densitometric evaluation:

Wavelength: A and B—280 nm; HR—294 nm
Scanning mode: Reflectance/Absorbance
HRF: Antipyrin—22; Hexylresorcinol—35; Benzocaine—43
Linearity (ng/band): Antipyrin—50–500; Benzocaine—50–250; Hexylresorcinol—25–100
Recovery (%): 97.0–98.4 for all the three compounds

References: —

Comments:

- The method was optimized and analytical work carried out at **Anchrom's HPTLC Application Laboratory**, Mumbai, India.
- At the concentrations applied, hexylresorcinol could not be scanned. After scanning benzocaine and antipyrin, the plate was exposed to iodine vapours for 10 min, removed from iodine chamber and immediately scanned at 294 nm for hexylresorcinol.
- Several market samples of similar composition were analysed by the proposed method with reproducible results.

HPTLC : High Performance Thin Layer Chromatography
HPTLC Densitogram

No. 445

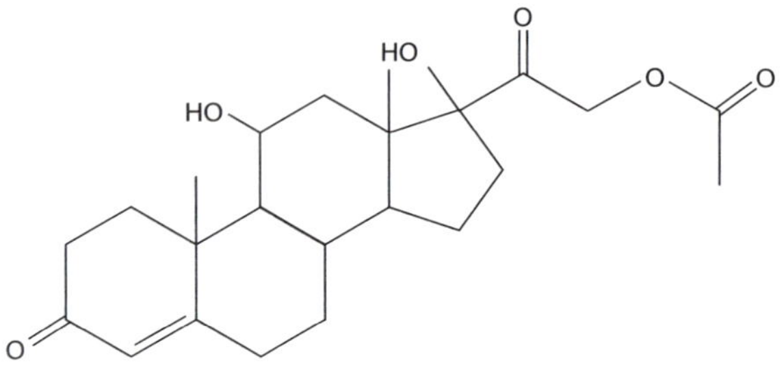

Hydrocortisone acetate

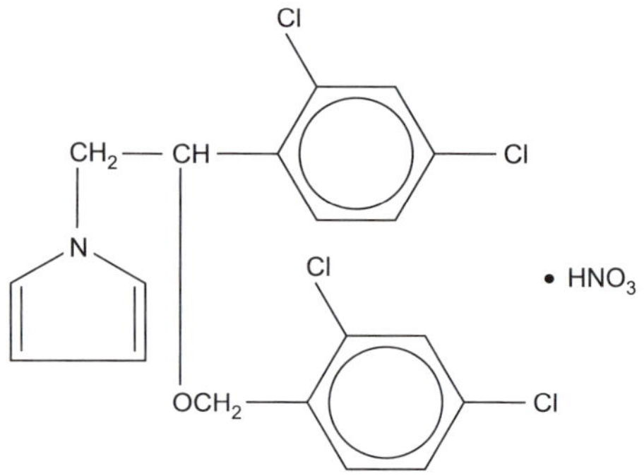

Miconazole nitrate

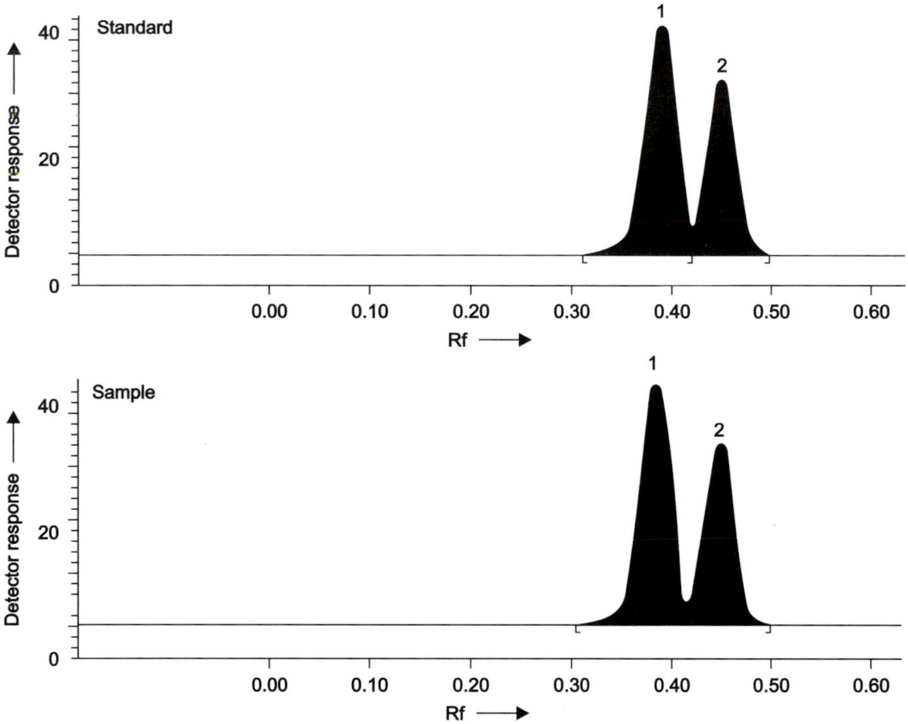

Typical densitogram of the sample and standard containing tinidazole and miconazole nitrate. For detailed experimental and chromatographic conditions, refer to Protocol No. 445. Peaks identification: 1. Tinidazole; 2. Miconazole nitrate.

PROTOCOL FOR HPTLC ANALYSIS OF PHARMACEUTICAL FORMULATION

Protocol No. 445

Formulation: Hydrocortisone acetate, Miconazole nitrate

Classification: External **Dosage form:** Cream, Gel

Standard preparation: Weigh about 20 mg of miconazole nitrate (M) and 10 mg of hydrocortisone acetate (H), add methanol, stir and dilute to 50 ml with methanol and use for analysis.

Sample preparation: Weigh homogenized sample equivalent to 10 mg of miconazole nitrate, add 20–30 ml methanol, vortex and make up to 25 ml, chill, filter and use the filtrate for analysis.

Chromatographic equipments:

Sample applicator: Camag Linomat–IV
Development chamber: Camag twin-trough glass chamber, 10 × 10 cm
Densitometric scanner: Camag TLC Scanner–II

Chromatographic conditions:

1. Stationary phase: Silica gel $60F_{254}$ pre-coated HPTLC plates, 7 × 10 cm (200 μm) – Merck
2. Mobile phase (MP): Toluene–acetone–25% ammonia (7 : 3 : 0.2 v/v)
3. Standard/Sample application:
   Band length: 10 mm Volume applied: 10 μl Spacing: 10 mm
4. Chamber saturation: 30 min (MP)
5. RH (%): 55 ± 5
6. Temperature °C: 22 ± 2
7. Separation technique: Ascending
8. Quantity of mobile phase: 10.2 ml
9. Migration distance: 50 mm
10. Migration time: 14 min

Densitometric evaluation:

Wavelength: UV–277 nm Scanning mode: Reflectance/Absorbance
HRF: Hydrocortisone acetate—38; Miconazole nitrate—45
Linearity (ng/band): Miconazole nitrate—100–500; Hydrocortisone acetate—25–150
Recovery (%): 100.50–102.50 for both the compounds

References: —

Comments:

- The method was optimized and analytical work carried out at **Anchrom's HPTLC Application Laboratory**, Mumbai, India.
- For extraction from cream, suspend the sample in methanol, store in refrigerator overnight and then decant for application.
- Several market samples of similar composition were analysed by the proposed method with reproducible results.

HPTLC : High Performance Thin Layer Chromatography
HPTLC Densitogram

No. 446

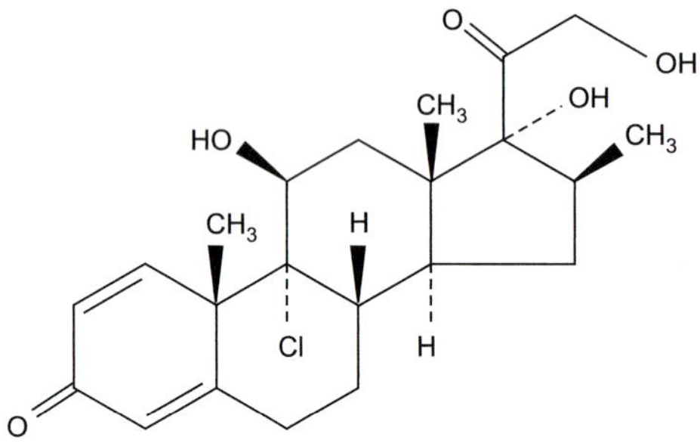

Beclomethasone

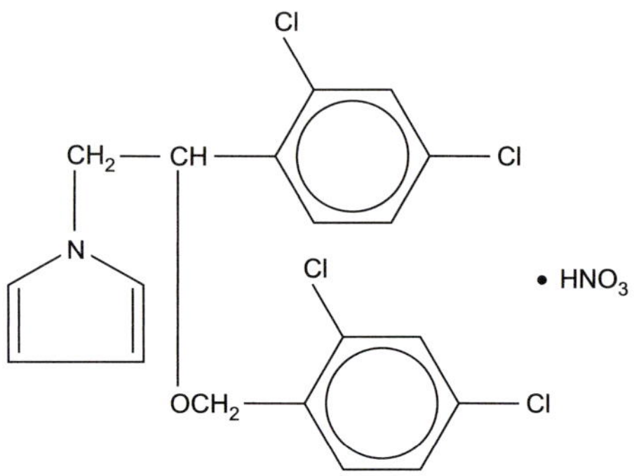

Miconazole nitrate

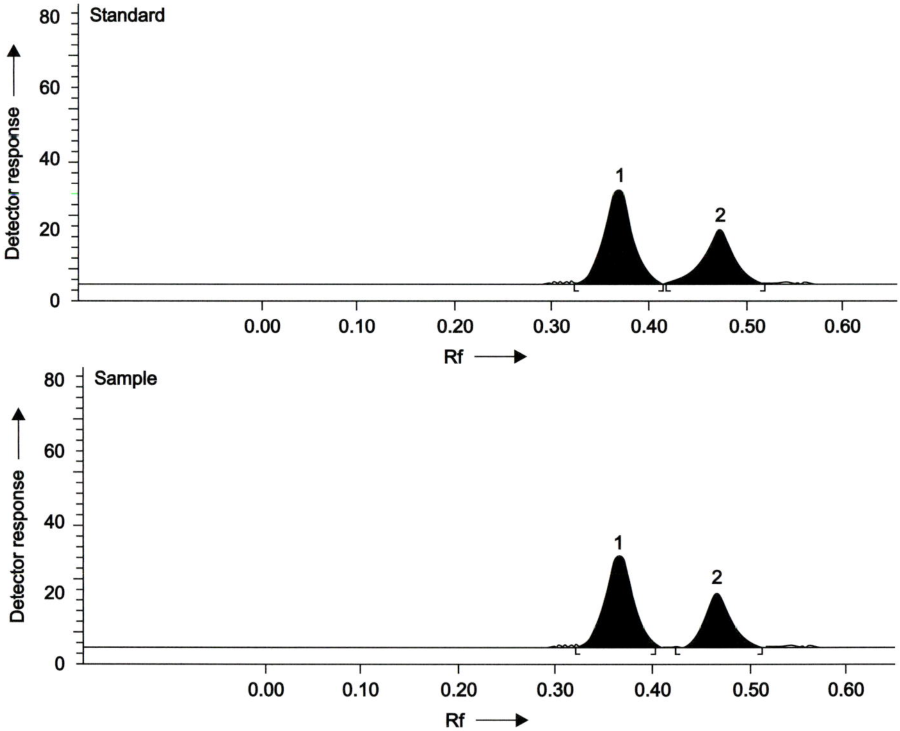

Typical densitogram of the sample and standard containing beclomethasone dipropionate and miconazole nitrate. For detailed experimental and chromatographic conditions, refer to Protocol No. 446. Peaks identification: 1. Miconazole nitrate; 2. Beclomethasone dipropionate.

PROTOCOL FOR HPTLC ANALYSIS OF PHARMACEUTICAL FORMULATION

Protocol No. 446

Formulation: Beclomethasone dipropionate, Miconazole nitrate

Classification: External **Dosage form:** Cream, Ointment

Standard preparation: Prepare 1 mg/ml solution of beclomethasone dipropionate in methanol (1), dilute 1 ml of solution (1) to 10 ml with methanol (2). Accurately weigh about 8 mg of miconazole nitrate, add 1 ml of solution (2) and dilute to 10 ml with methanol.

Sample preparation: Weigh accurately about 1 g of homogenised sample (cream), add methanol, warm slightly, dilute to 25 ml with methanol, chill, filter or decant and use for analysis.

Chromatographic equipments:

Sample applicator: Camag Nanomat–IV

Development chamber: Camag twin-trough glass chamber, 10 × 10 cm

Densitometric scanner: Camag TLC Scanner–II

Chromatographic conditions:

1. Stationary phase: Silica gel $60F_{254}$ pre-coated HPTLC plates, 10 × 10 cm (200 μm) – Merck
2. Mobile phase (MP): Toluene–acetone–25% ammonia (7 : 3 : 0.5 v/v)
3. Standard/Sample application:
   Band length: 5 mm Volume applied: 5 μl Spacing: 5 mm
4. Chamber saturation: 30 min (MP)
5. RH (%): 55 ± 5
6. Temperature °C: 22 ± 2
7. Separation technique: Ascending
8. Quantity of mobile phase: 10.5 ml
9. Migration distance: 50 mm
10. Migration time: 14 min

Densitometric evaluation:

Wavelength: UV–254 nm Scanning mode: Reflectance/Absorbance

HRF: Miconazole nitrate—37; Beclomethasone dipropionate—47

Linearity (ng/band): Miconazole nitrate—100–500; Beclomethasone dipropionate—25–100

Recovery (%): 98.02–100.75 for both the compounds

References: —

Comments:

- The method was optimized and analytical work carried out at **Anchrom's HPTLC Application Laboratory**, Mumbai, India.
- For extraction from cream, store the sample in methanol overnight in refrigerator, then decant and use for application.
- Several market samples of similar composition were analysed by the proposed method with reproducible results.

HPTLC : High Performance Thin Layer Chromatography
HPTLC Densitogram

No. 447

Beclomethasone

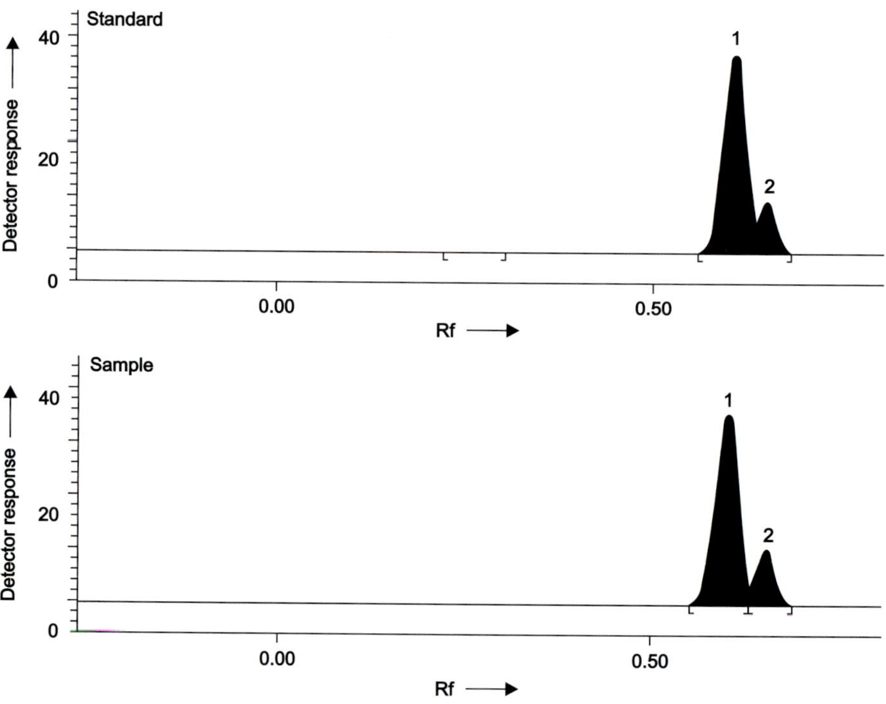

Typical densitogram of the sample and standard containing beclomethasone dipropionate and clotrimazole. For detailed experimental and chromatographic conditions, refer to Protocol No. 447. Peaks identification: 1. Clotrimazole; 2. Beclomethasone dipropionate.

PROTOCOL FOR HPTLC ANALYSIS OF PHARMACEUTICAL FORMULATION

Protocol No. 447

Formulation: Beclomethasone dipropionate, Clotrimazole
Classification: External **Dosage form:** Cream, Ointment
Standard preparation: (1) Prepare 100 μg/ml solution of beclomethasone dipropionate in chloroform. (2) Prepare 1 μg/ml solution of clotrimazole in chloroform. (3) To 2 ml of solution (2), add 0.5 ml of solution (1) and dilute to 10 ml with chloroform.
Sample preparation: Weigh sample accurately equivalent to 5 mg of clotrimazole, add 20 ml of chloroform, vortex for 10 min, dilute to 25 ml, filter and use the filtrate for analysis.
Chromatographic equipments:
Sample applicator: Camag Linomat–IV
Development chamber: Camag twin-trough glass chamber, 10 × 10 cm
Densitometric scanner: Camag TLC Scanner–II
Chromatographic conditions:
1. Stationary phase: Silica gel $60F_{254}$ pre-coated HPTLC plates, 10 × 10 cm (200 μm) – Merck
2. Mobile phase (MP): Toluene–acetone–ammonia (7 : 3 : 0.5 v/v)
3. Standard/Sample application:
   Band length: 10 mm Volume applied: 10 μl Spacing: 10 mm
4. Chamber saturation: 30 min (MP)
5. RH (%): 55 ± 5
6. Temperature °C: 22 ± 2
7. Separation technique: Ascending
8. Quantity of mobile phase: 10.5 ml
9. Migration distance: 50 mm
10. Migration time: 2 × 13 min

Densitometric evaluation:
Wavelength: UV–254 nm Scanning mode: Reflectance/Absorbance
HRF: Clotrimazole—60; Beclomethasone dipropionate—65
Linearity (ng/band): Clotrimazole—100–500; Beclomethasone dipropionate—25–100
Recovery (%): 98.80–100.80 for both the compounds
References: —
Comments:
- The method was optimized and analytical work carried out at **Anchrom's HPTLC Application Laboratory**, Mumbai, India.
- For proper resolution, the plate was developed twice (2 × 13 min) in the same mobile phase with drying after each development.
- Several market samples of similar composition were analysed by the proposed method with reproducible results.

HPTLC : High Performance Thin Layer Chromatography
HPTLC Densitogram

No. 448

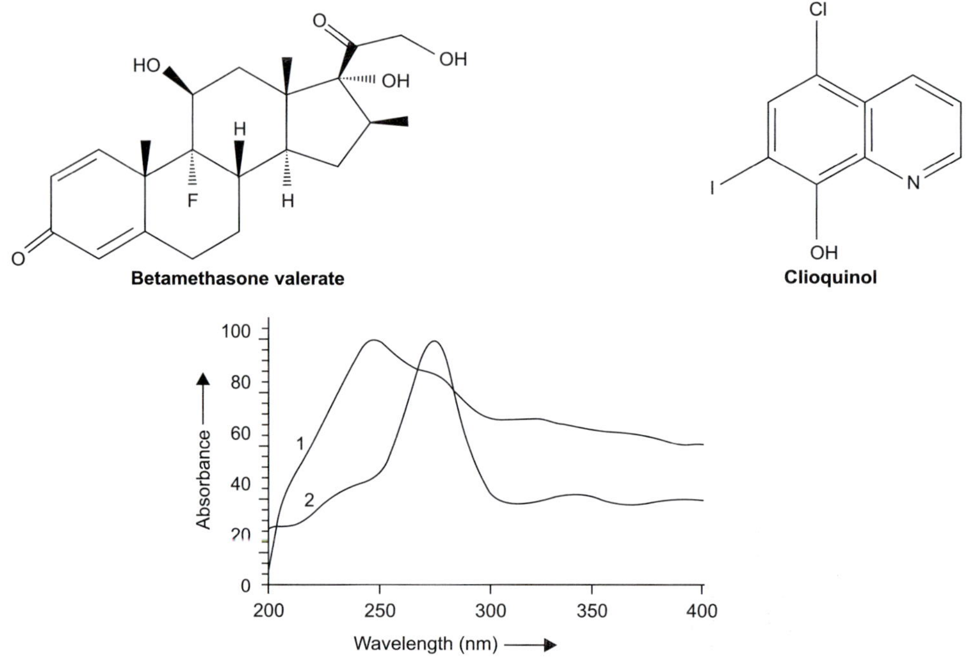

Overlaid UV-spectra of betamethasone valerate (1) and clioquinol (2) for selection of suitable wavelength for densitometric scanning

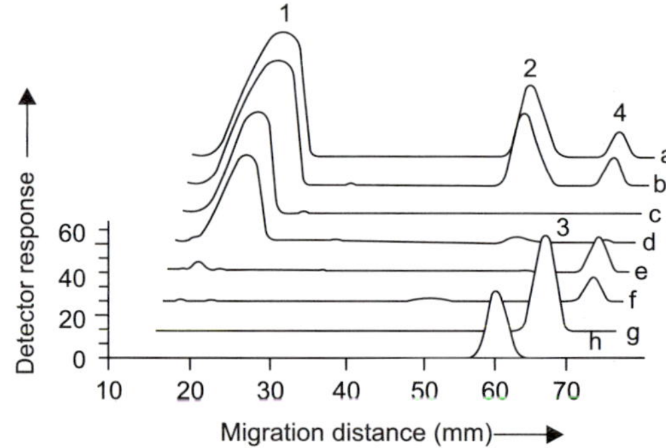

Typical densitogram obtained from: (a) Extract of one year old laboratory-made cream; (b) New laboratory-made cream; (c) and (d) Standard solutions of clioquinol (6 and 4 μg/band), respectively; (e) and (f) Betamethasone valerate (600 and 400 ng/band) respectively; (g) Betamethasone base (2 μg/band); (h) Excipients. For detailed experimental and chromatographic conditions, refer to Protocol No. 448. Peaks identification: 1. Clioquinol; 2. Nipagin and nipasol; 3. Betamethasone base; 4. Betamethasone valerate.

PROTOCOL FOR HPTLC ANALYSIS OF PHARMACEUTICAL FORMULATION

Protocol No. 448

Formulation: Betamethasone valerate, Clioquinol

Classification: External **Dosage form:** Cream

Standard preparation: Prepare solution of both the compounds in acetone to get 10–300 μg/ml (betamethasone valerate) and 300–2500 μg/ml (clioquinol). Apply 4 μl of each solution for linearity profile.

Sample preparation: Accurately weighed quantity of the sample suspended in acetone, sonicated for 10 min, diluted, centrifuged and filtered. The filtrate suitably diluted with acetone and 4 μl applied for assay.

Chromatographic equipments:

Sample applicator: Camag Nanomat–IV

Development chamber: Camag twin-trough glass chamber, 20 × 10 cm

Densitometric scanner: Camag TLC Scanner–II

Chromatographic conditions:

1. Stationary phase: Silica gel $60F_{254}$ pre-coated HPTLC plates, 10 × 10 cm (200 μm) – Merck
2. Mobile phase (MP): Ethyl acetate–n-butanol–25% ammonia (11 : 5 : 4 v/v)
3. Standard/Sample application:
   Band length: 10 mm Volume applied: 4 μl Spacing: 10 mm
4. Chamber saturation: 30 min (MP)
5. RH (%): 55 ± 5
6. Temperature °C: 25 ± 1
7. Separation technique: Ascending
8. Quantity of mobile phase: 20 ml
9. Migration distance: 80 mm
10. Migration time: 30 min

Densitometric evaluation:

Wavelength: UV–247 nm Scanning mode: Reflectance/Absorbance

HRF: Clioquinol—20; Betamethasone (base)—55; Betamethasone valerate—81

Linearity (ng/band): Betamethasone valerate—400–1200; Clioquinol—1200–10000

Recovery (%): 98.02–100.75 for both the compounds

References: G. Indrayanto, et al., *J. Planar Chromatogr.*, **10(3)**, 204–207, 1997.

Comments: The method is stability indicating (acid, base, oxidative, thermal, photolytic). The degradation products were separated from main compounds.

HPTLC : High Performance Thin Layer Chromatography
HPTLC Densitogram

No. 449

Beclomethasone

Salicylic acid

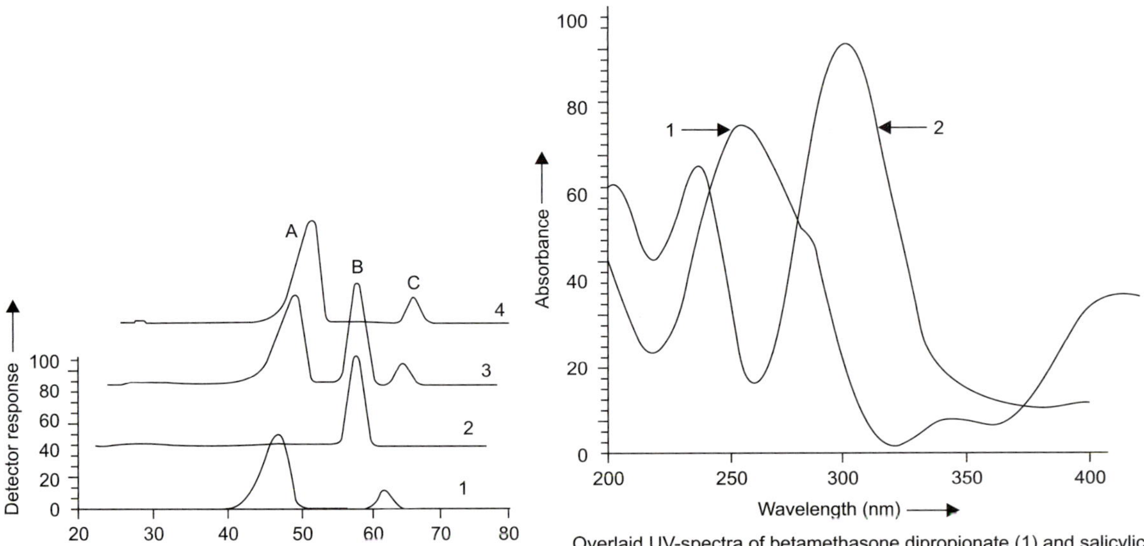

Overlaid UV-spectra of betamethasone dipropionate (1) and salicylic acid (2) for selection of suitable wavelength for densitometric scanning

Typical densitogram obtained from: (1) Solution of standards of betamethasone dipropionate and salicylic acid; (2) Extract of laboratory-made lotion; (3) Extract of excipients of laboratory-made lotion; (4) Extract of commercial lotion. For detailed experimental and chromatographic conditions, refer to Protocol No. 449. Peaks identification: (A) Salicylic acid; (B) Nipagin; (C) Betamethasone.

PROTOCOL FOR HPTLC ANALYSIS OF PHARMACEUTICAL FORMULATION

Protocol No. 449

Formulation: Betamethasone dipropionate, Salicylic acid

Classification: External **Dosage form:** Lotion

Standard preparation: Prepare 30 mg/ml solution of betamethasone dipropionate in methanol. Take 2 ml of this solution, add 400 mg of salicylic acid, dilute to 50 ml with methanol. Prepare solution containing 400–4000 μg/ml of salicylic acid and 65–650 μg/ml of betamethasone. Apply 1 μl for analysis.

Sample preparation: 1 ml of the lotion was diluted to 10 ml with methanol. Apply 1 μl for analysis of salicylic acid and 5 μl for analysis of betamethasone dipropionate.

Chromatographic equipments:

Sample applicator: Camag Nanomat–III

Development chamber: Camag twin-trough glass chamber, 20 × 10 cm

Densitometric scanner: Camag TLC Scanner–II

Chromatographic conditions:

1. Stationary phase: Silica gel $60F_{254}$ pre-coated TLC plates, 10 × 20 cm (200 μm) – Merck
2. Mobile phase (MP): Ethanol–toluene–chloroform–glacial acetic acid (6 : 20 : 14 : 0.5 v/v)
3. Standard/Sample application:
   Band length: 5 mm Volume applied: 1–5 μl Spacing: 10 mm
4. Chamber saturation: 120 min (MP)
5. RH (%): 60 ± 5
6. Temperature °C: 25 ± 2
7. Separation technique: Ascending
8. Quantity of mobile phase: 40 ml
9. Migration distance: 80 mm
10. Migration time: 30 min

Densitometric evaluation:

Wavelength: UV–250 nm (betamethasone); 310 nm (salicylic acid)

Scanning mode: Reflectance/Absorbance

HRF: Salicylic acid—30; Betamethasone dipropionate—52

Linearity (ng/band): Salicylic acid—1600–2400; Betamethasone propionate—260–390

Recovery (%): 98.1–101.3 for both the compounds

References: Listyo Wulandari and G. Indrayanto, *J. Planar Chromatogr.*, **16(6)**, 438–441, 2003.

Comments: The method validated for accuracy, precision, linearity, LOD, LOQ, specificity, robustness and ruggedness.

HPTLC : High Performance Thin Layer Chromatography
HPTLC Densitogram

No. 450

• HCl

Terbinafine hydrochloride

Triamcinolone acetonide

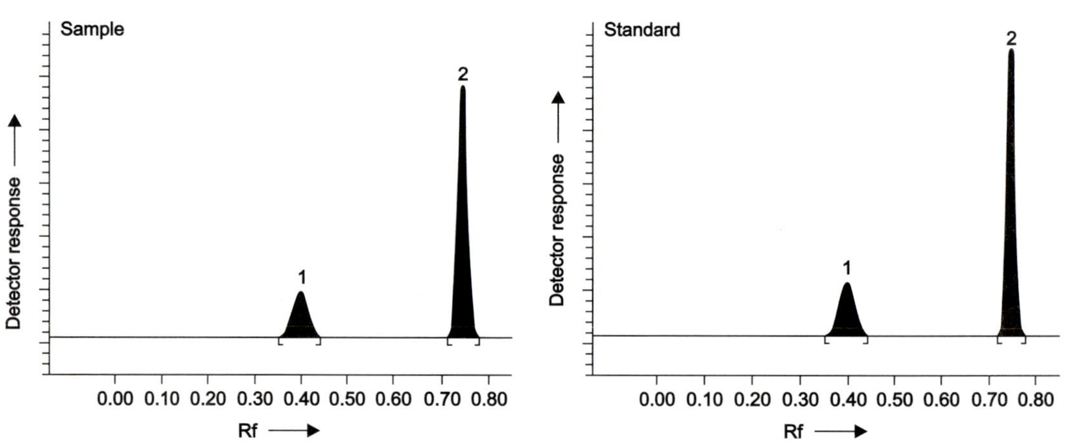

Typical densitogram of the sample and standard containing terbinafine HCl and triamcinolone acetonide. For detailed experimental and chromatographic conditions, refer to Protocol No. 450. Peaks identification: 1. Triamcinolone acetonide; 2. Terbinafine HCl.

PROTOCOL FOR HPTLC ANALYSIS OF PHARMACEUTICAL FORMULATION

Protocol No. 450

Formulation: Triamcinolone acetonide, Terbinafine hydrochloride

Classification: External **Dosage form:** Cream

Standard preparation: Prepare 1 mg/ml solution of each compound in methanol. Further serial dilutions are made for chromatographic application and linearity studies.

Sample preparation: Extract the sample with methanol, store in refrigerator overnight. Decant and dilute to get the concentration within linearity range. Apply 10 μl for analysis.

Chromatographic equipments:

Sample applicator: Hamilton microsyringe, 25 μl, calibrated at 0.2 μl per unit

Development chamber: Camag twin-trough glass chamber, 10 × 10 cm

Densitometric scanner: Shimadzu CS–9000 densitometer

Chromatographic conditions:

1. Stationary phase: Silica gel $60F_{254}$ pre-coated TLC plates, 10 × 10 cm (250 μm) – Merck
2. Mobile phase (MP): Ether–dichloromethane–methanol (5 : 19.5 : 0.5 v/v)
3. Standard/Sample application:
   Band length: 10 mm Volume applied: 10 μl Spacing: 10 mm
4. Chamber saturation: 30 min (MP)
5. RH (%): 55 ± 2
6. Temperature °C: 22 ± 2
7. Separation technique: Ascending
8. Quantity of mobile phase: 25 ml
9. Migration distance: 15 mm
10. Migration time: 40 min

Densitometric evaluation:

Wavelength: 238 nm (TA); 283 nm (TH) Scanning mode: Reflectance/Absorbance

HRF: Triamcinolone acetonide—40; Terbinafine HCl—75

Linearity (ng/band): Terbinafine HCl—5–25; Triamcinolone acetonide—2.5–22.5

Recovery (%): 99.93–100.32 for both the compounds

References: Yasser S. El-Saharty, Nagiba Y. Hassan and Fadia H. Metwally, *J. Pharm. Biomed. Anal.*, 2001.

Comments:

- The method validated for accuracy, precision, linearity, LOD, LOQ, specificity, robustness and ruggedness.
- The HPTLC method was comparable with UV-derivative spectrophotometric method.

HPTLC : High Performance Thin Layer Chromatography
HPTLC Densitogram

No. 451

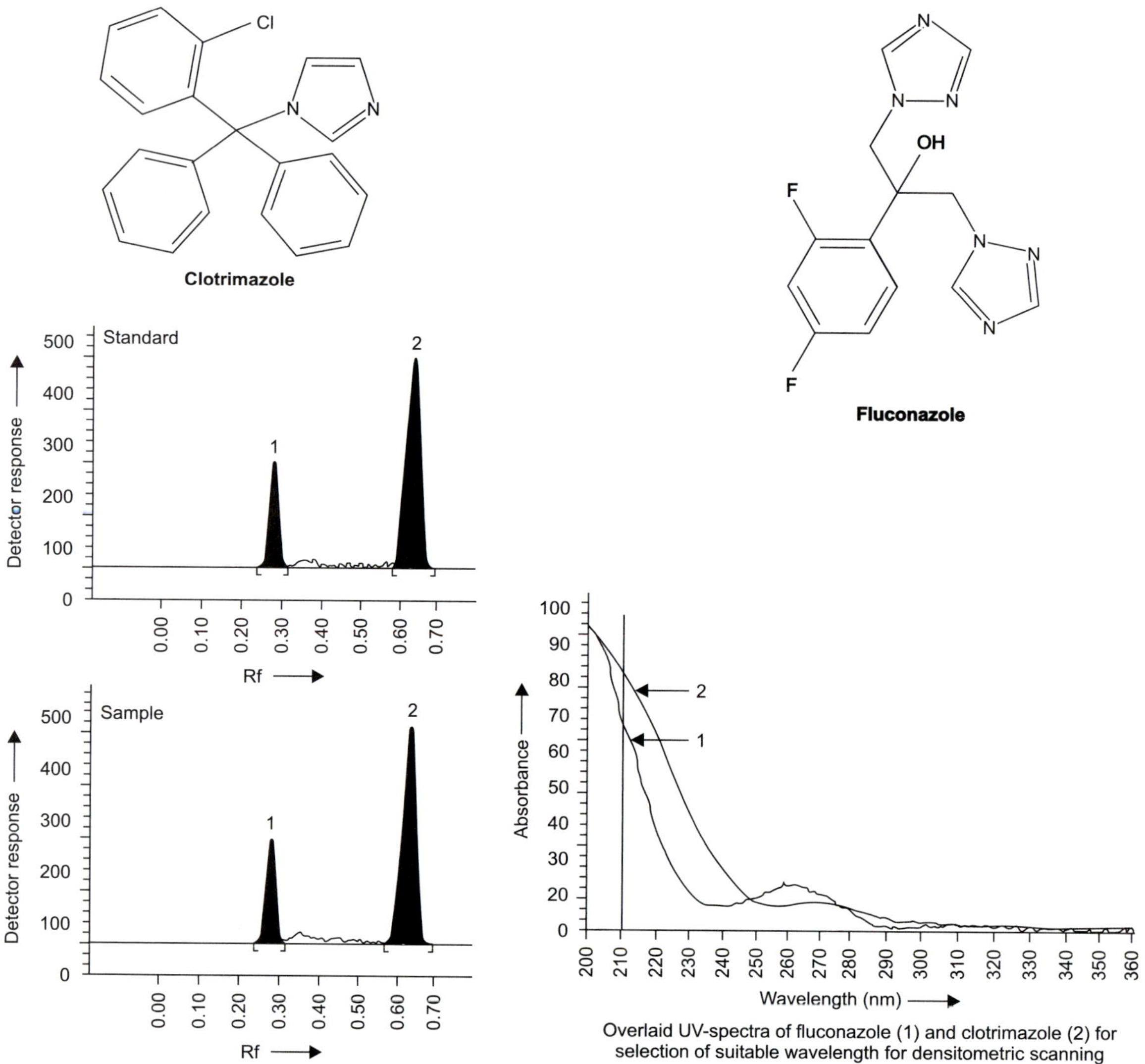

Overlaid UV-spectra of fluconazole (1) and clotrimazole (2) for selection of suitable wavelength for densitometric scanning

Typical densitogram of the sample and standard containing fluconazole and clotrimazole. For detailed experimental and chromatographic conditions, refer to Protocol No. 451. Peaks identification: 1. Fluconazole; 2. Clotrimazole.

PROTOCOL FOR HPTLC ANALYSIS OF PHARMACEUTICAL FORMULATION

Protocol No. 451

Formulation: Fluconazole, Clotrimazole

Classification: External **Dosage form:** Cream, Tablets

Standard preparation: Prepare 1 mg/ml solution of each compound in methanol. Further serial dilutions made to cover linearity range. Apply 5 μl of each solution for chromatographic separation.

Sample preparation: Powdered sample equivalent to 25 mg of fluconazole suspended in methanol, sonicated, diluted to 25 ml. Filtered and the filtrate suitably diluted. Apply 5 μl for assay.

Chromatographic equipments:

Sample applicator: Camag Linomat–V

Development chamber: Camag twin-trough glass chamber, 10 × 10 cm

Densitometric scanner: Camag TLC Scanner–III

Chromatographic conditions:

1. Stationary phase: Silica gel 60F_{254} pre-coated TLC plates, 10 × 10 cm (250 μm) – Merck
2. Mobile phase (MP): Toluene–chloroform–methanol (1.2 : 3.0 : 0.4 v/v)
3. Standard/Sample application:
   Band length: 4 mm Volume applied: 5 μl Spacing: 4 mm
4. Chamber saturation: 15 min (MP)
5. RH (%): 60 ± 5
6. Temperature °C: 20 ± 2
7. Separation technique: Ascending
8. Quantity of mobile phase: 15 ml
9. Migration distance: 70 mm
10. Migration time: 18 min

Densitometric evaluation:

Wavelength: UV–210 nm Scanning mode: Reflectance/Absorbance

HRF: Fluconazole—28; Clotrimazole—62

Linearity (ng/band): 600–1600 for both the compounds

Recovery (%): 98.30–100.72 for both the compounds

References: Dhananjay B. Meshram, Shashikant B. Bagade and Madhukar R. Tajne, *J. Planar Chromatogr.*, **21(3)**, 191–196, 2008.

Comments: The method validated for accuracy, precision, linearity, LOD, LOQ, specificity, robustness and ruggedness.

HPTLC : High Performance Thin Layer Chromatography
HPTLC Densitogram

No. 452

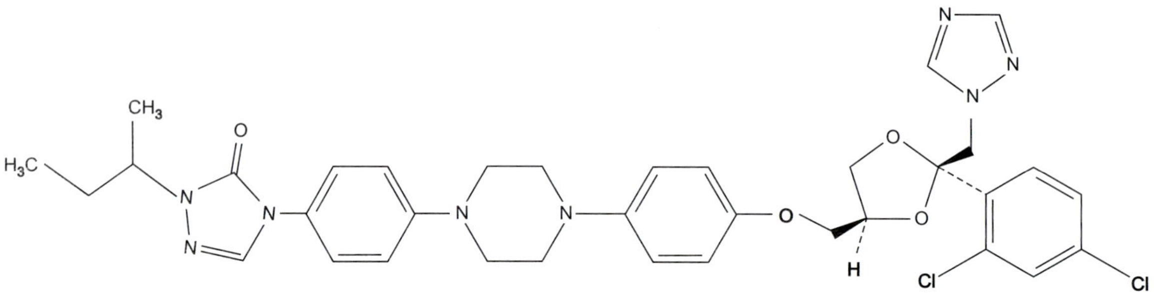

Itraconazole

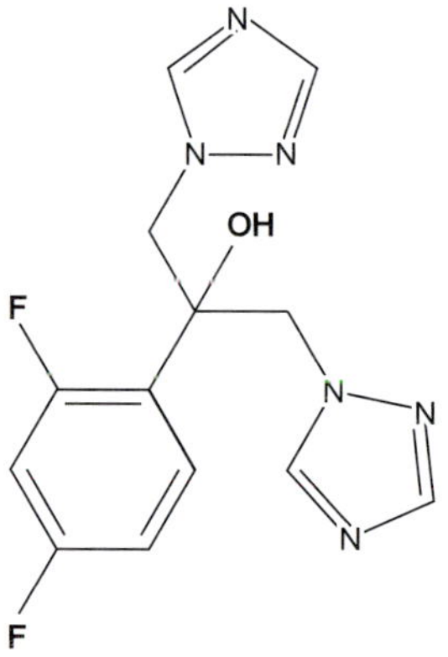

Fluconazole

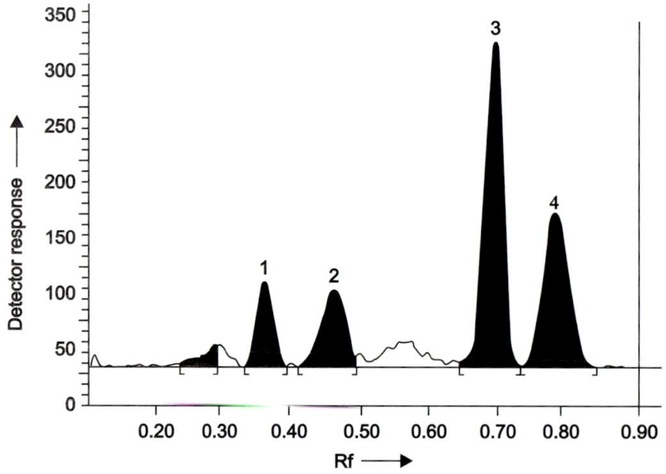

Typical densitogram for the mixture containing all the investigated compounds. For details experimental and chromatographic conditions, refer to Protocol No. 452. Peaks identification: 1. Ketoconazole; 2. Fluconazole; 3. Bifonazole; 4. Itraconazole.

PROTOCOL FOR HPTLC ANALYSIS OF PHARMACEUTICAL FORMULATION

Protocol No. 452

Formulation: **Fluconazole, Ketoconazole, Bifonazole, Itraconazole**

Classification: External **Dosage form:** Tablets

Standard preparation: Solutions of ketoconazole, bifonazole and fluconazole (1 mg/ml) were prepared in methanol. For itraconazole, the substance was first suspended in chloroform and then diluted with methanol to get final ratio of solvents (3 : 1).

Sample preparation: The powdered sample suspended in solvent, shaken for 30 min, diluted and filtered. The filtrate suitably diluted with the solvent for chromatographic analysis.

Solvent: Methanol–chloroform (3 : 1 v/v).

Chromatographic equipments:

Sample applicator: Camag Linomat–V

Development chamber: Sigma-Aldrich chromatographic chamber, 18 × 9 × 18 cm

Densitometric scanner: Camag TLC Scanner–III

Chromatographic conditions:

1. Stationary phase: Kieselgel 60F_{254} pre-coated TLC plates, 10 × 10 cm (250 μm) – Merck
2. Mobile phase (MP): n-hexane–ethyl acetate–methanol–water–glacial acetic acid (42 : 40 : 15 : 2 : 1 v/v)
3. Standard/Sample application:
   Band length: 8 mm Volume applied: 3–30 μl Spacing: 10 mm
4. Chamber saturation: 20 min (MP)
5. RH (%): 60 ± 5
6. Temperature °C: 22 ± 2
7. Separation technique: Ascending
8. Quantity of mobile phase: 20 ml
9. Migration distance: 60 mm
10. Migration time: 28 min

Densitometric evaluation:

Wavelength: UV–260 nm (B), 280 nm (F) and 230 nm (I & K)

Scanning mode: Reflectance/Absorbance

HRF: Ketoconazole (K)—35; Fluconazole (F)—45; Bifonazole (B)—70; Itraconazole (I)—79

Linearity: 100–1000 ng/band for all the four compounds

Recovery (%): 99.0–102.40 for all the compounds

References: Rodostaw J. Ekiert, Jan Krzek and Wtodzimier Rzeszu, *Chromatographia*, **67(11, 12)**, 995–997, 2008.

Comments: The method validated for accuracy, precision, linearity, LOD, LOQ, specificity, robustness and ruggedness.

HPTLC : High Performance Thin Layer Chromatography
HPTLC Densitogram

No. 453

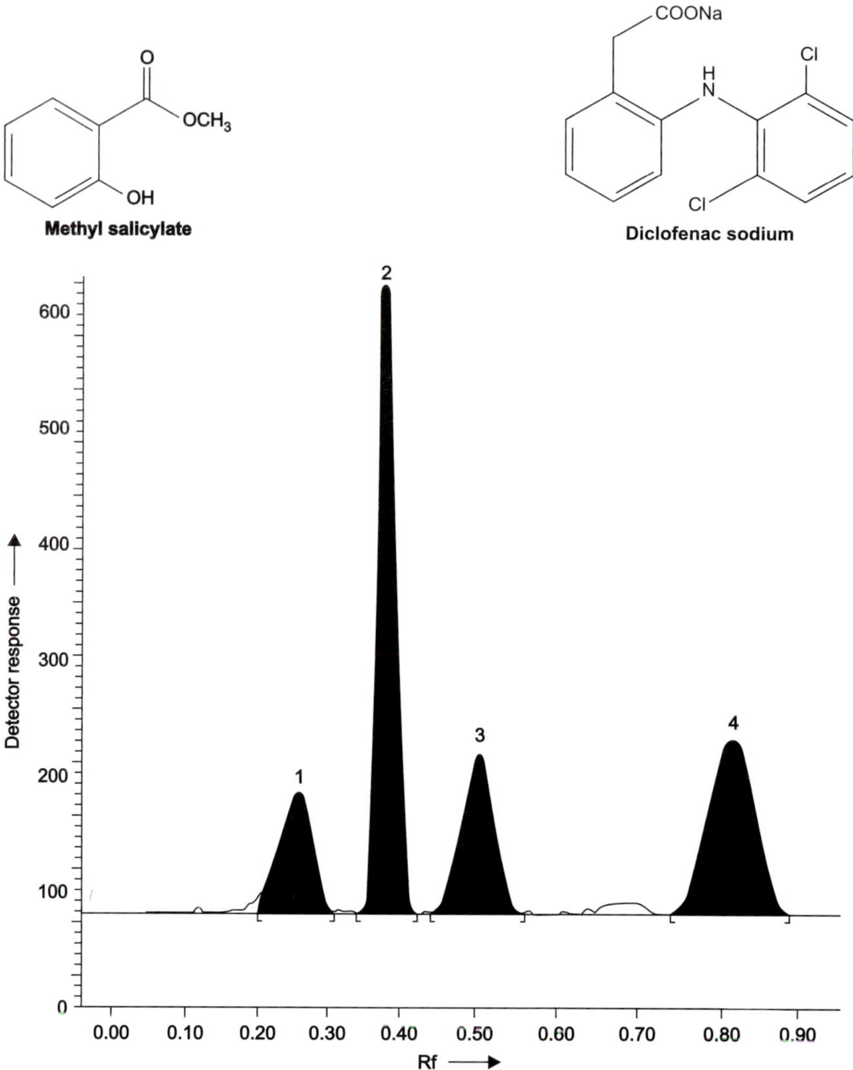

Typical densitogram of the sample containing diclofenac, salicylic acid and methyl salicylate. For detailed experimental and chromatographic conditions, refer to Protocol No. 453. Peaks identification: 1. Salicylic acid; 2. Diclofenac Na^+; 3. Unknown; 4. Methyl salicylate.

PROTOCOL FOR HPTLC ANALYSIS OF PHARMACEUTICAL FORMULATION

Protocol No. 453

Formulation: Diclofenac sodium, Salicylic acid, Methyl salicylate

Classification: External **Dosage form:** Gel

Standard preparation: Prepare 20 mg/ml solution of diclofenac sodium in methanol. Apply 10–30 μl of the solution for linearity profile.

Sample preparation: Weighed amount of gel was suspended in methanol, warmed, diluted, cooled and decanted. Clear solution suitably diluted. Apply 20 μl for assay.

Chromatographic equipments:

Sample applicator: Camag Linomat–IV

Development chamber: Camag twin-trough glass chamber, 10 × 10 cm

Densitometric scanner: Camag TLC Scanner–III

Chromatographic conditions:

1. Stationary phase: Silica gel $60F_{254}$ pre-coated HPTLC plates, 10 × 10 cm (200 μm) – Merck, pre-washed with methanol, dried at 60°C for 5 min prior to use
2. Mobile phase (MP): Toluene–ethyl acetate–glacial acetic acid (6 : 4 : 0.02 v/v)
3. Standard/Sample application:
   Band length: 5 mm Volume applied: 10 μl Spacing: 5 mm
4. Chamber saturation: 60 min (MP)
5. RH (%): 55 ± 5
6. Temperature °C: 22 ± 2
7. Separation technique: Ascending
8. Quantity of mobile phase: 10 ml
9. Migration distance: 70 mm
10. Migration time: 20 min

Densitometric evaluation:

Wavelength: UV–238 nm Scanning mode: Reflectance/Absorbance

HRF: Salicylic acid—29; Diclofenac Na^+—39; Methyl salicylate—81

Linearity (ng/band): Diclofenac Na^+—200–600

Recovery (%): 99.45–100.36 for diclofenac sodium

References: H.J. Panchal, I.S. Rathod and S.A. Shah, *Indian Drugs*, **45(4)**, 301–306, 2008.

Comments:

- The method validated for accuracy, precision, linearity, LOD, LOQ, specificity, robustness and ruggedness.
- The method is suitable for determination of diclofenac sodium; and for identification of other compounds often present in formulation.

HPTLC : High Performance Thin Layer Chromatography
HPTLC Densitogram

No. 454

Phenylephrine hydrochloride • HCl

Lignocaine hydrochloride • HCl

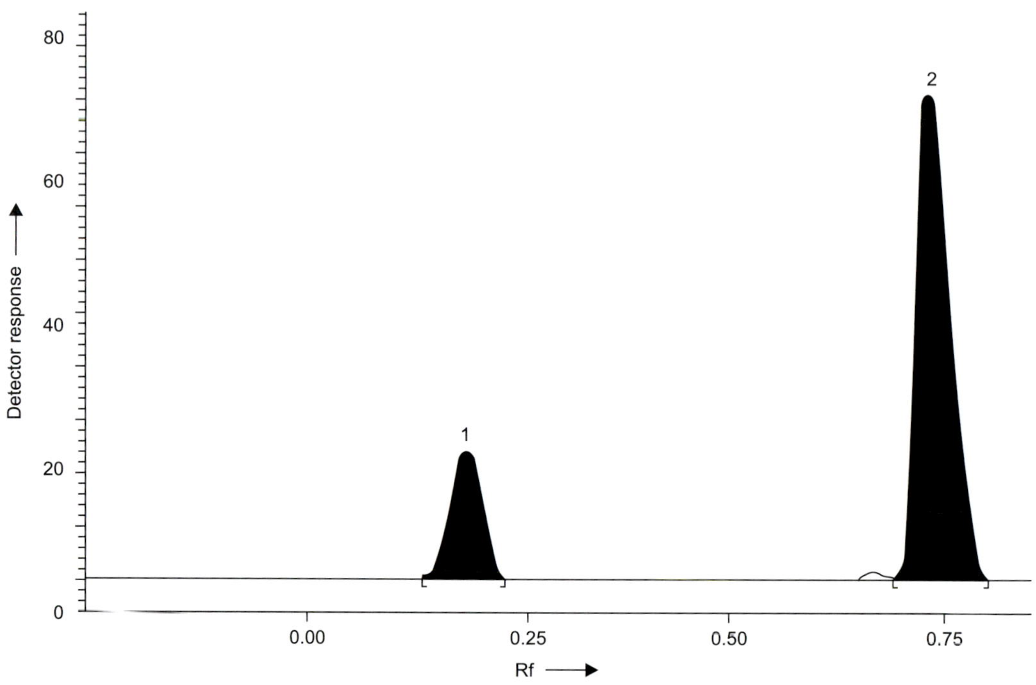

Typical densitogram of the sample containing phenylephrine hydrochloride and lignocaine hydrochloride. For detailed experimental and chromatographic conditions, refer to Protocol No. 454. Peaks identification: 1. Phenylephrine hydrochloride; 2. Lignocaine hydrochloride.

PROTOCOL FOR HPTLC ANALYSIS OF PHARMACEUTICAL FORMULATION

Protocol No. 454

Formulation: Phenylephrine hydrochloride, Lignocaine hydrochloride
Classification: External
Dosage form: Drug delivery system for local anaesthesia
Standard preparation: Prepare 1 mg/ml solution of lignocaine hydrochloride and 0.5 mg/ml solution of phenylephrine hydrochloride, both in water. Apply appropriate quantity of each solution to establish linearity range.
Sample preparation: The sample solution was prepared in water. Apply sufficient volume of the sample containing 14 μg of lignocaine HCl and 7 μg of phenylephrine for assay. Also see comments below.
Chromatographic equipments:
Sample applicator: Camag Linomat–IV
Development chamber: Normal flat bottom glass chamber, 20 × 20 cm
Densitometric scanner: Camag TLC Scanner–II
Chromatographic conditions:
1. Stationary phase: Silica gel $60F_{254}$ pre-coated HPTLC plates, 10 × 10 cm (200 μm) – Merck
2. Mobile phase (MP): Ethyl acetate–methanol–25% ammonia (8 : 2 : 0.8 v/v)
3. Standard/Sample application:
   Band length: 5 mm   Volume applied: —   Spacing: 5 mm
4. Chamber saturation: 30 min (MP)
5. RH (%): 55 ± 5
6. Temperature °C: 22 ± 2
7. Separation technique: Ascending
8. Quantity of mobile phase: 20 ml
9. Migration distance: 80 mm
10. Migration time: 20 min

Densitometric evaluation:
Wavelength: UV–262 nm (LIG) and 291 nm (PHE)
Scanning mode: Reflectance/Absorbance
HRF: Phenylephrine HCl—23; Lignocaine hydrochloride—75
Linearity (μg/band): Lignocaine HCl (LIG)—8–18; Phenylephrine HCl (PHE)—4–9
Recovery (%): 98.99–100.43 for both the compounds
References: Padma V. Devarajan, Manisha H. Adani, Anilkumar S. Gandhi, *J. Pharm. Biomed. Anal.*, **22**, 685–690, 2000.
Comments:
- The method validated for accuracy, precision, linearity, LOD, LOQ, specificity, robustness and ruggedness.
- Based on the concentration of LIG and PHE present in the formulation, two separate aliquots of the sample were spotted i.e. 3 μl (LIG) and 50 μl (PHE) to keep the drugs' concentration within linearity range.

HPTLC : High Performance Thin Layer Chromatography
HPTLC Densitogram

No. 455

H_3C CH_3 CH_3 CH_3 CH_3 COOH

Isotretinoin

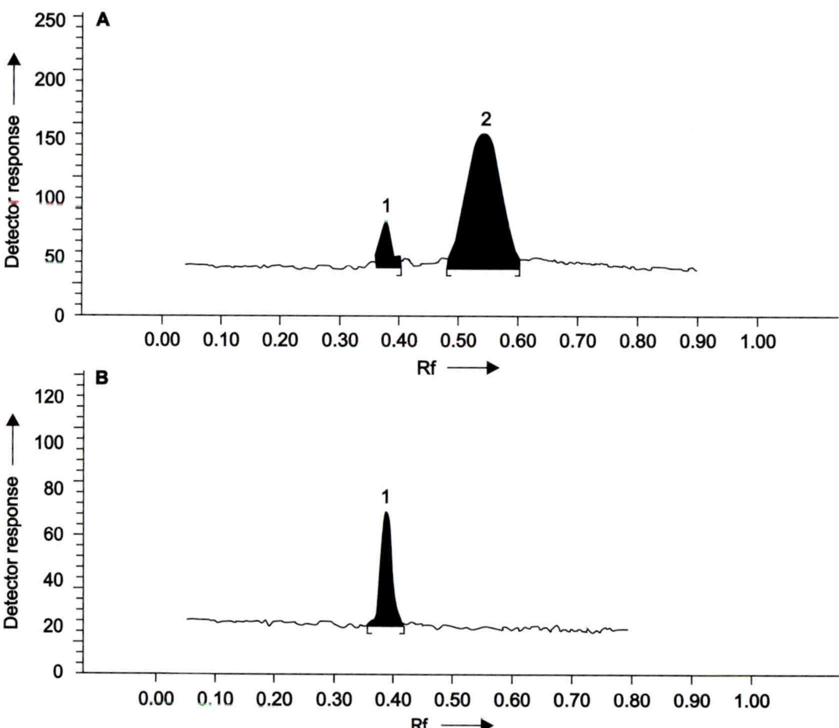

Typical densitogram of the sample containing isotretinoin and erythromycin. For detailed experimental and chromatographic conditions, refer to Protocol No. 455. Peaks identification: 1. Isotretinoin; 2. Erythromycin.

A. Densitogram of erythromycin scanned at 410 nm after derivatization.

B. Densitogram of isotretinoin scanned at 340 nm prior to derivatization.

PROTOCOL FOR HPTLC ANALYSIS OF PHARMACEUTICAL FORMULATION

Protocol No. 455

Formulation: Isotretinoin, Erythromycin

Classification: External **Dosage form:** Gel

Standard preparation: Prepare solution of both the drugs in methanol to get 150 μg/ml of isotretinoin and 6000 μg/ml of erythromycin. Further dilutions made with methanol to get 15 μg/ml of isotretinoin and 600 μg/ml of erythromycin. Apply 2–10 μl of each solution for linearity profile.

Sample preparation: Weigh the sample equivalent to 0.5 mg of isotretinoin and 20 mg of erythromycin, suspend in 8 ml of methanol, sonicate for 30 min, dilute to 10 ml, filter through 0.45 μm nylon filter and apply 2 μl of the resulting solution for assay.

Chromatographic equipments:

Sample applicator: Camag Linomat–IV
Development chamber: Camag flat solution glass chamber, 20 × 10 cm
Densitometric scanner: Camag TLC Scanner–III

Chromatographic conditions:

1. Stationary phase: Silica gel $60F_{254}$ pre-coated TLC plates, 20 × 10 cm (250 μm) – Merck, pre-washed with methanol, activated at 110°C for 5 min prior to use
2. Mobile phase (MP): Toluene–DMSO–methanol (6.5 : 0.2 : 2.5 v/v)
3. Standard/Sample application:
   Band length: 6 mm Volume applied: 2–10 μl Spacing: 6 mm
4. Chamber saturation: 30 min (MP)
5. RH (%): 60 ± 5
6. Temperature °C: 25 ± 2
7. Separation technique: Ascending
8. Quantity of mobile phase: 18 ml
9. Migration distance: 80 mm
10. Migration time: 45 min

Densitometric evaluation:

Wavelength: 340 nm (isotretinoin), 410 nm (erythromycin)
Scanning mode: Reflectance/Absorbance
HRF: Isotretinoin—38; Erythromycin—55
Linearity (ng/band): Isotretinoin—30–150; Erythromycin—1200–6000
Recovery (%): Isotretinoin—98.26–99.72; Erythromycin—98.07–101.55

References: Atul S. Rathor, L. Sathiyanarayanan and K.R. Mahadik, *Am. J. Anal. Chem.*, **1**, 144–149, 2010.

Comments:

- The method validated for accuracy, precision, linearity, LOD, LOQ, specificity, robustness and ruggedness.
- After scanning the plate at 340 nm for isotretinoin, the plate was treated with 10% H_2SO_4 in methanol, heated at 100°C for 15 min, and then scanned at 410 nm for erythromycin.

HPTLC : High Performance Thin Layer Chromatography
HPTLC Densitogram

No. 456

Brimonidine tartrate **Timolol maleate**

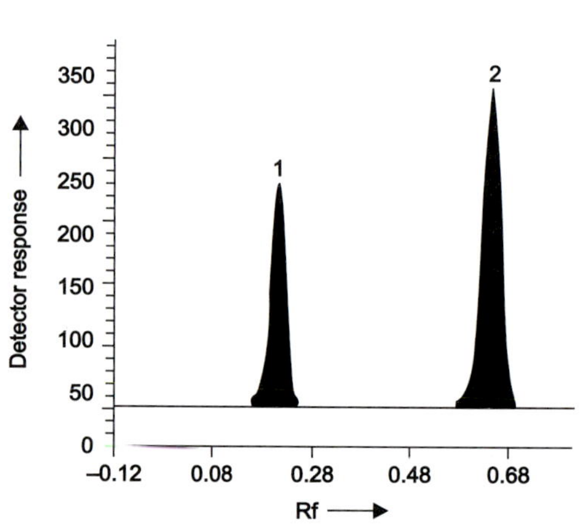

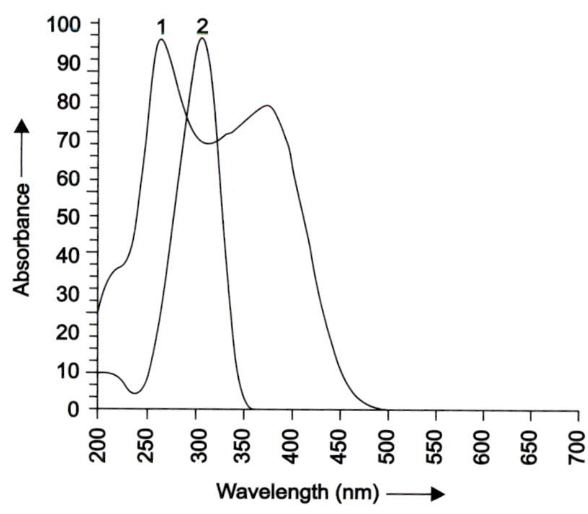

Overlaid UV-spectra of brimonidine tartrate (1) and timolol maleate (2) for selection of suitable wavelength for densitometric scanning

Typical densitogram of the standard containing brimonidine tartrate and timolol maleate. For detailed experimental and chromatographic conditions, refer to Protocol No. 456. Peaks identification: 1. Brimonidine tartrate; 2. Timolol maleate.

PROTOCOL FOR HPTLC ANALYSIS OF PHARMACEUTICAL FORMULATION

Protocol No. 456

Formulation: Brimonidine tartrate, Timolol maleate

Classification: External **Dosage form:** Eye drops

Standard preparation: Prepare 1 mg/ml solution of each compound in methanol. Further dilute 3 ml of brimonidine tartrate to 10 ml and use both the solutions for linearity profile by applying 1–5 μl of each solution.

Sample preparation: Eye drops are suitably diluted to get 300 μg/ml of BT and 1000 μg/ml of TM. Apply 3 μl for chromatographic separation and analysis.

Chromatographic equipments:

Sample applicator: Camag Linomat–V

Development chamber: Camag twin-trough glass chamber, 20 × 10 cm

Densitometric scanner: Camag TLC Scanner–III

Chromatographic conditions:

1. Stationary phase: Silica gel RP–18F_{254s} pre-coated HPTLC plate, 20 × 10 cm (200 μm) – Merck
2. Mobile phase (MP): Methanol–water–triethylamine (2 : 2 : 0.2 v/v)
3. Standard/Sample application:
   Band length: 6 mm Volume applied: 1–5 μl Spacing: 15 mm
4. Chamber saturation: 20 min (MP)
5. RH (%): 60 ± 5
6. Temperature °C: 25 ± 2
7. Separation technique: Ascending
8. Quantity of mobile phase: 23 ml
9. Migration distance: 80 mm
10. Migration time: 18 min

Densitometric evaluation:

Wavelength: UV–264 nm

Scanning mode: Reflectance/Absorbance

HRF: Brimonidine tartrate—23; Timolol maleate—63

Linearity (ng/band): Brimonidine tartrate—300–1800; Timolol maleate—1000–6000

Recovery (%): Brimonidine tartrate—99.24–100.18; Timolol maleate—99.11–99.87

References: Pritam S. Jain, Rahul N. Khatal, Hardik N. Jivani and Sanjay J. Surana, *J. Chromatographic Separation Techniques*, **2(3)**, 1–5, 2011.

Comments: The method validated for accuracy, precision, linearity, LOD, LOQ, specificity, robustness and ruggedness.

HPTLC : High Performance Thin Layer Chromatography
HPTLC Densitogram

No. 457

Ketorolac tromethamine

Ofloxacin

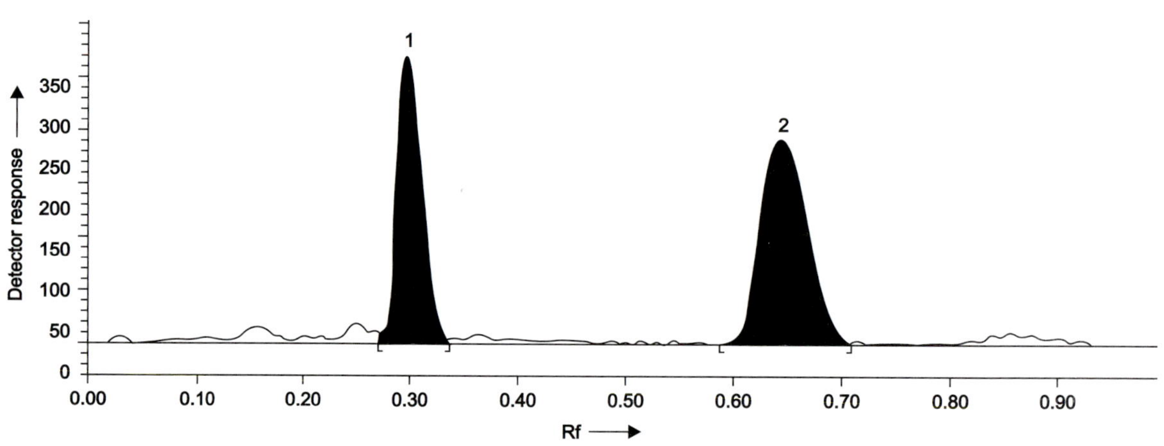

Typical densitogram of the standard containing ofloxacin and ketorolac. For detailed experimental and chromatographic conditions, refer to Protocol No. 457. Peaks identification: 1. Ofloxacin; 2. Ketorolac.

PROTOCOL FOR HPTLC ANALYSIS OF PHARMACEUTICAL FORMULATION

Protocol No. 457

Formulation: Ofloxacin, Ketorolac tromethamine

Classification: External **Dosage form:** Eye drops

Standard preparation: Prepare 100 μg/ml solution of both the compounds separately in methanol. Further serial dilutions made for linearity profile.

Sample preparation: Eye drops containing 3 mg/ml of ofloxacin and 5 mg/ml of ketorolac were suitably diluted with methanol to get 30 μg/ml of ofloxacin and 50 μg/ml of ketorolac and the solution used for analysis.

Chromatographic equipments:

Sample applicator: Camag Linomat–V

Development chamber: Camag twin-trough glass chamber, 20 × 20 cm

Densitometric scanner: Camag TLC Scanner–III

Chromatographic conditions:

1. Stationary phase: Silica gel $60F_{254}$ pre-coated HPTLC plates, 20 × 20 cm (200 μm) – Merck
2. Mobile phase (MP): n-butanol–ethanol–25% ammonia (6 : 1 : 3 v/v)
3. Standard/Sample application:
   Band length: — Volume applied: 10 μl Spacing: —
4. Chamber saturation: —
5. RH (%): 55 ± 5
6. Temperature °C: Ambient
7. Separation technique: Ascending
8. Quantity of mobile phase: 20 ml
9. Migration distance: —
10. Migration time: —

Densitometric evaluation:

Wavelength: UV–310 nm Scanning mode: Reflectance/Absorbance

HRF: Ofloxacin—30; Ketorolac—65

Linearity (ng/band): Ofloxacin—30–150; Ketorolac—50–250

Recovery (%): 99.01–101.69 for both the compounds

References: Sejal P. Gandhi, Mohit G. Dewani, Tejas C. Borole and Mrinalini C. Damle, *J. Advanced Scientific Res.*, **2(3)**, 77–82, 2011.

Comments:

- The method validated for accuracy, precision, linearity, LOD, LOQ, specificity and robustness.
- The method is stability indicating (acid, base, hydrolytic, oxidative, thermolytic and photolytic).
- The compound degraded under all stress conditions except photolytic.
- For analysis of ophthalmic preparations containing ketorolac tromethamine with moxifloxacin, authors have suggested the use of chloroform–methanol–formic acid (8.5 : 1.5 : 0.05 v/v) as MP and detection at 305 nm (R.S. Kakde et al., Abstract No. F-294, 63rd IPC, 2011).

HPTLC : High Performance Thin Layer Chromatography
HPTLC Densitogram

No. 458

Capsaicin

Standard

Sample

UV-spectra of capsaicin showing different maxima (210 nm, 280 nm) used for densitometric scanning

Typical densitogram of the sample and standard containing capsaicin. For detailed experimental and chromatographic conditions, refer to Protocol No. 458. Peaks Identification: 5. Capsaicin.

PROTOCOL FOR HPTLC ANALYSIS OF PHARMACEUTICAL FORMULATION

Protocol No. 458

Formulation: Capsaicin in oleoresin

Classification: External **Dosage form:** Cream, Ointment

Standard preparation: Prepare 2 mg/ml solution of capsaicin in methanol or ethyl acetate. Further dilutions made suitably for application on plate.

Sample preparation: Weigh sample equivalent to 20 mg of capsaicin, suspend in 5–7 ml methanol, sonicate for 5 min and dilute to 20 ml with methanol. Filter and use the filtrate for chromatographic analysis.

Chromatographic equipments:

Sample applicator: Camag Linomat–IV
Development chamber: Camag twin-trough glass chamber, 10 × 10 cm
Densitometric scanner: Camag TLC Scanner–II

Chromatographic conditions:

1. Stationary phase: Silica gel $60F_{254}$ pre-coated HPTLC plates, 10 × 10 cm (200 μm) – Merck
2. Mobile phase (MP): Toluene–acetone–chloroform (4 : 3.5 : 2.5 v/v) or toluene–methanol (9 : 1 v/v)
3. Standard/Sample application:
   Band length: 5 mm Volume applied: 2 μl Spacing: 5 mm
4. Chamber saturation: 15 min (MP)
5. RH (%): 55 ± 5
6. Temperature °C: 22 ± 2
7. Separation technique: Ascending
8. Quantity of mobile phase: 10 ml
9. Migration distance: 15 mm
10. Migration time: 14 min

Densitometric evaluation:

Wavelength: UV–210 nm; 280 nm or 590 nm
Scanning mode: Reflectance/Absorbance
HRF: Capsaicin—65
Linearity (μg/band): Capsaicin—2–8
Recovery (%): 100.25–101.75 for both the compounds

References: A. Aezel, *J. Planar Chromatogr.*, **2**, 151, 1989.

Comments:

1. This method is described for estimation of capsaicin in oleoresin. Usually content of capsaicin is 20–25%. In pharmaceutical preparations (creams and ointments), the sample can be extracted with ethyl acetate, the extract evaporated to dryness in CO_2 atmosphere with the help of rotary evaporator. Residue is taken up in ethyl acetate to get 2 mg/ml in respect of capsaicin.
2. The chromatogram can be sprayed with Gibbs reagent (1% solution of 2,6-dichloroquinone-4-chloromide in methanol and scanned at 590 nm.

HPTLC : High Performance Thin Layer Chromatography
HPTLC Densitogram

No. 459

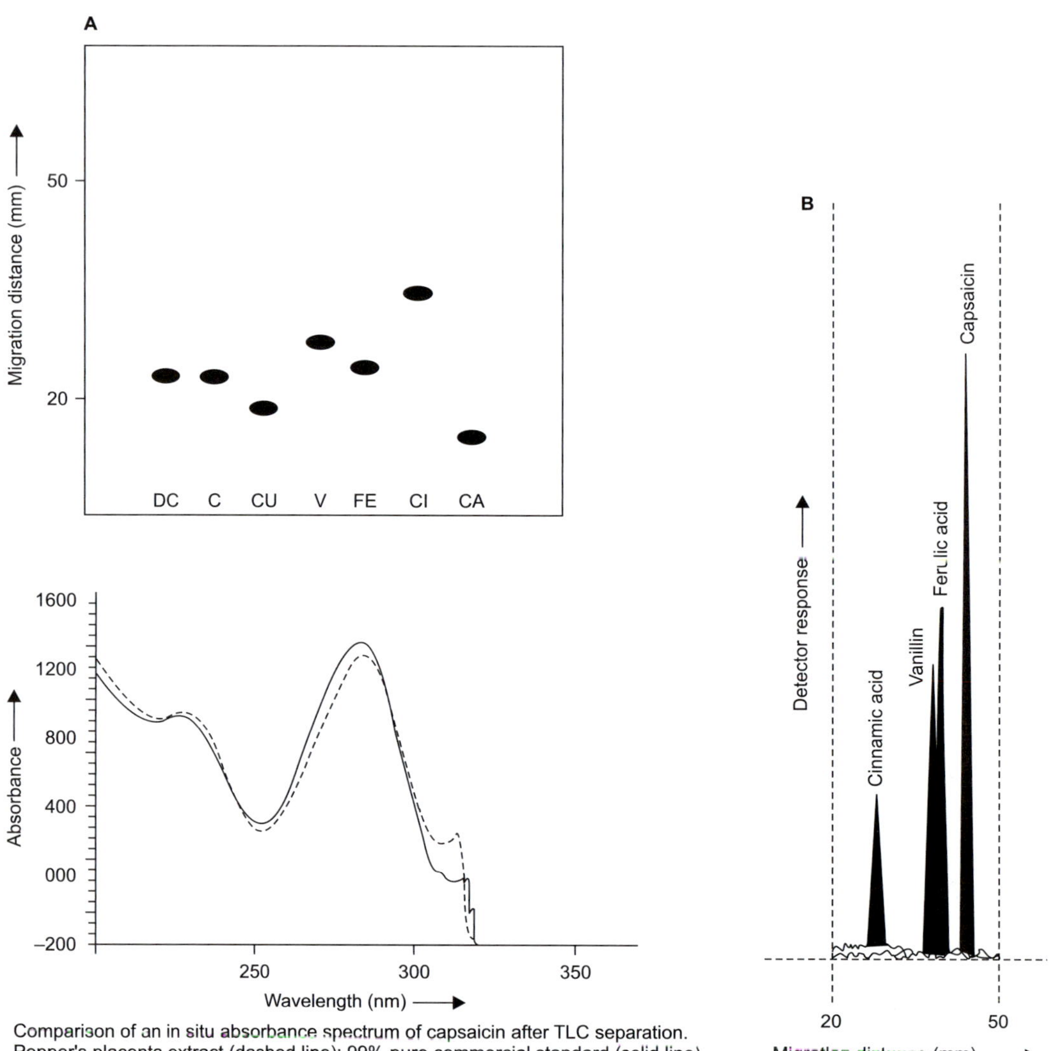

Comparison of an in situ absorbance spectrum of capsaicin after TLC separation. Pepper's placenta extract (dashed line); 99% pure commercial standard (solid line).

Chromatographic separation of capsaicinoids from their biosynthetic intermediaries. (A) Chromatogram visualized under UV light (254 nm). DC, dihydrocapsaicin; C. capsaicin; Cu, coumaric acid; V. vanillin, FE, ferulic acid, CA, cinnamic acid. Mobile phase; cyclohexane–chloroform–acetic acid (70 : 20 : 10). (B) Densitometric estimation of the chromatographic spots. For detailed experimental and chromatographic conditions, refer to Protocol No. 459.

PROTOCOL FOR HPTLC ANALYSIS OF PHARMACEUTICAL FORMULATION

Protocol No. 459

Formulation: **Capsaicinoids (capsaicin) and its biosynthetic intermediates**

Classification: External **Dosage form:** Extract

Standard preparation: Standard solutions of different compounds were prepared in methanol or acetone for identification.

Sample preparation: Powdered pepper was extracted with acetone by incubating for 5 hrs in glass desiccator at room temperature with orbital shaking (50 rpm), organic phase evaporated and residue taken up in methanol for analysis.

Chromatographic equipments:

Sample applicator: Micropipette (digital) fitted with ultramicrotips, 0.5–10 μl
Development chamber: Flat bottom glass chamber, 10 × 10 cm
Densitometric scanner: Shimadzu CS–930 dual wavelength scanner

Chromatographic conditions:

1. Stationary phase: Silica gel 60F_{254} pre-coated TLC plates, 10 × 10 cm (250 μm) – Merck
2. Mobile phase (MP): (a) Cyclohexane–chloroform–acetic acid (7 : 2 : 1 v/v), (b) Chloroform–methanol–acetic acid (95 : 1 : 5 v/v); (c) cyclohexane–acetone (4 : 5 v/v)
3. Standard/Sample application:
   Band length: 2 mm Volume applied: 2 μl Spacing: 5 mm
4. Chamber saturation: 15 min (MP)
5. RH (%): 60 ± 5
6. Temperature °C: 22 ± 2
7. Separation technique: Ascending
8. Quantity of mobile phase: 20 ml
9. Migration distance: 90 mm
10. Migration time: 30 min

Densitometric evaluation:

Wavelength: UV–281 nm Scanning mode: Reflectance/Absorbance
HRF: See densitogram
Linearity (ng/band): —
Recovery (%): —

References: Miriam Monforte-González, Fatima Medina–Lara, Guadalupe Gutierrez-Carbajal and Felipe Vázquez-Flota, *J. Liq. Chromatogr. and Related Technol.*, **30**, 1697–1704, 2004.

Comments:

- Plates in MP (a) were developed twice to obtain better resolution.
- Capsaicin and dihydrocapsaicin could not be separated.

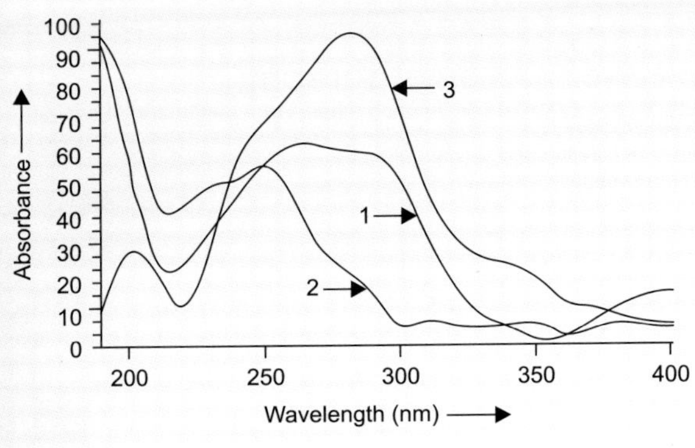

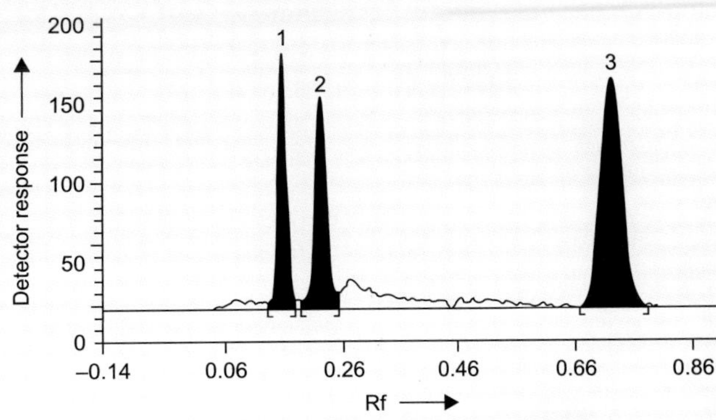

Miscellaneous

- Hypolipidaemic agents
- Antidiabetics
- Anticoagulants and Antithrombotics
- Antivirals
- Oral contraceptives
- Others

Protocols and Densitograms from 460 to 528

Anything worth having takes blood, sweat and toil.

HPTLC : High Performance Thin Layer Chromatography
HPTLC Densitogram

No. 460

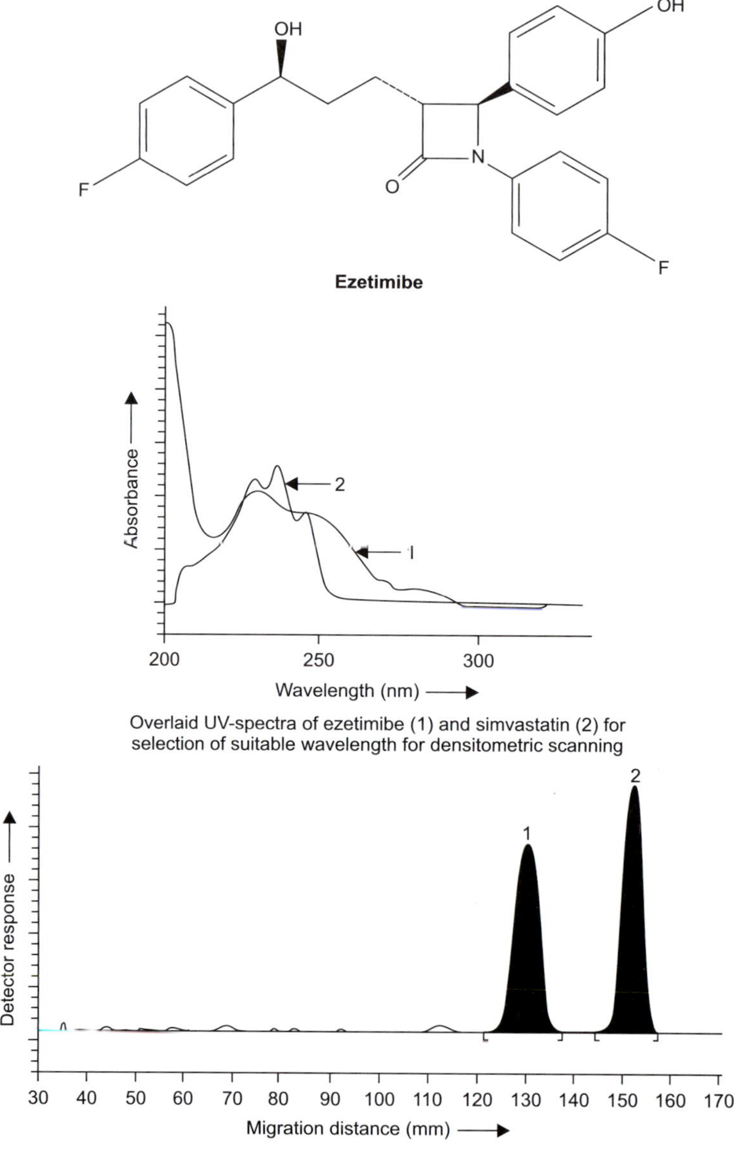

Overlaid UV-spectra of ezetimibe (1) and simvastatin (2) for selection of suitable wavelength for densitometric scanning

Typical densitogram of the sample containing simvastatin and ezetimibe. For detailed experimental and chromatographic conditions, refer to Protocol No. 460. Peaks identification: 1. Simvastatin; 2. Ezetimibe.

PROTOCOL FOR HPTLC ANALYSIS OF PHARMACEUTICAL FORMULATION

Protocol No. 460

Formulation: Simvastatin, Ezetimibe

Classification: Miscellaneous **Dosage form:** Tablets

Standard preparation: Prepare 1 mg/ml solution of each compound separately in methanol. Further serial dilutions made to get different concentrations. Apply 5 μl of each solution for linearity profile.

Sample preparation: Powdered sample equivalent to 10 mg of simvastatin suspended in methanol, sonicated, diluted and filtered. The filtrate suitably diluted with methanol for chromatographic analysis.

Chromatographic equipments:

Sample applicator: Camag Linomat–IV

Development chamber: Camag twin-trough glass chamber, 10 × 10 cm

Densitometric scanner: Camag TLC Scanner–III

Chromatographic conditions:

1. Stationary phase: Silica gel $60F_{254}$ pre-coated HPTLC plates, 10 × 10 cm (200 μm) – Merck
2. Mobile phase (MP): Ethyl acetate–chloroform (8 : 2 v/v)
3. Standard/Sample application:
   Band length: 16 mm Volume applied: 5 μl Spacing: 10 mm
4. Chamber saturation: 10 min MP)
5. RH (%): 55 ± 5
6. Temperature °C: 20 ± 2
7. Separation technique: Ascending
8. Quantity of mobile phase: 10 ml
8. Migration distance: 70 mm
9. Migration time: 15 min

Densitometric evaluation:

Wavelength: UV–220 nm Scanning mode: Reflectance/Absorbance

HRF: Simvastatin—76; Ezetimibe—89

Linearity: 600–1400 ng/band for both the compounds

Recovery (%): 98.68–99.34 for both the compounds

References: K. Shivshanker, N. Sreekanth, N. Harikrishnan, C. Roosewelt, P. Shanmuga Pandiyan, G. Srinivasa Rao and V. Gunasekaran, *Asian J. Chem.*, **19(5)**, 3627–3632, 2007.

Comments: The method validated for accuracy, precision, linearity, LOD, LOQ, specificity, robustness and ruggedness.

HPTLC : High Performance Thin Layer Chromatography
HPTLC Densitogram

No. 461

Ezetimibe

Simvastatin

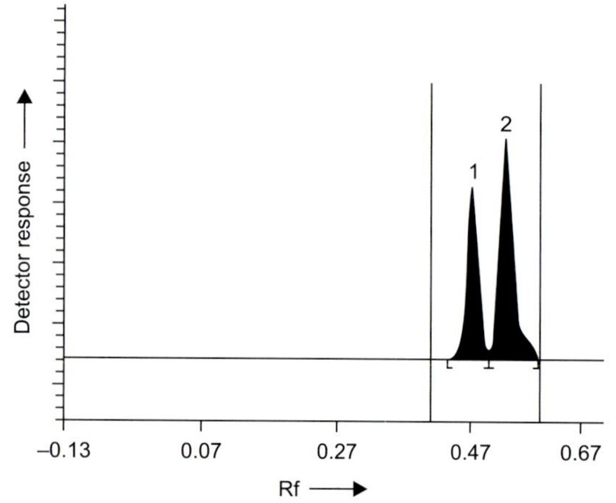

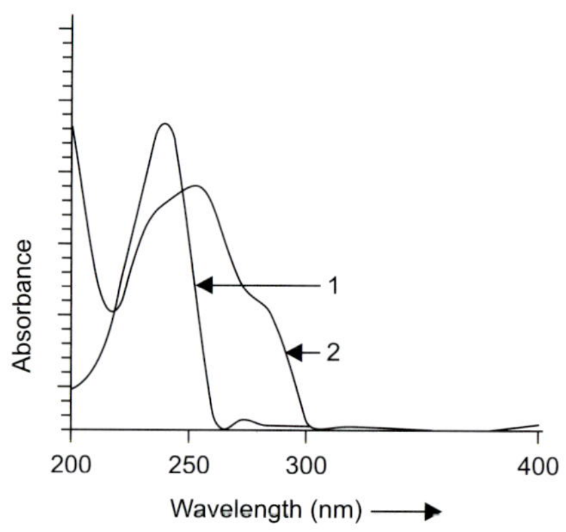

Overlaid UV-spectra of simvastatin (1) and ezetimibe (2) for selection of suitable wavelength for densitometric scanning

Typical densitogram of the sample containing simvastatin and ezetimibe. For detailed experimental and chromatographic conditions, refer to Protocol No. 461. Peaks identification: 1. Simvastatin; 2. Ezetimibe.

PROTOCOL FOR HPTLC ANALYSIS OF PHARMACEUTICAL FORMULATION

Protocol No. 461

Formulation: Simvastatin, Ezetimibe

Classification: Miscellaneous **Dosage form:** Tablets

Standard preparation: Prepare 1 mg/ml solution of each compound separately in methanol. Further serial dilutions made for linearity studies. Apply 4 μl of each solution for linearity profile.

Sample preparation: Powdered sample equivalent to 10 mg of simvastatin suspended in methanol, sonicated for 10 min, centrifuged, filtered and the filtrate suitably diluted with methanol. Apply 4 μl for chromatographic separation and evaluation.

Chromatographic equipments:

Sample applicator: Camag Linomat–IV

Development chamber: Camag twin-trough glass chamber, 20 × 10 cm

Densitometric scanner: Camag TLC Scanner–III

Chromatographic conditions:

1. Stationary phase: Silica gel 60F_{254} pre-coated HPTLC plates, 20 × 10 cm (200 μm) – Merck, pre-washed with methanol, activated at 105°C (20 min) prior to use
2. Mobile phase (MP): Toluene–isopropanol (8 : 2 v/v)
3. Standard/Sample application:
   Band length: 8 mm Volume applied: 4 μl Spacing: 12 mm
4. Chamber saturation: 20 min (MP)
5. RH (%): 55 ± 5
6. Temperature °C: 25 ± 2
7. Separation technique: Ascending
8. Quantity of mobile phase: 20 ml
8. Migration distance: 150 mm
9. Migration time: 35 min

Densitometric evaluation:

Wavelength: UV–240 nm Scanning mode: Reflectance/Absorbance

HRF: Simvastatin—48; Ezetimibe—53

Linearity: 400–200 ng/band for both the compounds

Recovery (%): 98.14–99 for both the compounds

References: S.S. Dhaneshwar, P. Deshpande, M. Patel, G. Vadnerkar and S.R. Dhaneshwar, *Acta Chromatographica*, **20(1)**, 71–79, 2008.

Comments: The method validated for accuracy, precision, linearity, LOD, LOQ, specificity, robustness and ruggedness.

HPTLC : High Performance Thin Layer Chromatography
HPTLC Densitogram

No. 462

Ezetimibe

Simvastatin

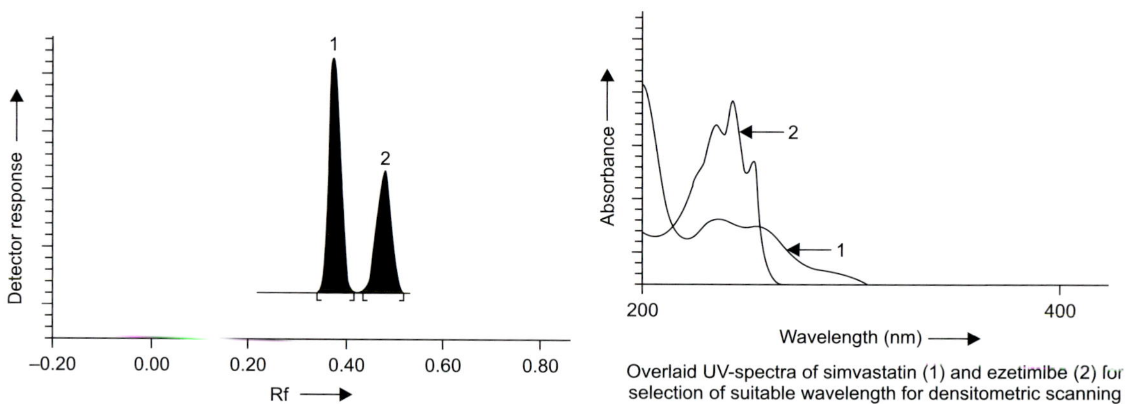

Overlaid UV-spectra of simvastatin (1) and ezetimibe (2) for selection of suitable wavelength for densitometric scanning

Typical densitogram of the sample containing simvastatin and ezetimibe. For detailed experimental and chromatographic conditions, refer to Protocol No. 462. Peaks identification: 1. Simvastatin; 2. Ezetimibe.

PROTOCOL FOR HPTLC ANALYSIS OF PHARMACEUTICAL FORMULATION

Protocol No. 462

Formulation: Simvastatin, Ezetimibe

Classification: Miscellaneous **Dosage form:** Tablets

Standard preparation: Prepare 1 mg/ml solution of each compound in methanol. Further serial dilutions made for linearity profile. Apply 1 μl of each solution for analysis.

Sample preparation: Powdered sample equivalent to 10 mg simvastatin suspended in methanol, sonicated, centrifuged and clear supernatant solution suitably diluted for assay.

Chromatographic equipments:

Sample applicator: Camag Linomat–IV

Development chamber: Camag twin-trough glass chamber, 10 × 10 cm

Densitometric scanner: Camag TLC Scanner–III

Chromatographic conditions:

1. Stationary phase: Silica gel $60F_{254}$ pre-coated TLC plates, 10 × 10 cm (250 μm) – Merck, pre-washed with methanol, dried at 105°C (15 min) prior to use
2. Mobile phase (MP): n-hexane–acetone (6 : 4 v/v)
3. Standard/Sample application:
   Band length: 5 mm Volume applied: 1 μl Spacing: 5 mm
4. Chamber saturation: 20 min (MP)
5. RH (%): 55 ± 5
6. Temperature °C: 22 ± 2
7. Separation technique: Ascending
8. Quantity of mobile phase: 10 ml
8. Migration distance: 80 mm
9. Migration time: 20 min

Densitometric evaluation:

Wavelength: UV–234 nm Scanning mode: Reflectance/Absorbance

HRF: Simvastatin—39; Ezetimibe—50

Linearity: 200–1600 ng/band for both the compounds

Recovery (%): 96.44–98.5 for both the drugs

References: Rahul P. Dixit, Chandrasekhar R. Barhate and Mangal S. Nagarsenker, *Chromatographia*, **67(1–2)**, 101–107, 2008.

Comments:

- The method validated for accuracy, precision, linearity, LOD, LOQ, specificity, robustness and ruggedness.
- The method is stability indicating (acid, base, oxidative, thermal, photolytic). The degradation products were separated from main compounds.

HPTLC : High Performance Thin Layer Chromatography
HPTLC Densitogram

No. 463

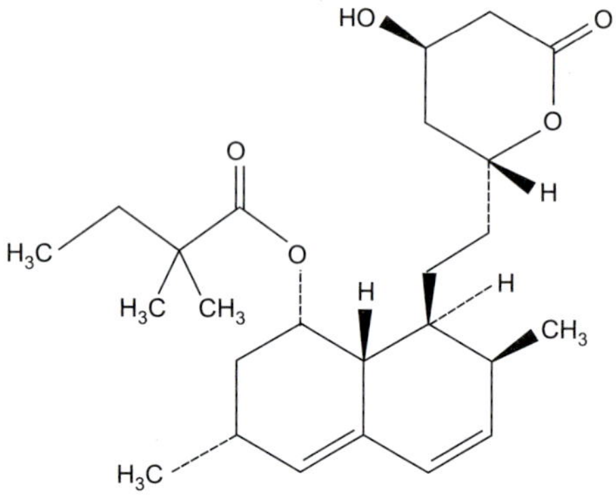

Simvastatin

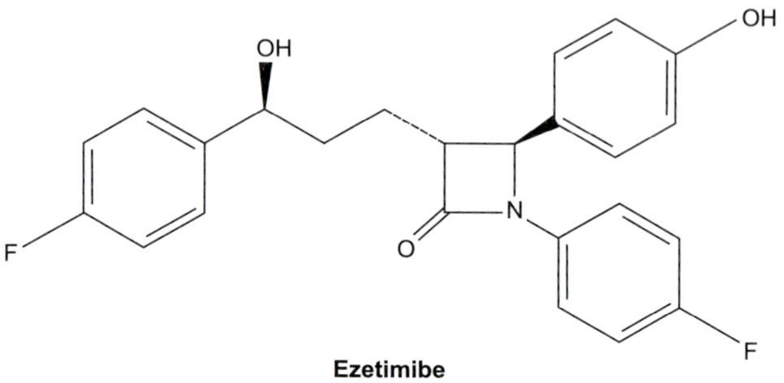

Ezetimibe

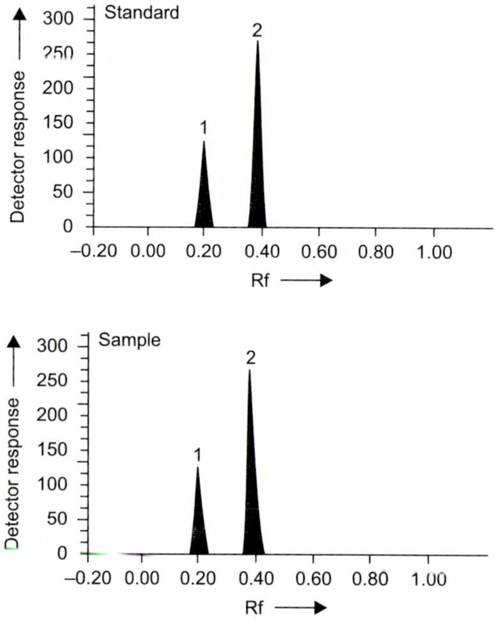

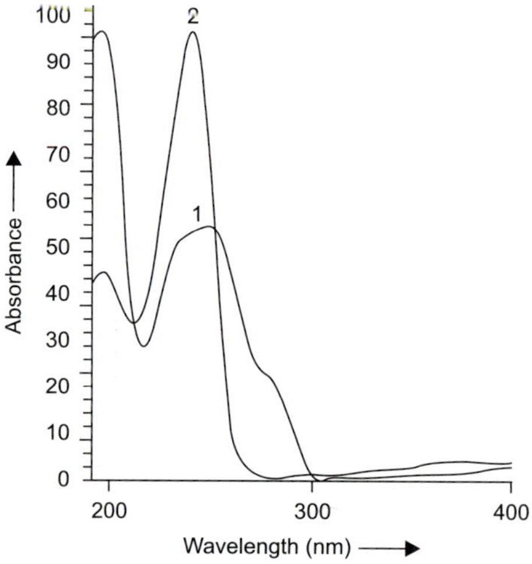

Overlaid UV spectra of ezetimibe (1) and simvastatin (2) for selection of suitable wavelength for densitometric scanning

Typical densitogram of the standard and sample containing ezetimibe and simvastatin. For detailed experimental and chromatographic conditions, refer to Protocol No. 463. Peaks identification: 1. Ezetimibe; 2. Simvastatin.

PROTOCOL FOR HPTLC ANALYSIS OF PHARMACEUTICAL FORMULATION

Protocol No. 463

Formulation: Simvastatin, Ezetimibe

Classification: Miscellaneous **Dosage form:** Tablets

Standard preparation: Prepare 1 mg/ml solution of each compound in methanol. Further serial dilutions made for linearity profile. Apply 10 µl of each solution.

Sample preparation: Powdered sample equivalent to 10 mg of simvastatin suspended in 8 ml of methanol, sonicated for 10 min, diluted to 10 ml and filtered. 1 ml of the filtrate diluted to 10 ml with methanol and used for analysis by applying 10 µl.

Chromatographic equipments:

Sample applicator: Camag Linomat–V

Development chamber: Camag ADC-2, saturated with Camag saturation pad

Densitometric scanner: Camag TLC Scanner–III

Chromatographic conditions:

1. Stationary phase: Silica gel $60F_{254}$ pre-coated TLC plates, 20 × 10 cm (250 µm) – Merck
2. Mobile phase (MP): n-hexane–acetone (12 : 8 v/v)
3. Standard/Sample application:
   Band length: 8 mm Volume applied: 10 µl Spacing: 10.6 mm
4. Chamber saturation: 20 min (MP)
5. RH (%): 55 ± 5
6. Temperature °C: 25 ± 1
7. Separation technique: Ascending
8. Quantity of mobile phase: 20 ml
8. Migration distance: 70 mm
9. Migration time: 8 min

Densitometric evaluation:

Wavelength: UV–251 nm Scanning mode: Reflectance/Absorbance

HRF: Ezetimibe—33; Simvastatin—42

Linearity: 0.5–5 µg/band for both the compounds

Recovery (%): 99.06–99.72 for both the compounds

References: —

Comments:

- The method was optimized and analytical work was carried out at **Anchrom HPTLC Application Laboratory**, Mumbai, India.
- Although MP in protocol No. 3 and 4 is the same but the retention order is reversed, needs verification.

HPTLC : High Performance Thin Layer Chromatography
HPTLC Densitogram

No. 464

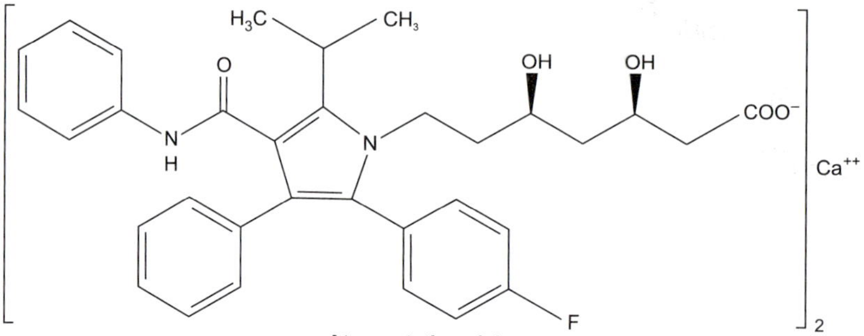

Atorvastatin calcium

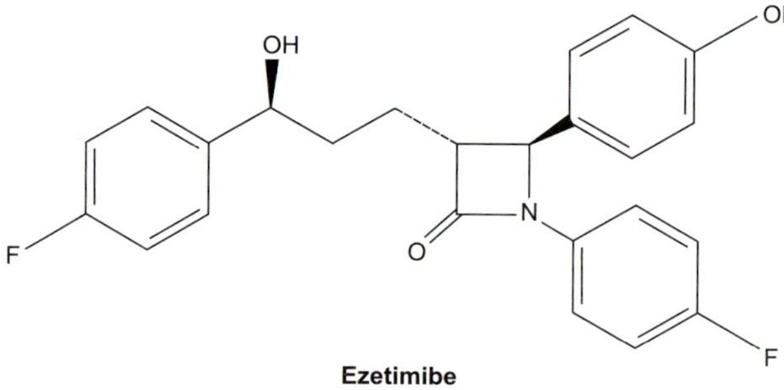

Ezetimibe

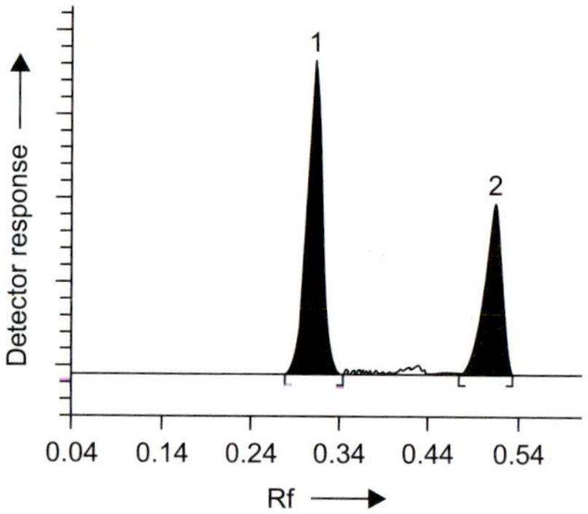

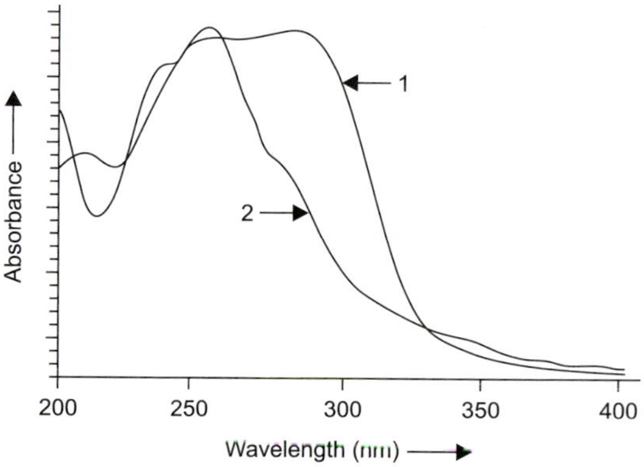

Overlaid UV-spectra of atorvastatin calcium (1) and ezetimibe (2) for selection of suitable wavelength for densitometric scanning

Typical densitogram of the sample containing atorvastatin calcium and ezetimibe. For detailed experimental and chromatographic conditions, refer to Protocol No. 464. Peaks identification: 1. Atorvastatin Ca^{++}; 2. Ezetimibe.

PROTOCOL FOR HPTLC ANALYSIS OF PHARMACEUTICAL FORMULATION

Protocol No. 464

Formulation: Atorvastatin calcium, Ezetimibe

Classification: Miscellaneous **Dosage form:** Tablets

Standard preparation: Prepare 1 mg/ml solution of atorvastatin calcium and 100 μg/ml solution of ezetimibe, both in methanol. Apply 0.8–4 μl of atorvastatin calcium and 1–10 μl of ezetimibe solution for linearity studies.

Sample preparation: Powdered sample equivalent to 25 mg of atorvastatin suspended in methanol, sonicated for 15 min, diluted and filtered. The filtrate suitably diluted with methanol. Apply 2 μl and 5 μl of the sample solution for chromatographic analysis.

Chromatographic equipments:

Sample applicator: Camag Linomat–V

Development chamber: Camag twin-trough glass chamber, 20 × 10 cm

Densitometric scanner: Camag TLC Scanner–III

Chromatographic conditions:

1. Stationary phase: Silica gel 60F_{254} pre-coated TLC plates, 20 × 10 cm (250 μm) – Merck, pre-washed with methanol, dried at 50°C for 5 min
2. Mobile phase (MP): Chloroform–benzene–methanol–acetic acid (6 : 3 : 1 : 0.1 v/v)
3. Standard/Sample application:
   Band length: 5 mm Volume applied: 1–10 μl Volume applied: 5 mm
4. Chamber saturation: 30 min (MP)
5. RH (%): 55 ± 5
6. Temperature °C: 22 ± 2
7. Separation technique: Ascending
8. Quantity of mobile phase: 20 ml
8. Migration distance: 72 mm
9. Migration time: 15 min

Densitometric evaluation:

Wavelength: UV–250 nm Scanning mode: Reflectance/Absorbance

HRF: Atorvastatin Ca^{++}—30; Ezetimibe—53

Linearity (ng/band): Atorvastatin Ca^{++}—800–4000; Ezetimibe—100–1000

Recovery (%): 9987–102.65 for both the compounds

References: G. Chaudhari, N.M. Patel, P.B. Shah and K.P. Modi, *Ind. J. Pharm. Sci.*, **68(6)**, 793–796, 2006.

Comments: The method validated for accuracy, precision, linearity, LOD, LOQ, specificity, robustness and ruggedness.

HPTLC : High Performance Thin Layer Chromatography
HPTLC Densitogram

No. 465

Ezetimibe

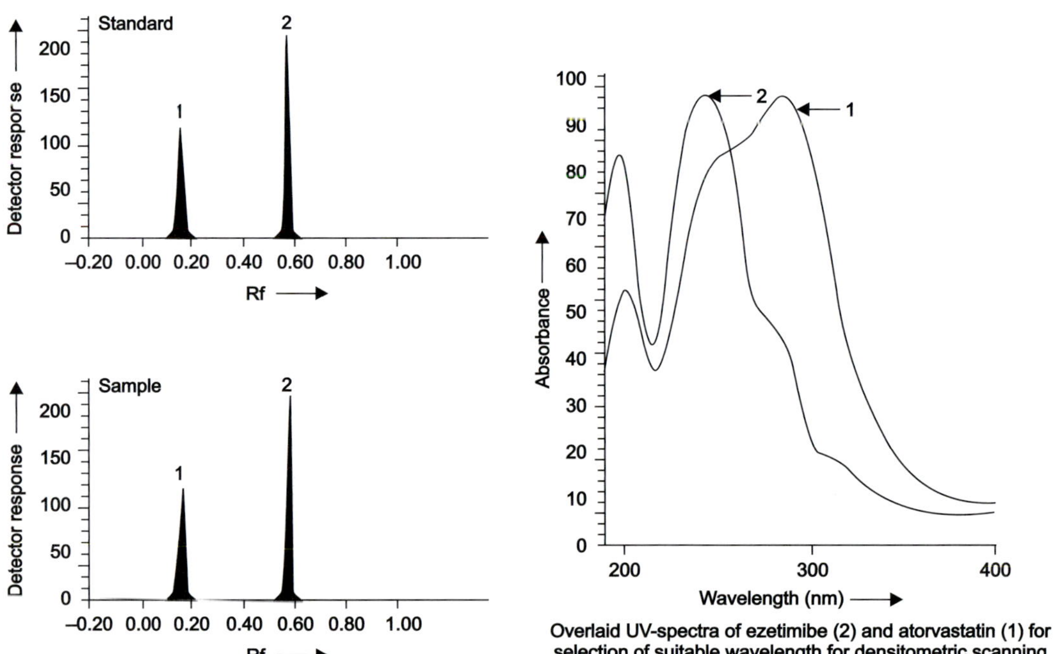

Overlaid UV-spectra of ezetimibe (2) and atorvastatin (1) for selection of suitable wavelength for densitometric scanning

Typical densitogram of the standard and sample containing atorvastatin calcium and ezetimibe. For detailed experimental and chromatographic conditions, refer to Protocol No. 465. Peaks identification: 1. Atorvastatin; 2. Ezetimibe.

PROTOCOL FOR HPTLC ANALYSIS OF PHARMACEUTICAL FORMULATION

Protocol No. 465

Formulation: Atorvastatin calcium, Ezetimibe

Classification: Miscellaneous **Dosage form:** Tablets

Standard preparation: Prepare 1 mg/ml solution of each compound in methanol. Make serial dilutions of each solution for linearity studies. Apply 10 μl of each solution.

Sample preparation: Accurately weighed quantity of the powdered sample equivalent to 10 mg of atorvastatin suspended in methanol, sonicated, diluted to 10 ml with methanol, filtered and the filtrate suitably diluted for analysis. Apply 10 μl for analysis.

Chromatographic equipments:

Sample applicator: Camag Linomat–V

Development chamber: Camag ADC–2, saturated with Camag saturation pads

Densitometric scanner: Camag TLC Scanner–III

Chromatographic conditions:

1. Stationary phase: Silica gel $60F_{254}$ pre-coated TLC plates glass, 20 × 10 cm Merck
2. Mobile phase (MP) (MP): Toluene–methanol–acetone–triethylamine (7 : 2 : 1 : 0.2 v/v)
3. Standard/Sample application:
   Band length: 8 mm Volume applied: 10 μl Spacing: 10.6 mm
4. Chamber saturation: 20 min (MP)
5. RH (%): 50 ± 5
6. Temperature °C: 25 ± 1
7. Separation technique: Ascending
8. Quantity of mobile phase: 20 ml
8. Migration distance: 70 mm
9. Migration time: 6 min

Densitometric evaluation:

Wavelength: UV–257 nm Scanning mode: Reflectance/Absorbance

HRF: Atorvastatin—16; Ezetimibe—58

Linearity: 0.5–5 μg/band for both the drugs

Recovery (%): 97.76–99.0 for both the compounds

References: —

Comments: The method was optimized and analytical work carried out at **Anchrom's HPTLC Application Laboratory**, Mumbai, India.

HPTLC : High Performance Thin Layer Chromatography
HPTLC Densitogram

No. 466

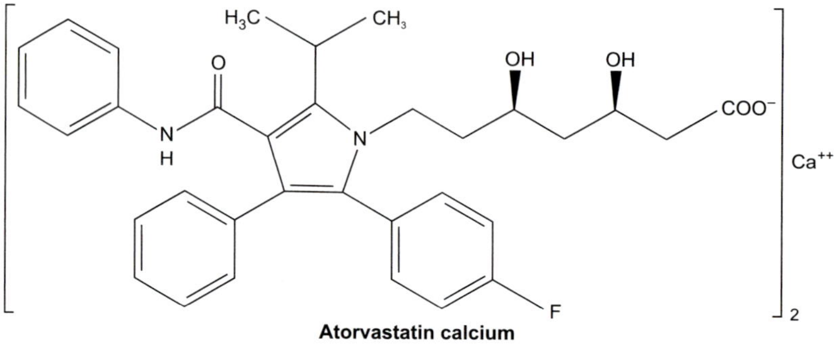

Atorvastatin calcium

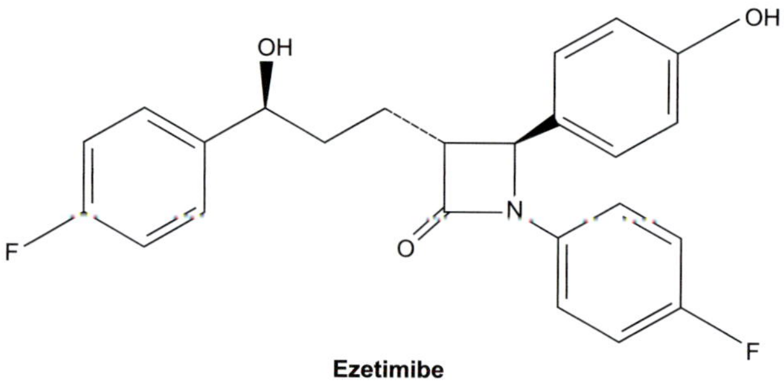

Ezetimibe

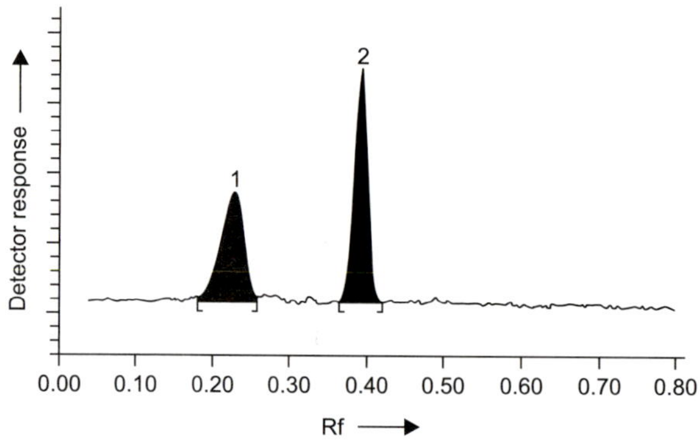

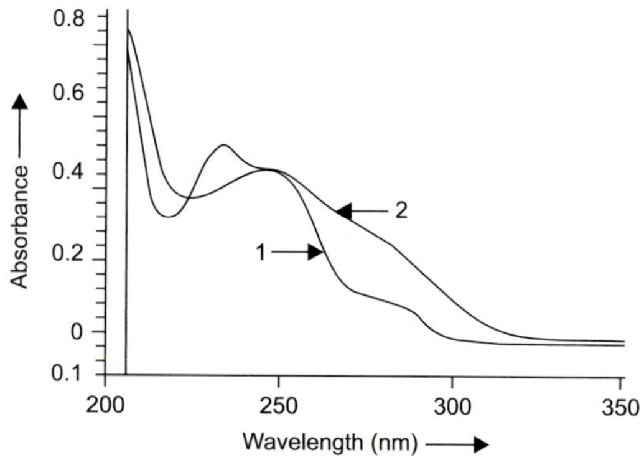

Overlaid UV-spectra of atorvastatin calcium (1) and ezetimibe (2) for selection of suitable wavelength for densitometric scanning

Typical densitogram of the sample containing atorvastatin calcium and ezetimibe. For detailed experimental and chromatographic conditions, refer to Protocol No. 466. Peaks identification: 1. Atorvastatin Ca^{++}; 2. Ezetimibe.

PROTOCOL FOR HPTLC ANALYSIS OF PHARMACEUTICAL FORMULATION

Protocol No. 466

Formulation: **Atorvastatin calcium, Ezetimibe**

Classification: Miscellaneous **Dosage form:** Tablets

Standard preparation: Prepare 1 mg/ml solution of each compound separately in methanol. Further dilutions made with methanol to get final concentration of 200 ng/μl. Apply varying volumes for linearity profile.

Sample preparation: Powdered sample equivalent to 10 mg of atorvastatin suspended in methanol, sonicated, diluted and centrifuged (600 rpm), clear supernatant liquid suitably diluted. Apply 4 μl for chromatographic analysis.

Chromatographic equipments:

Sample applicator: Camag Linomat–IV

Development chamber: Camag twin-trough glass chamber, 20 × 10 cm

Densitometric scanner: Camag TLC Scanner–IV

Chromatographic conditions:

1. Stationary phase: Silica gel $60F_{254}$ pre-coated TLC plates, 20 × 10 cm (250 μm) – Merck
2. Mobile phase (MP): Toluene–methanol (8 : 2 v/v)
3. Standard/Sample application:
   Band length: 6 mm Volume applied: 1–6 μl Spacing: 6 mm
4. Chamber saturation: 20 min (MP)
5. RH (%): 55 ± 5
6. Temperature °C: 22 ± 2
7. Separation technique: Ascending
8. Quantity of mobile phase: 20 ml
8. Migration distance: 150 mm
9. Migration time: 20 min

Densitometric evaluation:

Wavelength: UV–240 nm Scanning mode: Reflectance/Absorbance

HRF: Atorvastatin Ca^{++}—23; Ezetimibe—39

Linearity: 400–25400 ng/band for both the compounds

Recovery (%): 98.51–99.01 for both the drugs

References: S.S. Dhaneshwar, S.R. Dhaneshwar, P. Deshpande and M. Paul, *Acta Chromatographica*, **19**, 141–148, 2007.

Comments: The method validated for accuracy, precision, linearity, LOD, LOQ, specificity, robustness and ruggedness.

HPTLC : High Performance Thin Layer Chromatography
HPTLC Densitogram

No. 467

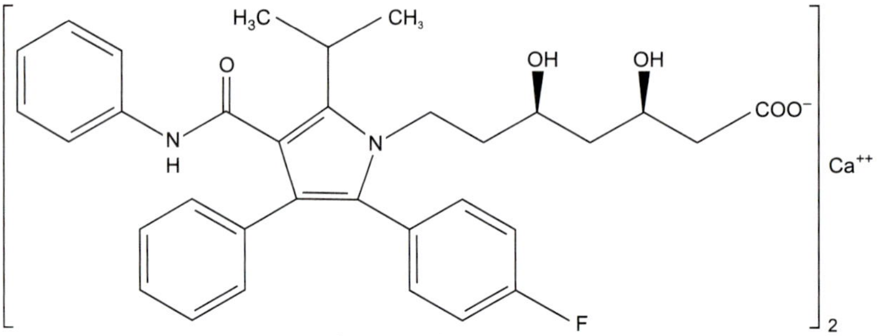

H$_3$C CH$_3$ O OH OH N N H COO$^-$ Ca^{++} F 2

Atorvastatin calcium

OH OH N F O F

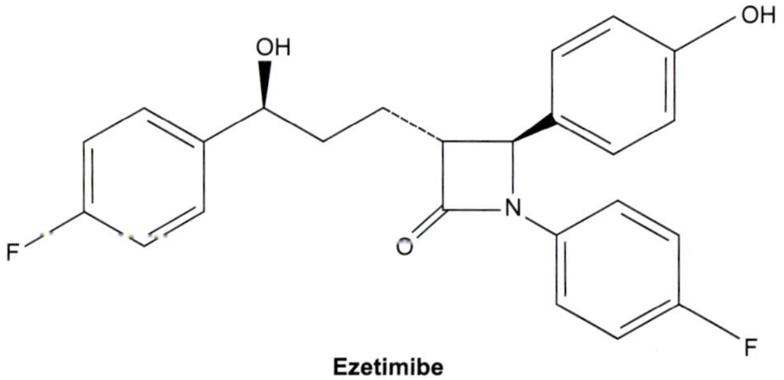

Ezetimibe

Detector response → 0 50 100 150 200 250 300 350 1 2 0.00 0.10 0.20 0.30 0.40 0.50 0.60 0.70 0.80 Rf →

Absorbance → 1 2 220 240 260 280 300 Wavelength (nm) →

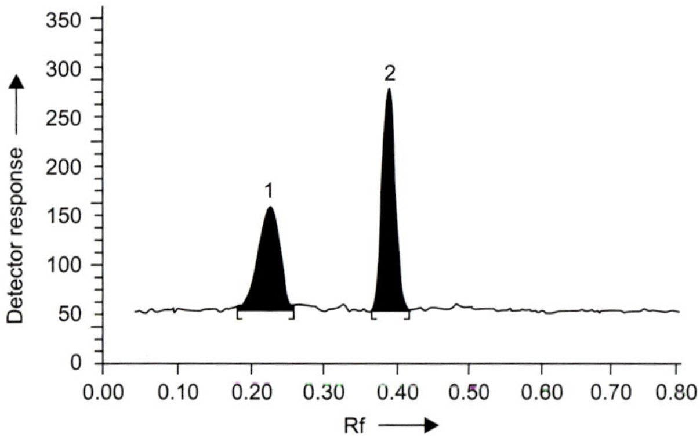

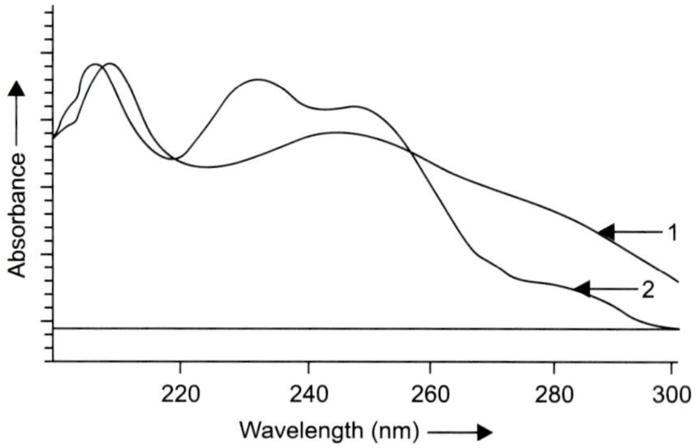

Overlaid UV-spectra of atorvastatin calcium (1) and ezetimibe (2) for selection of suitable wavelength for densitometric scanning

Typical densitogram of the standard containing atorvastatin calcium and ezetimibe. For detailed experimental and chromatographic conditions, refer to Protocol No. 467. Peaks identification: 1. Atorvastatin Ca^{++}; 2. Ezetimibe.

PROTOCOL FOR HPTLC ANALYSIS OF PHARMACEUTICAL FORMULATION

Protocol No. 467

Formulation: Atorvastatin calcium, Ezetimibe

Classification: Miscellaneous **Dosage form:** Tablets

Standard preparation: Prepare 1 mg/ml solution of each compound in methanol. Further dilutions made to get 100 μg/ml of each compound. Apply varying volumes of each solution for linearity profile.

Sample preparation: Powdered sample equivalent to 10 mg of ezetimibe suspended in methanol, stirred for 30 min to dissolve, dilute to 10 ml, filter and dilute 1 ml of the filtrate to 10 ml with methanol and apply 5 μl for assay.

Chromatographic equipments:

Sample applicator: Camag Linomat–IV

Development chamber: Camag twin-trough glass chamber, 20 × 20 cm

Densitometric scanner: Camag TLC Scanner–III

Chromatographic conditions:

1. Stationary phase: Silica gel $60F_{254}$ pre-coated TLC plates, 20 × 20 cm (250 μm) – Merck, pre-washed with methanol, activated at 105°C for 20 min prior to use
2. Mobile phase (MP): Benzene–methanol–acetone–triethylamine (7 : 2 : 1 : 0.2 v/v)
3. Standard/Sample application:
   Band length: 6 mm Volume applied: 1–7 μl Spacing: 6 mm
4. Chamber saturation: 20 min (MP)
5. RH (%): 55 ± 5
6. Temperature °C: 25 ± 2
7. Separation technique: Ascending
8. Quantity of mobile phase: 20 ml
8. Migration distance: 150 mm
9. Migration time: 25 min

Densitometric evaluation:

Wavelength: UV–266 nm Scanning mode: Reflectance/Absorbance

HRF: Atorvastatin Ca^{++}—22; Ezetimibe—39

Linearity: 100–700 ng/band for both the compounds

Recovery (%): Atorvastatin Ca^{++}—98.77–100.07; Ezetimibe—99.12–100.11

References: V. Rajamanickam, A. Rajasekaran, B. Stephen Rathinaraj and K. Ananadarajagopal, *World Applied Sciences Journal*, **9(12)**, 1424–1429, 2010.

Comments:

- The method validated for accuracy, precision, linearity and specificity.
- The method was comparable with UV-spectrophotometric and RP-HPLC.

HPTLC : High Performance Thin Layer Chromatography
HPTLC Densitogram

No. 468

Atorvastatin calcium

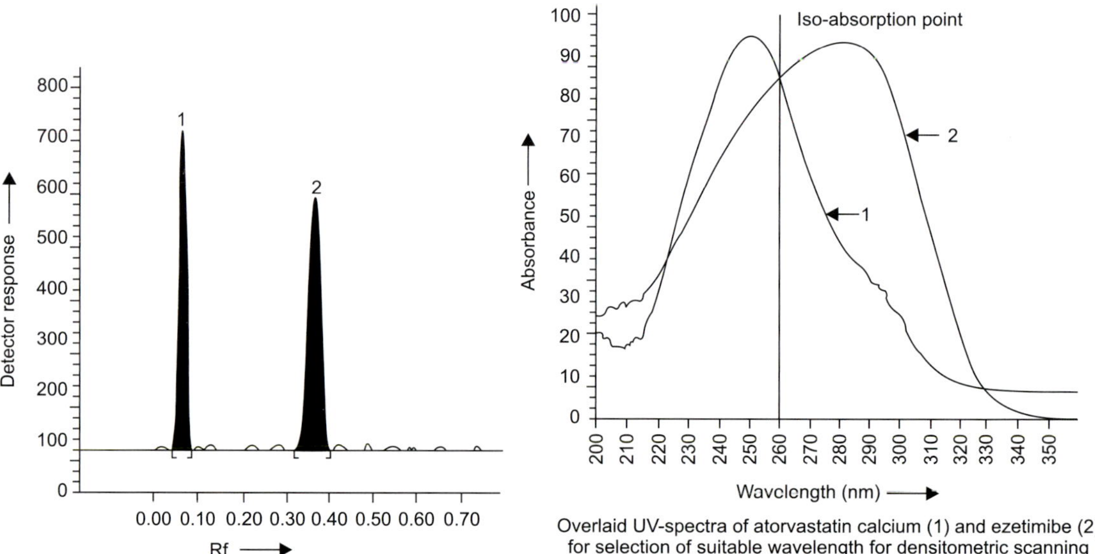

Overlaid UV-spectra of atorvastatin calcium (1) and ezetimibe (2) for selection of suitable wavelength for densitometric scanning

Typical densitogram of the sample containing atorvastatin calcium and ezetimibe. For detailed experimental and chromatographic conditions, refer to Protocol No. 468. Peaks identification: 1. Atorvastatin Ca^{++}; 2. Ezetimibe.

PROTOCOL FOR HPTLC ANALYSIS OF PHARMACEUTICAL FORMULATION

Protocol No. 468

Formulation: Atorvastatin calcium, Ezetimibe

Classification: Miscellaneous **Dosage form:** Tablets

Standard preparation: Prepare 1 mg/ml solution of each compound separately in methanol. Further serial dilutions are made with methanol. Apply 5 μl of each solution for linearity profile.

Sample preparation: Composite powdered sample equivalent to 10 mg of ezetimibe suspended in 8 ml of methanol, sonicated for 15 min, diluted to 10 ml with methanol, filtered and 1.8 ml of filtrate diluted to 10 ml with methanol and used for chromatographic analysis.

Chromatographic equipments:

Sample applicator: Camag Linomat–IV

Development chamber: Camag twin-trough glass chamber, 20 × 10 cm

Densitometric scanner: Camag TLC Scanner–III

Chromatographic conditions:

1. Stationary phase: Silica gel $60F_{254}$ pre-coated HPTLC plates, 20 × 10 cm (250 μm) – Merck, pre-washed with methanol, activated at 110°C for 15 min prior to use
2. Mobile phase (MP): Toluene–chloroform–methanol–triethylamine (8 : 0.5 : 1 : 0.5 v/v)
3. Standard/Sample application:
   Band length: 5 mm Volume applied: 5 μl Spacing: —
4. Chamber saturation: 10 min (MP)
5. RH (%): 60 ± 5
6. Temperature °C: 20 ± 2
7. Separation technique: Ascending
8. Quantity of mobile phase: 20 ml
8. Migration distance: 70 mm
9. Migration time: 15 min

Densitometric evaluation:

Wavelength: UV–259 nm (iso-absorption point)

Scanning mode: Reflectance/Absorbance

HRF: Atorvastatin Ca^{++}—07; Ezetimibe—37

Linearity: 500–1500 ng/band for both the compounds

Recovery (%): 99.54–99.83 for both the compounds

References: Sanjay G. Walode, A.V. Kasture and S.G. Wadodkar, *J. Planar Chromatogr.*, **25(1)**, 81–84, 2012.

Comments:

- The method validated for accuracy, precision, linearity, LOD, LOQ, specificity, robustness and ruggedness.
- The method is stability indicating (acid, base, oxidative, thermal, photolytic). The degradation products were separated from main compounds.

HPTLC : High Performance Thin Layer Chromatography
HPTLC Densitogram

No. 469

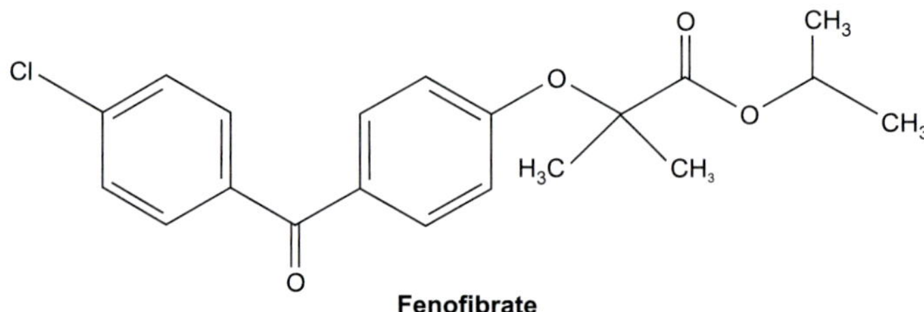

Fenofibrate

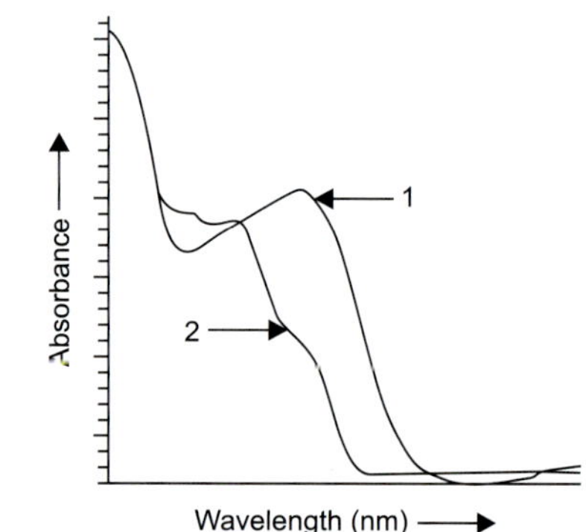

Overlaid UV-spectra of atorvastatin calcium (1) and fenofibrate (2) for selection of suitable wavelength for densitometric scanning

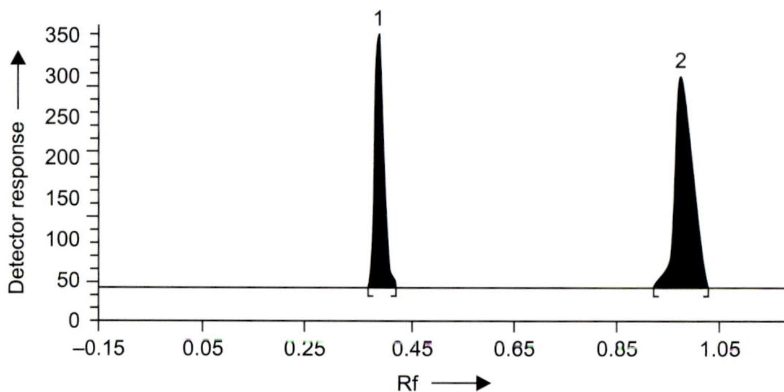

Typical densitogram of the sample containing atorvastatin calcium and fenofibrate. For detailed experimental and chromatographic conditions, refer to Protocol No. 469. Peaks identification: 1. Atorvastatin Ca^{++}; 2. Fenofibrate.

PROTOCOL FOR HPTLC ANALYSIS OF PHARMACEUTICAL FORMULATION

Protocol No. 469

Formulation: Atorvastatin calcium, Fenofibrate

Classification: Miscellaneous **Dosage form:** Tablets

Standard preparation: Prepare standard stock solution of both the compounds separately in methanol to get 100 μg/ml (atorvastatin calcium) and 1 mg/ml (fenofibrate). Further serial dilutions made for linearity studies. Apply 2 μl of each solution.

Sample preparation: Powdered sample equivalent to 10 mg of atorvastatin calcium suspended in methanol, sonicated for 20 min, suitably diluted and filtered. Apply 2 μl of the resulting solution for chromatographic separation and analysis.

Chromatographic equipments:

Sample applicator: Camag Linomat–V

Development chamber: Camag twin-trough glass chamber, 20 × 10 cm

Densitometric scanner: Camag TLC Scanner–III

Chromatographic conditions:

1. Stationary phase: Silica gel $60F_{254}$ pre-coated TLC plates, 10 × 10 cm (250 μm) – Merck, pre-washed with methanol, dried at 105°C for 5 min prior to use
2. Mobile phase (MP): Toluene–methanol–acetic acid (8 : 2 : 0.2 v/v)
3. Standard/Sample application:
   Band length: 5 mm Volume applied: 2 μl Spacing: 5 mm
4. Chamber saturation: 30 min (MP)
5. RH (%): 60 ± 5
6. Temperature °C: 25 ± 2
7. Separation technique: Ascending
8. Quantity of mobile phase: 20 ml
8. Migration distance: 75 mm
9. Migration time: 15 min

Densitometric evaluation:

Wavelength: UV–294 nm Scanning mode: Reflectance/Absorbance

HRF: Atorvastatin Ca^{++}—40; Fenofibrate—88

Linearity (ng/band): Atorvastatin Ca^{++}—60–700; Fenofibrate 100–700

Recovery (%): 100.30–100.9 for both the drugs

References: B.G. Chaudhari and N.M. Patel, *Indian Drugs*, **44(5)**, 378–384, 2007.

Comments: The method validated for accuracy, precision, linearity, LOD, LOQ, specificity, robustness and ruggedness.

HPTLC : High Performance Thin Layer Chromatography
HPTLC Densitogram

No. 470

Fenofibrate

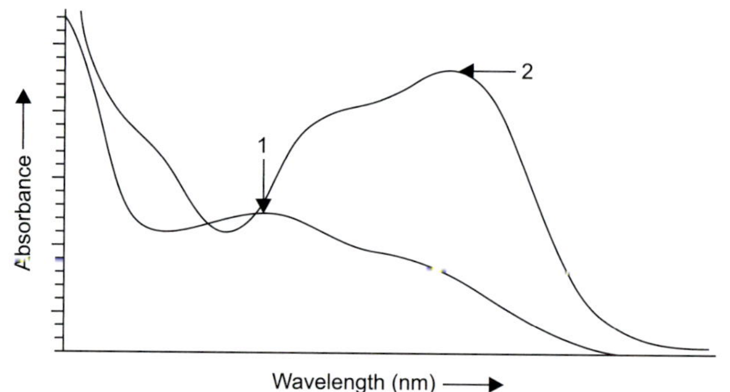

Overlaid UV-spectra of atorvastatin calcium (1) and fenofibrate (2) for selection of suitable wavelength for densitometric scanning

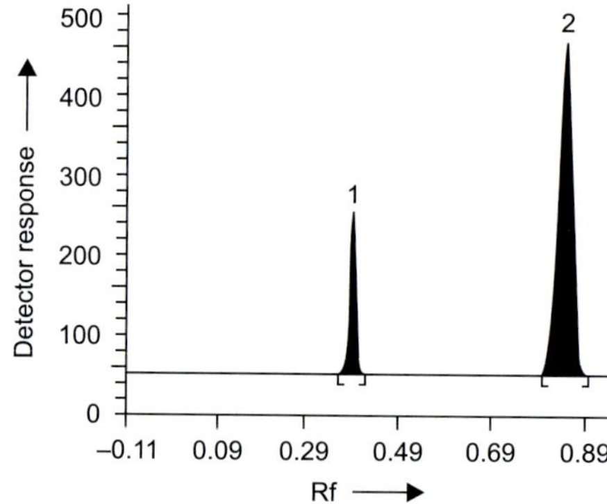

Typical densitogram of the sample containing atorvastatin calcium and fenofibrate. For detailed experimental and chromatographic conditions, refer to Protocol No. 470. Peaks identification: 1. Atorvastatin Ca^{++}; 2. Fenofibrate.

PROTOCOL FOR HPTLC ANALYSIS OF PHARMACEUTICAL FORMULATION

Protocol No. 470

Formulation: Atorvastatin calcium, Fenofibrate

Classification: Miscellaneous **Dosage form:** Tablets

Standard preparation: Prepare standard stock solution of both the compounds separately in methanol to get 100 μg/ml (atorvastatin calcium) and 1 mg/ml (fenofibrate). Further serial dilutions made for linearity studies. Apply 2 μl of each solution.

Sample preparation: Powdered sample equivalent to 10 mg of atorvastatin calcium suspended in methanol, sonicated for 20 min, suitably diluted and filtered. Apply 2 μl of the resulting solution for chromatographic separation for analysis.

Chromatographic equipments:

Sample applicator: Camag Linomat–V

Development chamber: Camag twin-trough glass chamber, 20 × 10 cm

Densitometric scanner: Camag TLC Scanner–III

Chromatographic conditions:

1. Stationary phase: Silica gel $60F_{254}$ pre-coated HPTLC plates, 20 × 10 cm (200 μm) – Merck, pre-washed with methanol, dried at 105°C for 5 min prior to use
2. Mobile phase (MP): Toluene–methanol–triethylamine (7 : 3 : 0.2 v/v)
3. Standard/Sample application:
   Band length: 6 mm Volume applied: 2 μl Spacing: 15 mm
4. Chamber saturation: 25 min (MP)
5. RH (%): 60 ± 5
6. Temperature °C: 25 ± 2
7. Separation technique: Ascending
8. Quantity of mobile phase: 20 ml
8. Migration distance: 80 mm
9. Migration time: 20 min

Densitometric evaluation:

Wavelength: UV–258 nm Scanning mode: Reflectance/Absorbance

HRF: Atorvastatin Ca^{++}—36; Fenofibrate—84

Linearity (ng/band): Atorvastatin Ca^{++}—100–800; Fenofibrate—1000–8000

Recovery (%): 99.41–100.86 for both the compound

References: Atul A. Shirkhedkar and Sanjay J. Surana, *J. Planar Chromatogr.*, **22(5)**, 355–358, 2009.

Comments: The method validated for accuracy, precision, linearity, LOD, LOQ, specificity, robustness and ruggedness.

HPTLC : High Performance Thin Layer Chromatography
HPTLC Densitogram

No. 471

Cl, O, O, O, O, H_3C, CH_3, CH_3, CH_3

Fenofibrate

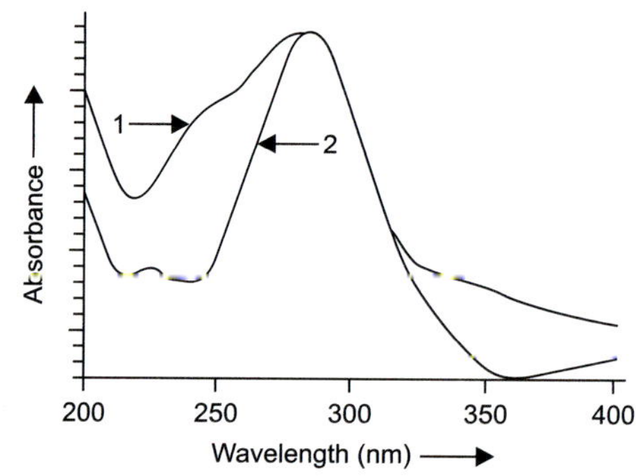

Overlaid UV-spectra of atorvastatin calcium (1) and finofibrate (2) for selection of suitable wavelength for densitometric scanning

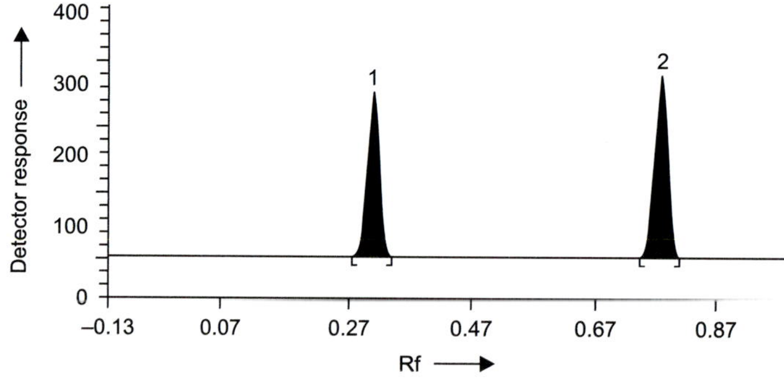

Typical densitogram of the sample containing atorvastatin calcium and fenofibrate. For detailed experimental and chromatographic conditions, refer to Protocol No. 471. Peaks identification: 1. Atorvastatin Ca^{++}; 2. Fenofibrate.

PROTOCOL FOR HPTLC ANALYSIS OF PHARMACEUTICAL FORMULATION

Protocol No. 471

Formulation: Atorvastatin calcium, Fenofibrate

Classification: Miscellaneous **Dosage form:** Tablets

Standard preparation: Prepare 1 mg/ml solution of each compound in methanol. Further dilutions made to get 100 μg/ml of atorvastatin and 160 μg/ml of fenofibrate. Apply 1–4 μl of each solution for linearity profile.

Sample preparation: Powdered sample suspended in methanol, sonicated, centrifuged, clear liquid diluted suitably with methanol and used for chromatographic application.

Chromatographic equipments:

Sample applicator: Camag Linomat–V

Development chamber: Camag twin-trough glass chamber, 20 × 20 cm

Densitometric scanner: Camag TLC Scanner–III

Chromatographic conditions:

1. Stationary phase: Silica gel $60F_{254}$ pre-coated HPTLC plates, 20 × 20 cm (200 μm) – Merck, pre-washed with methanol, dried at 105°C for 5 min prior to use
2. Mobile phase (MP): Chloroform–methanol (8 : 2 v/v)
3. Standard/Sample application:
   Band length: 8 mm Volume applied: 1–4 μl Spacing: 10 mm
4. Chamber saturation: 20 min (MP)
5. RH (%): 55 ± 5
6. Temperature °C: 25 ± 2
7. Separation technique: Ascending
8. Quantity of mobile phase: 20 ml
8. Migration distance: 150 mm
9. Migration time: 25 min

Densitometric evaluation:

Wavelength: UV–285 nm Scanning mode: Reflectance/Absorbance

HRF: Atorvastatin Ca^{++}—29; Fenofibrate—77

Linearity (ng/band): Atorvastatin Ca^{++}—200–1000; Fenofibrate—320–1600

Recovery (%): 98.30–99.10 for both the compounds

References: P.B. Deshpande, G. Shridharan, Libi Anandi, D. Yadav, M.C. Damle and S.V. Gandhi, *Pharma Review*, 151, May 2009.

Comments: The method validated for accuracy, precision, linearity, LOD, LOQ, specificity, robustness and ruggedness.

HPTLC : High Performance Thin Layer Chromatography
HPTLC Densitogram

No. 472

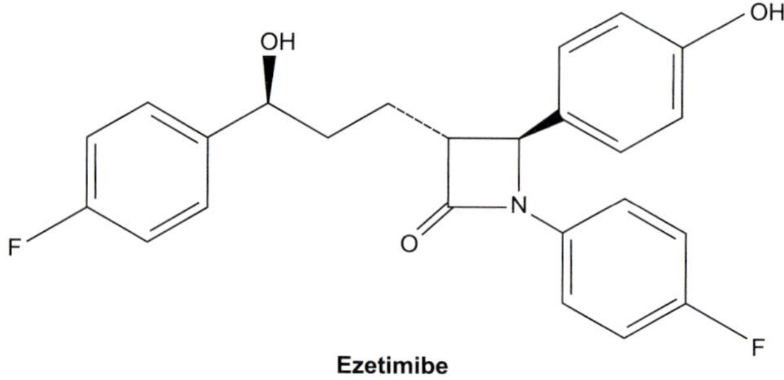

Ezetimibe

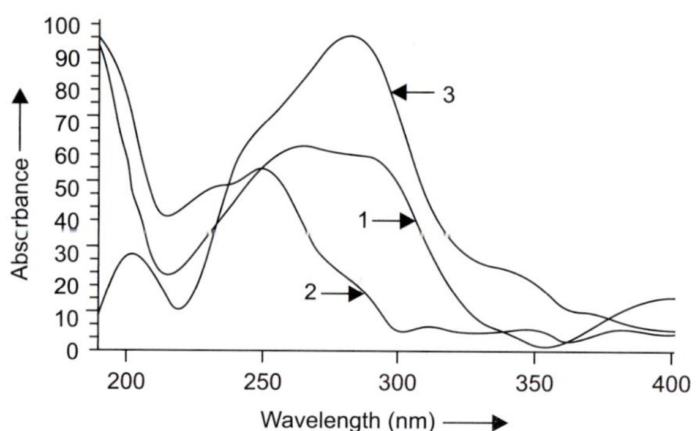

Overlaid UV-spectra of atorvastatin Ca^{++} (1), ezetimibe (2) and fenofibrate (3) for selection of suitable wavelength for densitometric scanning

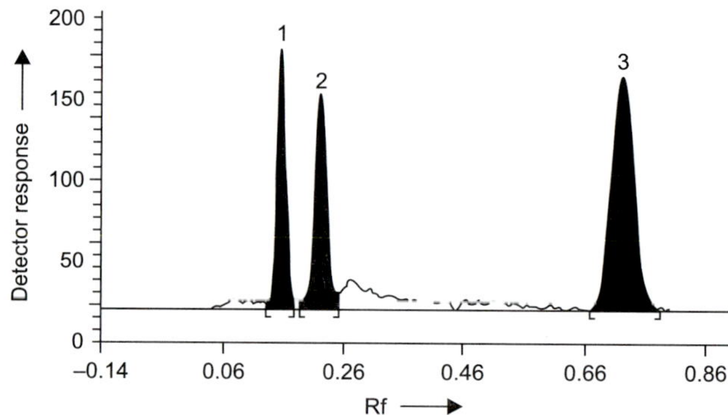

Typical densitogram of the sample containing atorvastatin calcium, fenofibrate and ezetimibe. For detailed experimental and chromatographic conditions, refer to Protocol No. 472. Peaks identification: 1. Atorvastatin calcium; 2. Ezetimibe; 3. Fenofibrate.

PROTOCOL FOR HPTLC ANALYSIS OF PHARMACEUTICAL FORMULATION

Protocol No. 472

Formulation: Atorvastatin calcium, Fenofibrate, Ezetimibe

Classification: Miscellaneous **Dosage form:** Tablets

Standard preparation: Prepare solution of each compound in methanol to get 1 mg/ml each of atorvastatin calcium and ezetimibe and 10 mg/ml of fenofibrate. Further serial dilutions of each solution made with methanol for linearity profile.

Sample preparation: Composite powdered sample equivalent to 10 mg of atorvastatin calcium suspended in 20 ml of methanol, sonicated for 30 min, diluted to 50 ml with methanol, centrifuged (6000 rpm) for 5 min and supernatant suitably diluted to get 100 μg/ml of atorvastatin and ezetimibe and 64 μg/ml of fenofibrate and used for chromatographic analysis.

Chromatographic equipments:

Sample applicator: Camag Linomat–V

Development chamber: Camag twin-trough glass chamber, 20 × 10 cm

Densitometric scanner: Camag TLC Scanner–III

Chromatographic conditions:

1. Stationary phase: Silica gel $60F_{254}$ pre-coated TLC plates, 20 × 10 cm (250 μm) – Merck, pre-washed with methanol and activated at 110°C for 5 min prior to chromatography
2. Mobile phase (MP): Toluene–chloroform–methanol–acetic acid (3 : 6 : 0.5 : 0.15 v/v)
3. Standard/Sample application:
   Band length: 10 mm Volume applied: 2–3 μl Spacing: 11.2 mm
4. Chamber saturation: 30 min (MP)
5. RH (%): 60 ± 5
6. Temperature °C: 22 ± 2
7. Separation technique: Ascending
8. Quantity of mobile phase: 19 ml
8. Migration distance: 80 mm
9. Migration time: 20 min

Densitometric evaluation:

Wavelength: UV–263 nm Scanning mode: Reflectance/Absorbance

HRF: Atorvastatin Ca^{++}—16; Ezetimibe—22; Fenofibrate—76

Linearity (ng/band): Atorvastatin Ca^{++}—75–375; Fenofibrate—66–330; Ezetimibe—99–693

Recovery (%): Atorvastatin Ca^{++}—99.11–101.80; Fenofibrate—100.50–101.64; Ezetimibe—100.90–101.47

References: A.G. Nikalje and U.P. Choudhari, *Acta Chromatographica*, **23(2)**, 267–280, 2011.

Comments: The method validated for accuracy, precision, linearity, LOD, LOQ, specificity, robustness and ruggedness.

HPTLC : High Performance Thin Layer Chromatography
HPTLC Densitogram

No. 473

Fenofibrate

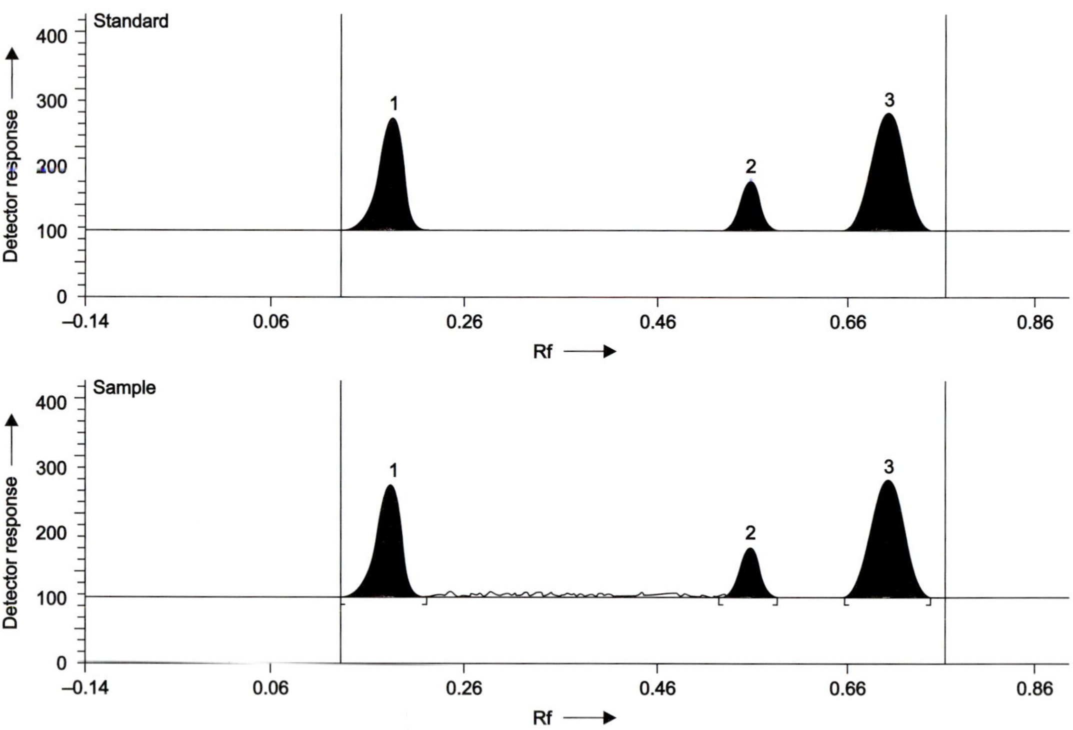

Typical densitogram of the sample and standard containing atorvastatin calcium, ezetimibe and fenofibrate. For detailed experimental and chromatographic conditions, refer to Protocol No. 473. Peaks identification: 1. Atorvastatin Ca^{++}; 2. Ezetimibe; 3. Fenofibrate.

PROTOCOL FOR HPTLC ANALYSIS OF PHARMACEUTICAL FORMULATION

Protocol No. 473

Formulation: Atorvastatin calcium, Ezetimibe, Fenofibrate

Classification: Miscellaneous **Dosage form:** Tablets

Standard preparation: Prepare 1 mg/ml solution of each drug in methanol. Dilute 0.5 ml of fenofibrate standard solution to 10 ml. Mixed standard: Take 0.5 ml each of standard solution of atorvastatin and ezetimibe, add 5 ml of fenofibrate solution and dilute to 10 ml with methanol.

Sample preparation: Weigh powdered sample equivalent to 10 mg of atorvastatin, suspend in 5 ml of methanol, sonicate for 30 min, dilute to 10 ml with methanol. Centrifuge (2000 rpm) for 10 min, use supernatant for further dilution. Dilute 0.5 ml to 10 ml with methanol and use for assay of atorvastatin and ezetimibe. Dilute 0.25 ml to 10 ml and use for assay of fenofibrate.

Chromatographic equipments:

Sample applicator: Camag Linomat–V

Development chamber: Camag twin-trough glass chamber, 20 × 20 cm

Densitometric scanner: Camag TLC Scanner–III

Chromatographic conditions:

1. Stationary phase: Silica gel $60F_{254}$ pre-coated TLC plates, 20 × 20 cm (250 μm) – Merck
2. Mobile phase (MP): Toluene–methanol–chloroform (6 : 3 : 4 v/v)
3. Standard/Sample application:
   Band length: 10 mm Volume applied: 2–12 μl Spacing: 11.30 mm
4. Chamber saturation: 20 min (MP)
5. RH (%): 55 ± 5
6. Temperature °C: 22 ± 2
7. Separation technique: Ascending
8. Quantity of mobile phase: 26 ml
8. Migration distance: 80 mm
9. Migration time: 20 min

Densitometric evaluation:

Wavelength: UV–280 nm Scanning mode: Reflectance/Absorbance

HRF: Atorvastatin calcium—20; Ezetimibe—56; Fenofibrate—70

Linearity (ng/band): Atorvastatin Ca^{++} and Ezetimibe—100–600; Fenofibrate—50–300

Recovery (%): 99.11–100.66 for all the three drugs

References: A.A. Naik, S.A. Naik and M.G. Pai, Abstract No. F-246, 62nd IPC, 2010; Personal communication, Prof. M.G. Pai, Goa College of Pharmacy.

Comments: The method validated for accuracy, precision, linearity, LOD, LOQ, specificity, robustness and ruggedness.

HPTLC : High Performance Thin Layer Chromatography
HPTLC Densitogram

No. 474

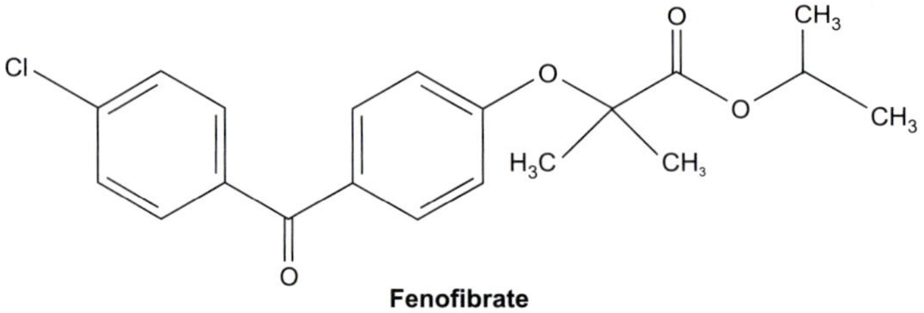

Fenofibrate

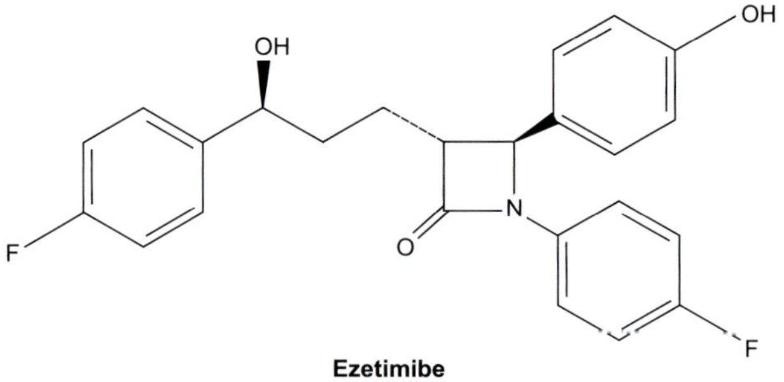

Ezetimibe

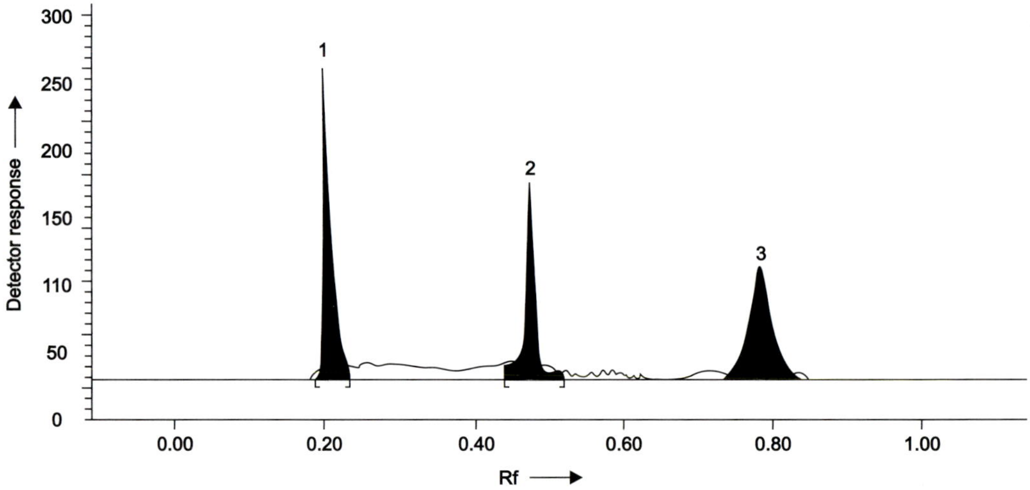

Typical densitogram of the standard containing atorvastatin calcium, ezetimibe and fenofibrate. For detailed experimental and chromatographic conditions, refer to Protocol No. 474. Peaks identification: 1. Atorvastatin Ca^{++}; 2. Ezetimibe; 3. Fenofibrate.

PROTOCOL FOR HPTLC ANALYSIS OF PHARMACEUTICAL FORMULATION

Protocol No. 474

Formulation: Atorvastatin calcium, Fenofibrate, Ezetimibe

Classification: Miscellaneous **Dosage form:** Tablets

Standard preparation: Prepare 1 mg/ml solution of each substance in methanol. Further dilutions of each solution made with methanol to get 100 μg/ml (atorvastatin Ca^{++}), 50 μg/ml (ezetimibe) and 25 μg/ml (fenofibrate). Apply appropriate volume of each solution for linearity profile.

Sample preparation: Powdered sample equivalent to 10 mg of atorvastatin suspended in 8 ml of methanol, sonicated, diluted to 10 ml, filtered and filtrate suitably diluted so that the final solution contains 2.5 μg/ml of atorvastatin Ca^{++}; 2.5 μg/ml of ezetimibe and 50 μg/ml of fenofibrate. Use the solution for assay.

Chromatographic equipments:

Sample applicator: Camag Linomat–V
Development chamber: Camag twin-trough glass chamber, 10 × 10 cm
Densitometric scanner: Camag TLC Scanner–III

Chromatographic conditions:

1. Stationary phase: Silica gel $60F_{254}$ pre-coated TLC plates, 10 × 10 cm (250 μm) – Merck, pre-washed with methanol, activated at 110°C for 5 min prior to use
2. Mobile phase (MP): Toluene–methanol–acetone–triethylamine (7 : 2 : 1 : 0.2 v/v)
3. Standard/Sample application:
   Band length: 8 mm Volume applied: 5 μl Spacing: 5 mm
4. Chamber saturation: 20 min (MP)
5. RH (%): 55 ± 5
6. Temperature °C: Ambient
7. Separation technique: Ascending
8. Quantity of mobile phase: 10 ml
8. Migration distance: 80 mm
9. Migration time: 20 min

Densitometric evaluation:

Wavelength: UV–252 nm Scanning mode: Reflectance/Absorbance
HRF: Atorvastatin Ca^{++}—22; Ezetimibe—47; Fenofibrate—79
Linearity (ng/band): Atorvastatin Ca^{++}—200–1200; Ezetimibe—100–350; Fenofibrate—50–300
Recovery (%): —

References: Jitesh Jadav, Sugandha Mulgund, Ashwinin Badanikar and Manisha Phoujdar, Abstract No. F-280, 63rd IPC, 2011. Courtesy: Prof. K.S. Jain, Principal.

Comments: The method validated for accuracy, precision, linearity, LOD, LOQ, specificity, robustness and ruggedness.

HPTLC : High Performance Thin Layer Chromatography
HPTLC Densitogram

No. 475

Atorvastatin calcium

Aspirin

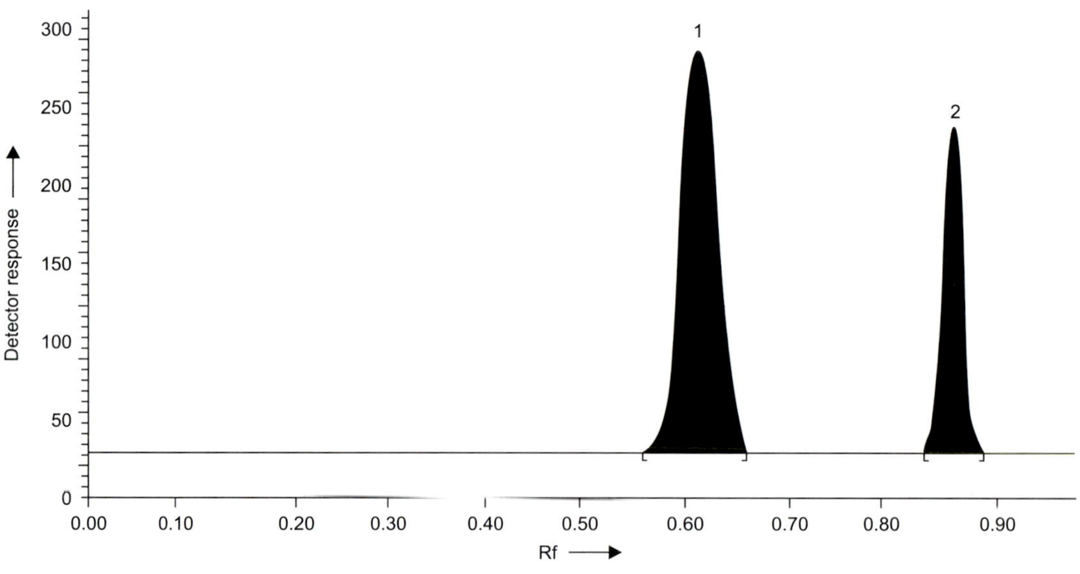

Typical densitogram of the standard containing atorvastatin calcium and aspirin. For detailed experimental and chromatographic conditions, refer to Protocol No. 475. Peaks identification: 1. Atorvastatin Ca^{++}; 2. Aspirin.

PROTOCOL FOR HPTLC ANALYSIS OF PHARMACEUTICAL FORMULATION

Protocol No. 475

Formulation: Atorvastatin calcium, Aspirin

Classification: Miscellaneous **Dosage form:** Tablets

Standard preparation: Prepare solution of both the drugs in methanol to get 500 µg/ml of atorvastatin calcium (AST) and 750 µg/ml of aspirin (ASP). Apply varying volumes of each solution for linearity profile.

Sample preparation: Powdered sample equivalent to 20 mg of AST suspended in 40 ml of methanol, sonicated for 30 min, filtered and diluted to 50 ml with methanol and used for chromatographic evaluation.

Chromatographic equipments:

Sample applicator: Camag Linomat-V

Development chamber: Camag twin-trough glass chamber, 10 × 10 cm

Densitometric scanner: Camag TLC Scanner–III

Chromatographic conditions:

1. Stationary phase: Silica gel $60F_{254}$ pre-coated TLC plates, 10 × 10 cm (250 µm) – Merck
2. Mobile phase (MP): Chloroform–toluene–methanol–glacial acetic acid (4 : 5.6 : 0.4 : 0.5 v/v)
3. Standard/Sample application:
   Band length: — Volume applied: 1–3 µl (AST); 1.5–5 µl (ASP)
   Spacing: —
4. Chamber saturation: 30 min (MP)
5. RH (%): 55 ± 5
6. Temperature °C: Ambient
7. Separation technique: Ascending
8. Quantity of mobile phase: 10 ml
8. Migration distance: 70 mm
9. Migration time: 20 min

Densitometric evaluation:

Wavelength: UV–247 nm Scanning mode: Reflectance/Absorbance

HRF: Atorvastatin Ca^{++}—61; Aspirin—84

Linearity (ng/band): Atorvastatin Ca^{++}—500–1500; Aspirin—1125–4125

Recovery (%): 99.39–99.46 for both the compounds

References: B.V. Suman, K. Kannan, V. Mahadevan and Chandini R. Nayar, Abstract No. F-389, 63rd IPC, 2011, Personal communication with the authors.

Comments: The method validated for accuracy, precision, linearity, LOD, LOQ, specificity, robustness and ruggedness.

HPTLC : High Performance Thin Layer Chromatography
HPTLC Densitogram

No. 476

Rosuvastatin calcium

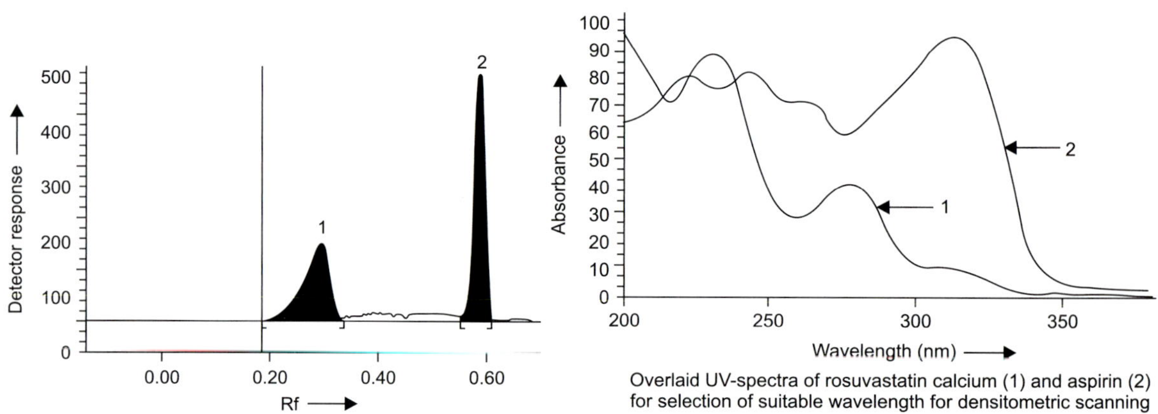

Overlaid UV-spectra of rosuvastatin calcium (1) and aspirin (2) for selection of suitable wavelength for densitometric scanning

Typical densitogram of the standard containing rosuvastatin calcium and aspirin. For detailed experimental and chromatographic conditions, refer to Protocol No. 476. Peaks identification: 1. Rosuvastatin Ca^{++}; 2. Aspirin.

PROTOCOL FOR HPTLC ANALYSIS OF PHARMACEUTICAL FORMULATION

Protocol No. 476

Formulation: Rosuvastatin calcium, Aspirin

Classification: Miscellaneous **Dosage form:** Capsules

Standard preparation: Prepare solution of both the drugs separately in methanol to get 75 μg/ml of aspirin and 10 μg/ml of rosuvastatin. Apply varying volumes of each solution for linearity profile.

Sample preparation: Composite sample equivalent to 75 mg of aspirin and 10 mg of rosuvastatin calcium suspended in 80 ml of methanol, sonicated for 5 min, diluted to 100 ml with methanol. Filtered and filtrate suitably diluted with methanol to get 75 μg/ml of aspirin and 10 μg/ml of rosuvastatin. Apply 5 μl for assay.

Chromatographic equipments:

Sample applicator: Camag Linomat–V

Development chamber: Camag twin-trough glass chamber, 10 × 10 cm

Denistometric scanner: Camag TLC Scanner–III

Chromatographic conditions:

1. Stationary phase: Silica gel $60F_{254}$ pre-coated HPTLC plates, 10 × 10 cm (200 μm) – Merck, pre-washed with methanol and dried prior to use
2. Mobile phase (MP): Toluene–ethylacetate–acetone–glacial acetic acid (4 : 4 : 2 : 0.1 v/v)
3. Standard/Sample application:
   Band length: 7 mm Volume applied: 4–10 μl Spacing: 10 mm
4. Chamber saturation: 30 min (MP)
5. RH (%): 55 ± 5
6. Temperature °C: 25 ± 2
7. Separation technique: Ascending
8. Quantity of mobile phase: 10 ml
9. Migration distance: 85 mm
10. Migration time: 20 min

Densitometric evaluation:

Wavelength: UV–254 nm Scanning mode: Reflectance/Absorbance

HRF: Rosuvastatin Ca^{++}—30; Aspirin—58

Linearity (ng/band): Rosuvastatin Ca^{++}—40–100; Aspirin—300–750

Recovery (%): 99.10–101.94 for both the compounds

References: Pooja Ramanuj, Kashyap N. Thumar and Navin R. Sheth, Manuscript submitted for Dr. P.D. Sethi Award, 2011. Data courtesy, Prof. Kashyap Thumar.

Comments: The method validated for accuracy, precision, linearity, LOD, LOQ, specificity and robustness.

HPTLC : High Performance Thin Layer Chromatography
HPTLC Densitogram

No. 477

COOH O CH$_3$ O

Aspirin

O OCH$_3$ N S Cl

Clopidogrel

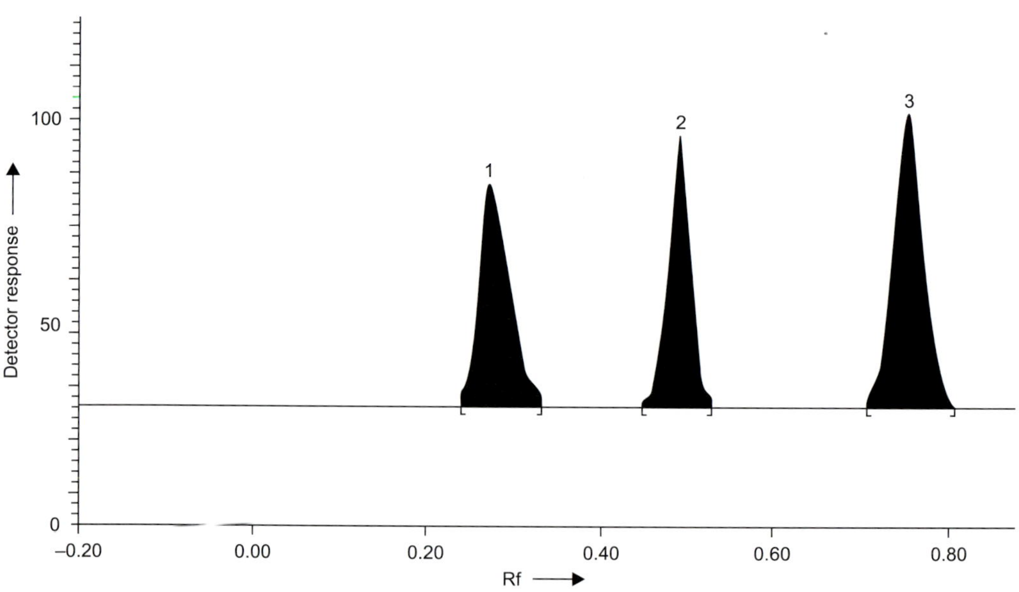

Typical densitogram of the sample containing atorvastatin, aspirin and clopidogrel bisulphate. For detailed experimental and chromatographic conditions, refer to Protocol No. 477. Peaks identification: 1. Aspirin; 2. Atorvastatin Ca^{++}; 3. Clopidogrel bisulphate.

PROTOCOL FOR HPTLC ANALYSIS OF PHARMACEUTICAL FORMULATION

Protocol No. 477

Formulation: Atorvastatin calcium, Aspirin, Clopidogrel bisulphate

Classification: Miscellaneous **Dosage form:** Capsules

Standard preparation: Prepare 100 μg/ml solution of each compound in methanol. Apply varying volumes (2–12 μl) of each solution for linearity profile.

Sample preparation: The sample equivalent to 75 mg of aspirin suspended in methanol, sonicated for 15 min, diluted to 100 ml with methanol, centrifuged for 10 min at 6000 rpm. Further diluted suitably. Apply 10 μl of resulting solution for chromatographic analysis.

Chromatographic equipments:

Sample applicator: Camag Linomat–V

Development chamber: Camag twin-trough glass chamber, 10 × 20 cm

Densitometric scanner: Camag TLC Scanner–III

Chromatographic conditions:

1. Stationary phase: Silica gel $60F_{254}$ pre-coated TLC plates, 10 × 20 cm (250 μm) – Merck, pre-washed with methanol and activated at 105°C for 20 min prior to use
2. Mobile phase (MP): Toluene–methanol–formic acid (6.5 : 3.5 : 0.1 v/v)
3. Standard/Sample application:
   Band length: 6 mm Volume applied: 2–12 μl Spacing: 6 mm
4. Chamber saturation: 20 min (MP)
5. RH (%): 55 ± 5
6. Temperature °C: 22 ± 2
7. Separation technique: Ascending
8. Quantity of mobile phase: 20 ml
8. Migration distance: 150 mm
9. Migration time: 35 min

Densitometric evaluation:

Wavelength: UV–254 nm Scanning mode: Reflectance/Absorbance

HRF: Aspirin—26; Atorvastatin Ca^{++}—47; Clopidogrel bisulphate—78

Linearity (ng/band): Atorvastatin Ca^{++}—150–300; Aspirin—500–3000; Clopidogrel bisulphate—500–3000

Recovery (%): 98.50–99.86 for all the three compounds

References: S.V. Londhe, S.V. Mulgund, R.S. Deshmukh and K.S. Jain, *Acta Chromatographica*, **22(2)**, 297–305, 2010.

Comments: The method validated for accuracy, precision, linearity, LOD, LOQ, specificity, robustness and ruggedness.

HPTLC : High Performance Thin Layer Chromatography
HPTLC Densitogram

No. 478

Rosuvastatin calcium

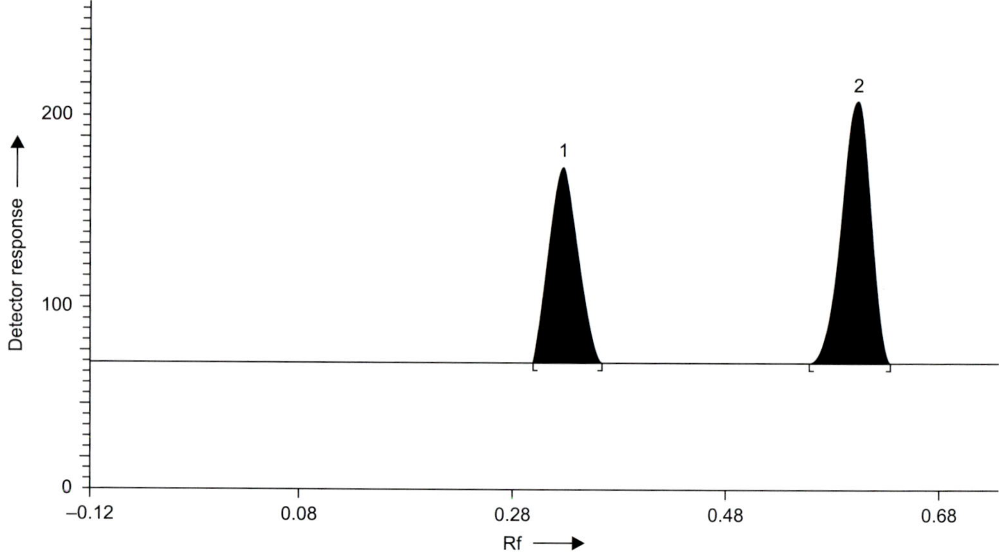

Typical densitogram of the standard containing rosuvastatin Ca^{++} and ezetimibe. For detailed experimental and chromatographic conditions, refer to Protocol No. 478. Peaks identification: 1. Rosuvastatin Ca^{++}; 2. Ezetimibe.

PROTOCOL FOR HPTLC ANALYSIS OF PHARMACEUTICAL FORMULATION

Protocol No. 478

Formulation: Rosuvastatin calcium, Ezetimibe

Classification: Miscellaneous **Dosage form:** Tablets

Standard preparation: Prepare 100 µg/ml solution of each drug in methanol. Apply 1–10 µl of each for linearity profile.

Sample preparation: Weigh powdered sample equivalent to 10 mg of rosuvastatin, suspend in 50 ml of methanol, shake for 10 min, dilute to 100 ml to get 100 µg/ml. Apply 5 µl of solution to carry out the chromatographic analysis.

Chromatographic equipments:

Sample applicator: Camag Linomat–V

Development chamber: Camag twin-trough glass chamber, 10 × 10 cm

Densitometric scanner: Camag TLC Scanner–III

Chromatographic conditions:

1. Stationary phase: Silica gel $60F_{254}$ pre-coated TLC plates, 10 × 10 cm (250 µm) – Merck
2. Mobile phase (MP): n-butyl acetate–chloroform–glacial acetic acid (1 : 8 : 1 v/v)
3. Standard/Sample application:
   Band length: 10 mm Volume applied: 1–10 µl Spacing: 10 mm
4. Chamber saturation: 30 min (MP)
5. RH (%): 55 ± 5
6. Temperature °C: 22 ± 2
7. Separation technique: Ascending
8. Quantity of mobile phase: 10 ml
8. Migration distance: 85 mm
9. Migration time: 25 mm

Densitometric evaluation:

Wavelength: UV–245 nm Scanning mode: Reflectance/Absorbance

HRF: Rosuvastatin Ca^{++}—30; Ezetimibe—58

Linearity: 100–900 ng/band for both the drugs

Recovery (%): 98–101% for both the drugs

References: Susheel John Verghese and T.K. Ravi, *J. AOAC Int.*, **93(4)**, 1222–1227, 2010.

Comments:

- The method validated for accuracy, precision, linearity, LOD, LOQ, specificity, robustness and ruggedness.
- The sample was simultaneous analysed by RP–HPLC. Both the methods were found to give comparable results.

HPTLC : High Performance Thin Layer Chromatography
HPTLC Densitogram

No. 479

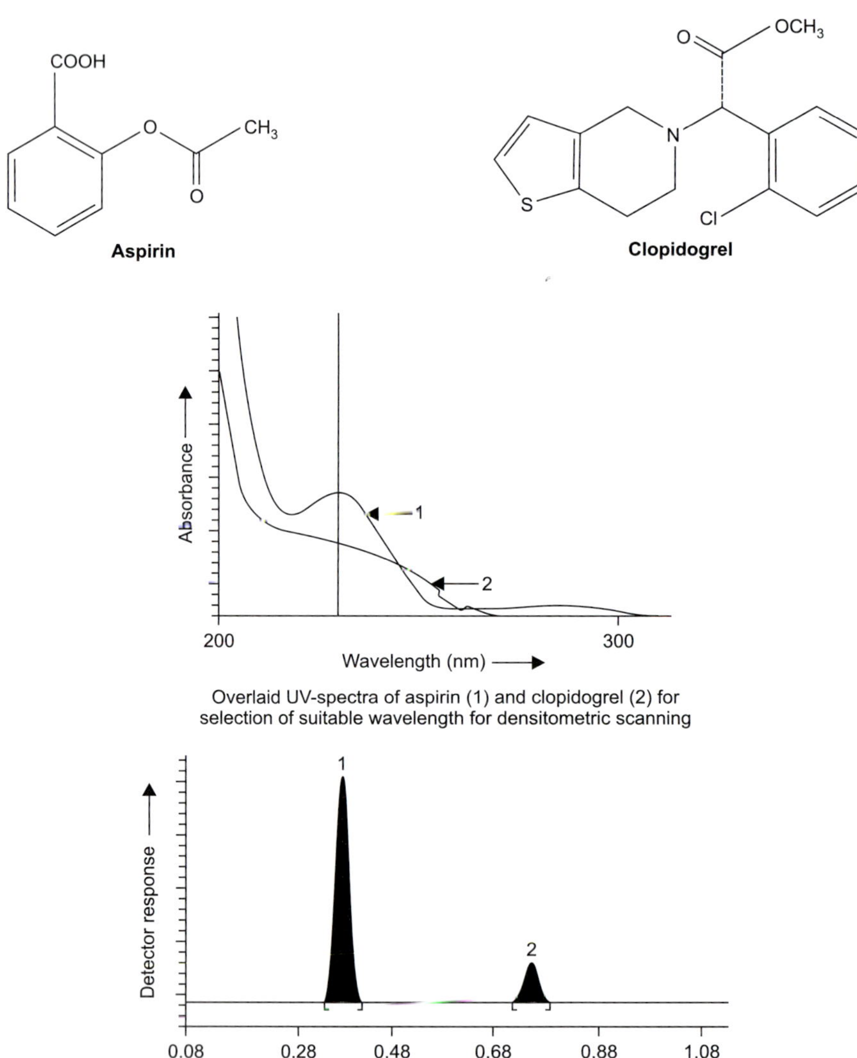

Overlaid UV-spectra of aspirin (1) and clopidogrel (2) for selection of suitable wavelength for densitometric scanning

Typical densitogram of the standard containing aspirin and clopidogrel bisulphate. For detailed experimental and chromatographic conditions, refer to Protocol No. 479. Peaks identification: 1. Aspirin; 2. Clopidogrel bisulphate.

PROTOCOL FOR HPTLC ANALYSIS OF PHARMACEUTICAL FORMULATION

Protocol No. 479

Formulation: Aspirin, Clopidogrel bisulphate

Classification: Miscellaneous **Dosage form:** Tablets

Standard preparation: Prepare 1 mg/ml solution of each compound separately in methanol. Apply 2–10 μl of each solution for linearity profile.

Sample preparation: Powdered sample equivalent to 10 mg of aspirin suspended in methanol, sonicated, diluted to 10 ml, filtered and 5 μl each of sample and standard solution applied for assay.

Chromatographic equipments:

Sample applicator: Camag Linomat–V

Development chamber: Camag twin-trough glass chamber, 10 × 10 cm

Densitometric scanner: Camag TLC Scanner–III

Chromatographic conditions:

1. Stationary phase: Silica gel $60F_{254}$ pre-coated HPTLC plates, 10 × 10 cm (200 μm) – Merck, pre-washed with methanol, dried at 110°C (30 min) prior to use
2. Mobile phase (MP): Toluene–ethyl acetate–glacial acetate acid (2 : 8 : 0.3 v/v)
3. Standard/Sample application:
   Band length: 4 mm Volume applied: 2–10 μl Spacing: 10 mm
4. Chamber saturation: 30 min (MP)
5. RH (%): 55 ± 5
6. Temperature °C: 22 ± 2
7. Separation technique: Ascending
8. Quantity of mobile phase: 10 ml
8. Migration distance: 82 mm
9. Migration time: 22 min

Densitometric evaluation:

Wavelength: UV–275 nm Scanning mode: Reflectance/Absorbance

HRF: Aspirin—37; Clopidogrel bisulphate—75

Linearity: 2–10 μg/band for both the compounds

Recovery (%): 100.50–103.0 for both the compounds

References: M. Gandhimathi, T.K. Ravi and N. Shukla, *Indian Drugs*, **5**, 397–399, 2006.

Comments: The method validated for accuracy, precision, linearity, LOD, LOQ, specificity, robustness and ruggedness.

HPTLC : High Performance Thin Layer Chromatography
HPTLC Densitogram

No. 480

Aspirin

Clopidogrel

Overlaid UV-spectra of aspirin (1) and clopidogrel bisulphate (2) for selection of suitable wavelength for densitometric scanning

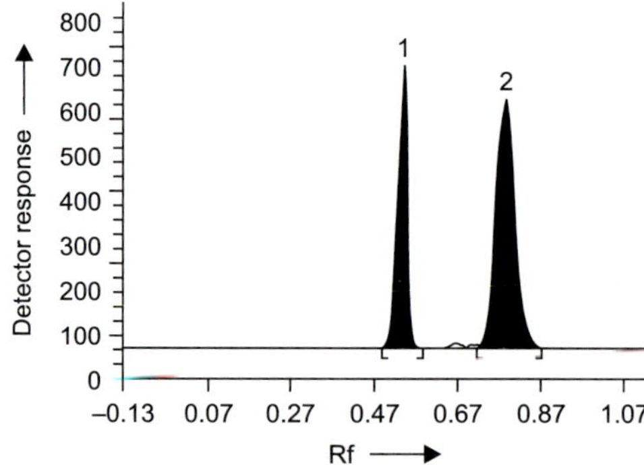

Typical densitogram of the standard containing aspirin and clopidogrel bisulphate. For detailed experimental and chromatographic conditions, refer to Protocol No. 480. Peaks identification: 1. Aspirin; 2. Clopidogrel bisulphate.

PROTOCOL FOR HPTLC ANALYSIS OF PHARMACEUTICAL FORMULATION

Protocol No. 480

Formulation: Aspirin, Clopidogrel bisulphate

Classification: Miscellaneous **Dosage form:** Tablets

Standard preparation: Prepare 100 μg/ml solution of each compound in methanol separately. Further dilutions made for linearity profile. Apply 10 μl of each solution for chromatographic evaluation.

Sample preparation: Powdered sample equivalent to 75 mg of aspirin suspended in methanol, sonicated for 10 min, diluted and filtered. The filtrate suitably diluted to get 12 μg/ml of each compound for assay.

Chromatographic equipments:

Sample applicator: Camag Linomat–V

Development chamber: Camag twin-trough glass chamber, 10 × 10 cm

Densitometric scanner: Camag TLC Scanner–III

Chromatographic conditions:

1. Stationary phase: Silica gel $60F_{254}$ pre-coated HPTLC plates, 10 × 10 cm (200 μm) – Merck
2. Mobile phase (MP): Ethyl acetate–methanol–toluene–glacial acetic acid (5 : 1 : 4 : 0.1 v/v)
3. Standard/Sample application:
   Band length: 6 mm Volume applied: 10 μl Spacing: 5 mm
4. Chamber saturation: 30 min (MP)
5. RH (%): 55 ± 5
6. Temperature °C: 22 ± 2
7. Separation technique: Ascending
8. Quantity of mobile phase: 10 ml
8. Migration distance: 80 mm
9. Migration time: 20 min

Densitometric evaluation:

Wavelength: UV–235 nm Scanning mode: Reflectance/Absorbance

HRF: Aspirin—55; Clopidogrel bisulphate—79

Linearity: 40–240 ng/band for both the drugs

Recovery (%): 99.98–100.16 for both the compounds

References: R.B. Patel and M.B. Shankar, *J. AOAC Int.*, **91(4)**, 750–754, 2008

Comments:

- The method validated for accuracy, precision, linearity, LOD, LOQ, specificity, robustness and ruggedness.
- The analytical results by HPTLC method were comparable with HPLC method.

HPTLC : High Performance Thin Layer Chromatography
HPTLC Densitogram

No. 481

Aspirin

Clopidogrel

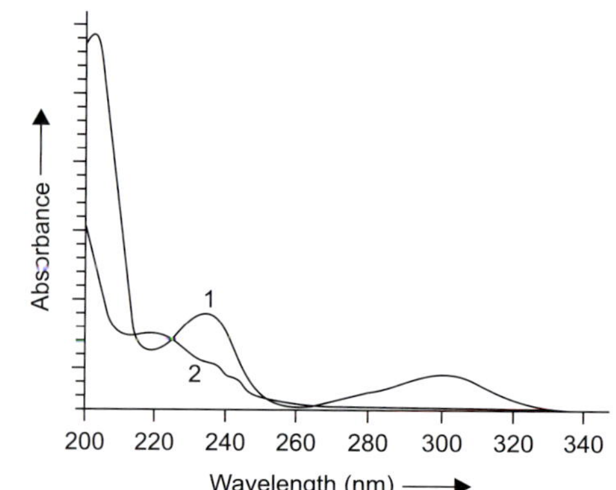

Overlaid UV-spectra of aspirin (1) and clopidogrel (2) for selection of suitable wavelength for densitometric scanning

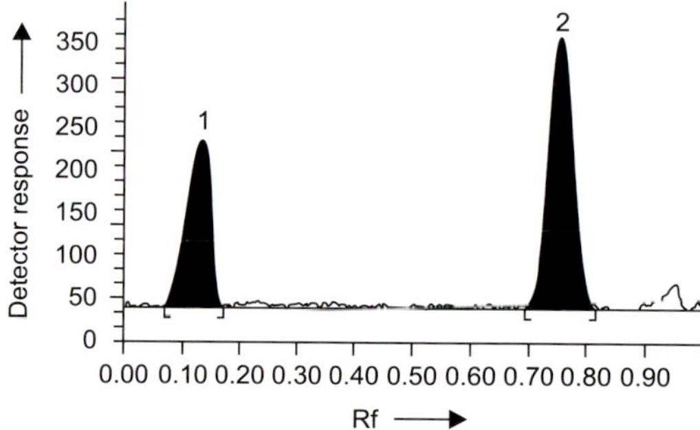

Typical densitogram of the standard containing aspirin and clopidogrel bisulphate. For detailed experimental and chromatographic conditions, refer to Protocol No. 481. Peaks identification: 1. Aspirin; 2. Clopidogrel bisulphate.

PROTOCOL FOR HPTLC ANALYSIS OF PHARMACEUTICAL FORMULATION

Protocol No. 481

Formulation: Aspirin, Clopidogrel bisulphate

Classification: Miscellaneous **Dosage form:** Tablets

Standard preparation: Prepare 1 mg/ml solution of each compound separately in methanol. Different volumes of each solution were spotted for linearity profile.

Sample preparation: Powdered sample equivalent to 75 mg of aspirin was dispersed in methanol, sonicated, diluted, filtered through Whatman No. 41 filter paper, the filtrate spotted for assay along with standard solution.

Chromatographic equipments:

Sample applicator: Camag Linomat–V

Development chamber: Camag twin-trough glass chamber, 10 × 10 cm

Densitometric scanner: Camag TLC Scanner–III

Chromatographic conditions:

1. Stationary phase: Silica gel $60F_{254}$ pre-coated TLC plates, 10 × 10 cm (250 μm) – Merck
2. Mobile phase (MP): Carbon tetrachloride–acetone (6 : 2.4 v/v)
3. Standard/Sample application:
   Band length: 4 mm   Volume applied: 5 μl   Spacing: 10 mm
4. Chamber saturation: 20 min (MP)
5. RH (%): 55 ± 5
6. Temperature °C: 22 ± 2
7. Separation technique: Ascending
8. Quantity of mobile phase: 16 ml
8. Migration distance: 70 mm
9. Migration time: 15 min

Densitometric evaluation:

Wavelength: UV–220 nm   Scanning mode: Reflectance/Absorbance

HRF: Aspirin—13; Clopidogrel bisulphate—78

Linearity (ng/band): Aspirin—200–600; Clopidogrel bisulphate—300–600

Recovery (%): Aspirin—97.5–102; Clopidogrel bisulphate—98.5–101.2

References: P.K. Sinha, M.C. Damle and K.G. Botha, *Eurasian J. Anal. Chem.*, **4(2)**, 152–160, 2009.

Comments:

- The method validated for accuracy, precision, linearity, LOD, LOQ, specificity, robustness and ruggedness.
- The method is stability indicating (acid, base, oxidative, thermal, photolytic). The degradation products were separated from main compounds.

HPTLC : High Performance Thin Layer Chromatography
HPTLC Densitogram

No. 482

COOH
O
CH_3
O
Aspirin

N N N N
H N O
Cilostazole

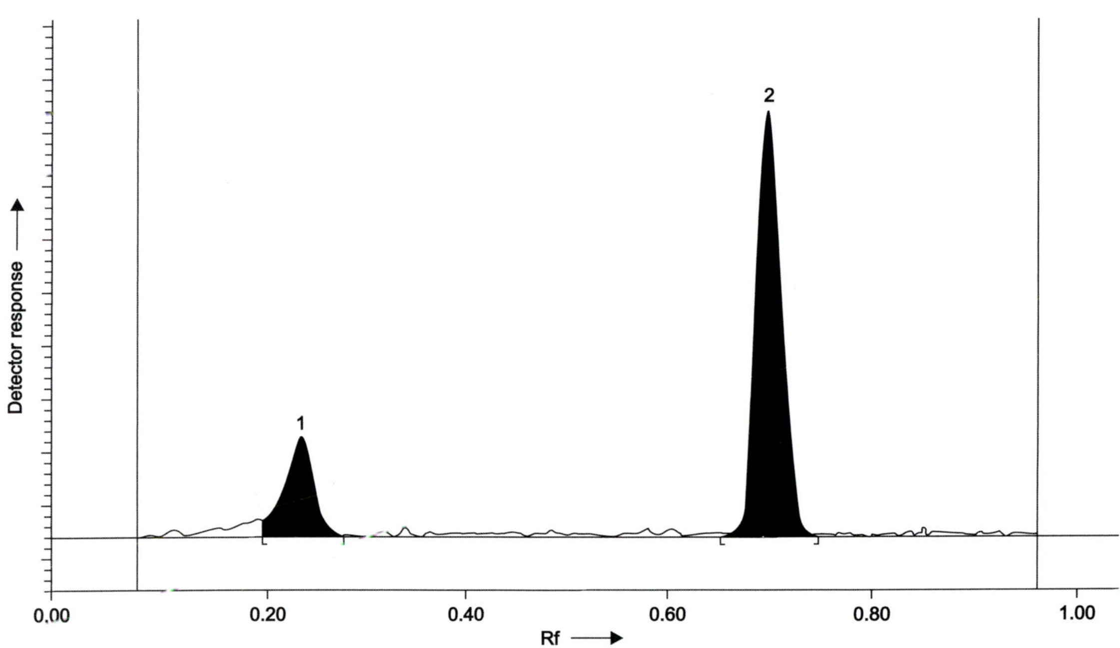

Typical densitogram of the analyte mixture containing aspirin and cilostazol. For detailed experimental and chromatographic conditions, refer to Protocol No. 482. Peaks identification: 1. Aspirin; 2. Cilostazol.

PROTOCOL FOR HPTLC ANALYSIS OF PHARMACEUTICAL FORMULATION

Protocol No. 482

Formulation: Aspirin, Cilostazol

Classification: Miscellaneous **Dosage form:** Analyte

Standard preparation: Prepare 1 mg/ml solution of each compound separately in methanol. Further serial dilutions are made with methanol. Apply 5 μl of each solution for linearity profile.

Sample preparation: Powdered sample equivalent to 10 mg of aspirin suspended in methanol, sonicated, diluted and filtered. The filtrate suitably diluted with methanol. Apply 5 μl for chromatographic analysis.

Chromatographic equipments:

Sample applicator: Camag Linomat–V

Development chamber: Camag twin-trough glass chamber, 10 × 10 cm

Densitometric scanner: Camag TLC Scanner–III

Chromatographic conditions:

1. Stationary phase: Silica gel 60F_{254} pre-coated TLC plates, 10 × 10 cm (250 μm) – Merck
2. Mobile phase (MP): Toluene–ethyl acetate–methanol–diethylether (2 : 2 : 1 : 0.5 v/v)
3. Standard/Sample application:
   Band length: 6 mm Volume applied: 5 μl Spacing: 6 mm
4. Chamber saturation: 15 min (MP)
5. RH (%): 55 ± 5
6. Temperature °C: 22 ± 2
7. Separation technique: Ascending
8. Quantity of mobile phase: 11 ml
8. Migration distance: 80 mm
9. Migration time: 20 min

Densitometric evaluation:

Wavelength: UV–257 nm Scanning mode: Reflectance/Absorbance

HRF: Aspirin—24; Cilostazol—72

Linearity (ng/band): Aspirin—75–525; Cilostazol—200–700

Recovery (%): Aspirin—98.4–99.80; Cilostazol—99.30–100.27

References: Personal communication, Jesh V. Patel, Shri Sarvajanik Pharmacy College, Gujarat.

Comments: The method validated for accuracy, precision, linearity, LOD and LOQ.

HPTLC : High Performance Thin Layer Chromatography
HPTLC Densitogram

No. 483

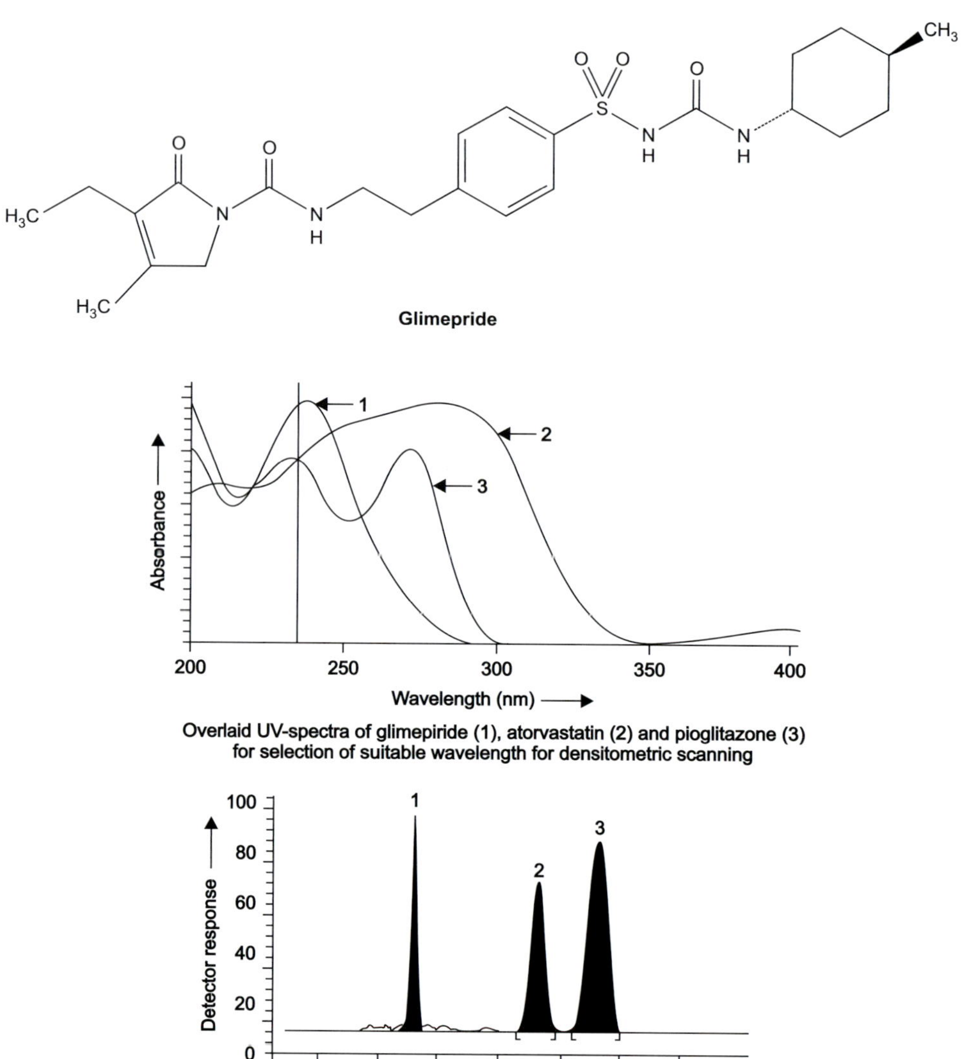

Typical densitogram of the standard containing glimepiride and pioglitazone. For detailed experimental and chromatographic conditions, refer to Protocol No. 483. Peaks identification: 1. Atorvastatin (IS); 2. Glimepiride; 3. Pioglitazone.

PROTOCOL FOR HPTLC ANALYSIS OF PHARMACEUTICAL FORMULATION

Protocol No. 483

Formulation: **Pioglitazone, Glimepiride**

Classification: Miscellaneous **Dosage form:** Tablets

Standard preparation: Prepare standard solutions of each compound including (IS) separately in MP to get final concentration of pioglitazone (1500 μg/ml); glimepiride (200 μg/ml); atorvastatin–IS (500 μg/ml). Prepare serial dilutions for linearity studies. Apply 10 μl of each solution.

Sample preparation: Powdered sample, accurately weighed, suspended in methanol, sonicated, diluted after adding required amount of (IS). Filtered and filtrate suitably diluted with methanol for assay. Apply 10 μl for chromatographic separation.

Chromatographic equipments:

Sample applicator: Camag Linomat–V

Development chamber: Camag twin-trough glass chamber, 10 × 10 cm

Densitometric scanner: Camag TLC Scanner–III

Chromatographic conditions:

1. Stationary phase: Silica gel $60F_{254}$ pre-coated HPTLC plates, 10 × 10 cm 200 μm) – Merck, pre-washed with methanol, dried at 105°C (60 min) prior to use
2. Mobile phase (MP): Toluene–methanol–ethyl acetate–formic acid (7 : 2 : 1.5 : 0.01 v/v)
3. Standard/Sample application:
   Band length: 10 mm Volume applied: 10 μl Spacing: 10 mm
4. Chamber saturation: 20 min (MP)
5. RH (%): 55 ± 5
6. Temperature °C: 22 ± 2
7. Separation technique: Ascending
8. Quantity of mobile phase: 20 ml
8. Migration distance: 90 mm
9. Migration time: 20 min

Densitometric evaluation:

Wavelength: UV–235 nm Scanning mode: Reflectance/Absorbance

HRF: Atorvastatin (IS)—26; Glimepiride—47; Pioglitazone—56

Linearity (ng/band): Pioglitazone—800–2500; Glimepiride—50–400

Recovery (%): 100.13–102.22 for both the compounds

References: R.T. Sane et al., *J. Planar Chromatogr.*, **17(2)**, 154–156, 2004.

Comments: The method validated for accuracy, precision, linearity, LOD, LOQ, specificity, robustness and ruggedness.

HPTLC : High Performance Thin Layer Chromatography
HPTLC Densitogram

No. 484

H_3C N O S O NH O

Pioglitazone

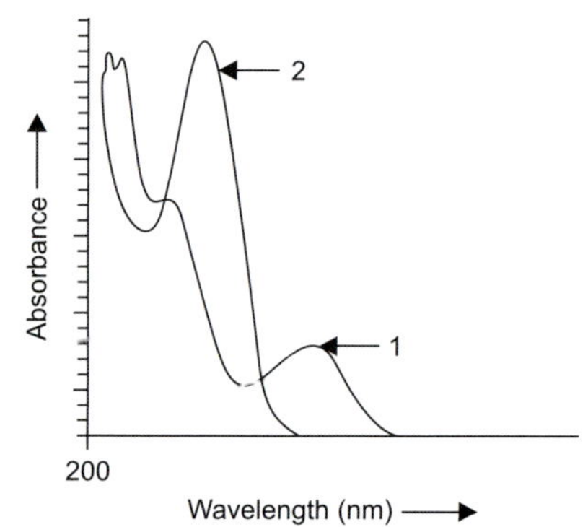

Overlaid UV-spectra of pioglitazone (1) and glimepiride (2) for selection of suitable wavelength for densitometric scanning

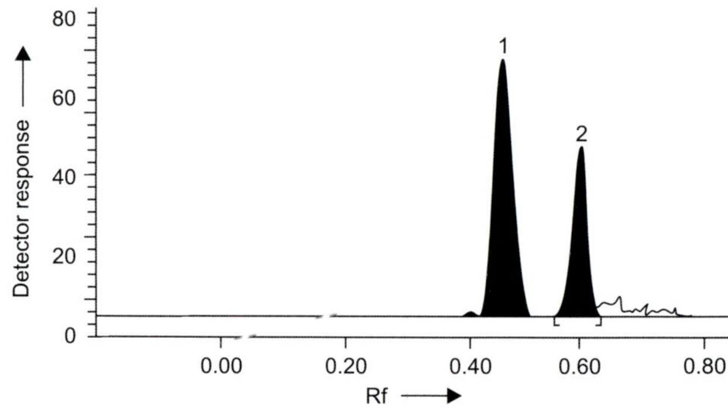

Typical densitogram of the sample containing glimepiride and pioglitazone. For detailed experimental and chromatographic conditions, refer to Protocol No. 484. Peaks identification: 1. Glimepiride; 2. Pioglitazone.

PROTOCOL FOR HPTLC ANALYSIS OF PHARMACEUTICAL FORMULATION

Protocol No. 484

Formulation: Pioglitazone, Glimepiride

Classification: Miscellaneous **Dosage form:** Tablets

Standard preparation: Prepare solution of each compound separately in methanol to get 100 μg/ml of glimepiride and 750 μg/ml of pioglitazone. Apply 2–7 μl of each solution for linearity profile.

Sample preparation: An appropriate quantity of powdered sample suspended in methanol, sonicated for 15 min, diluted and filtered. Filtrate suitably diluted with methanol. Apply 5 μl of the final solution for chromatographic separation and assay.

Chromatographic equipments:

Sample applicator: Camag Linomat–V

Development chamber: Camag twin-trough glass chamber, 10 × 10 cm

Densitometric scanner: Camag TLC Scanner–III

Chromatographic conditions:

1. Stationary phase: Silica gel $60F_{254}$ pre-coated HPTLC plates, 10 × 10 cm (200 μm) – Merck
2. Mobile phase (MP): Toluene–ethyl acetate–methanol (5 : 4.5 : 0.5 v/v)
3. Standard/Sample application:
   Band length: 6 mm Volume applied: 2–7 μl Spacing: 8 mm
4. Chamber saturation: 30 min (MP)
5. RH (%): 55 ± 5
6. Temperature °C: 22 ± 2
7. Separation technique: Ascending
8. Quantity of mobile phase: 10 ml
8. Migration distance: 80 mm
9. Migration time: 20 min

Densitometric evaluation:

Wavelength: UV–230 nm Scanning mode: Reflectance/Absorbance

HRF: Glimepiride—45; Pioglitazone—60

Linearity (ng/band): Glimepiride—200–700; Pioglitazone—1500–5250

Recovery (%): 98.40–98.75 for both the compounds

References: Jegnesh B. Patel et al., *Asian J. Chem.*, **18(4)**, 2875–2878, 2006

Comments: The method validated for accuracy, precision, linearity, LOD, LOQ, specificity, robustness and ruggedness.

HPTLC : High Performance Thin Layer Chromatography
HPTLC Densitogram

No. 485

Rosiglitazone

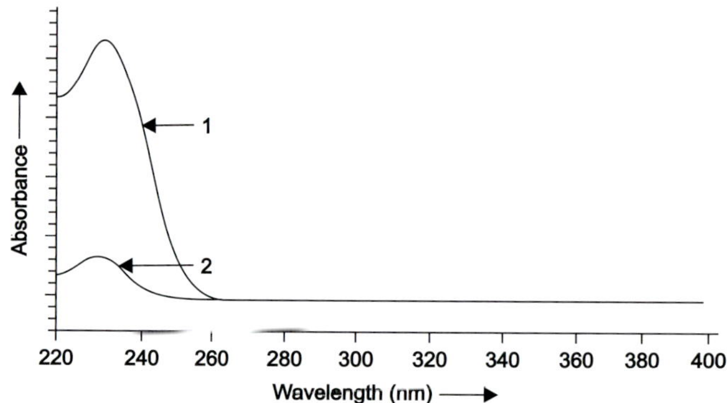

Overlaid UV-spectra of rosiglitazone (1) and gliclazide (2) for selection of suitable wavelength for densitometric scanning

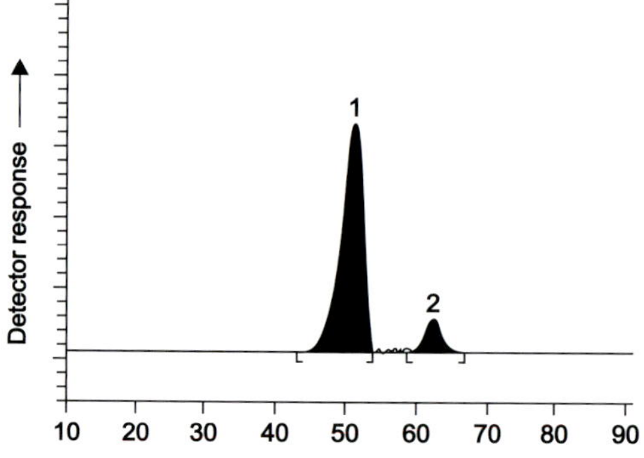

Typical densitogram of the sample containing gliclazide and rosiglitazone. For detailed experimental and chromatographic conditions, refer to Protocol No. 485. Peaks identification: 1. Gliclazide; 2. Rosiglitazone.

PROTOCOL FOR HPTLC ANALYSIS OF PHARMACEUTICAL FORMULATION

Protocol No. 485

Formulation: Rosiglitazone, Gliclazide

Classification: Miscellaneous **Dosage form:** Tablets

Standard preparation: Prepare 1 mg/ml solution of each compound separately in MP. Further serial dilutions are made with MP for linearity profile. Apply 10 μl of each solution for chromatographic evaluation.

Sample preparation: Powdered sample equivalent to 80 mg of gliclazide suspended in 50 ml of MP, sonicated, diluted, filtered and filtrate suitably diluted. Apply 10 μl for chromatographic separation and analysis.

Chromatographic equipments:

Sample applicator: Camag Linomat–IV

Development chamber: Camag twin-trough glass chamber, 10 × 10 cm

Densitometric scanner: Camag TLC Scanner–III

Chromatographic conditions:

1. Stationary phase: Silica gel $60F_{254}$ pre-coated HPTLC plates, 10 × 10 cm (200 μm) – Merck
2. Mobile phase (MP): Toluene–ethyl acetate–methanol (8.5 : 0.5 : 1 v/v)
3. Standard/Sample application:
   Band length: 6 mm Volume applied: 10 μl Spacing: 15 mm
4. Chamber saturation: 30 min (MP)
5. RH (%): 55 ± 5
6. Temperature °C: 22 ± 2
7. Separation technique: Ascending
8. Quantity of mobile phase: 10 ml
8. Migration distance: 120 mm
9. Migration time: 50 min

Densitometric evaluation:

Wavelength: UV–230 nm Scanning mode: Reflectance/Absorbance

HRF: Gliclazide—36; Rosiglitazone—47

Linearity (ng/band): Pioglitazone—50–100; Gliclazide—1000–3000

Recovery (%): 98.15–99.50 for both the compounds

References: S. Gayatri, A. Shantha and V. Vaidya, *Ind. J. Pharm Sci.*, **65(6)**, 503, 2003.

Comments: The method validated for accuracy, precision, linearity, LOD, LOQ, specificity, robustness and ruggedness.

HPTLC : High Performance Thin Layer Chromatography
HPTLC Densitogram

No. 486

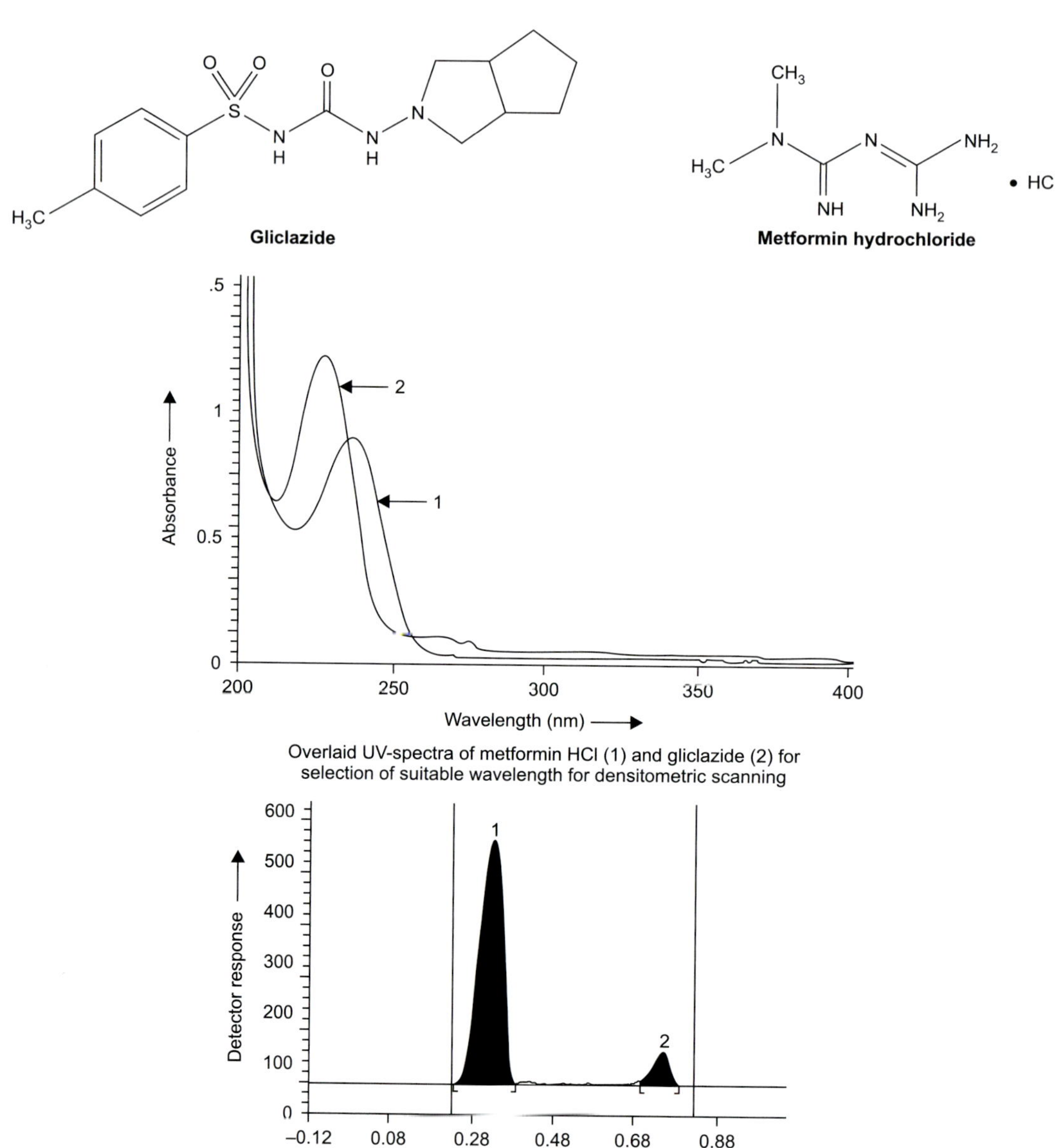

Overlaid UV-spectra of metformin HCl (1) and gliclazide (2) for selection of suitable wavelength for densitometric scanning

Typical densitogram of the standard containing metformin and gliclazide. For detailed experimental and chromatographic conditions, refer to Protocol No. 486. Peaks identification: 1. Metformin HCl; 2. Gliclazide.

PROTOCOL FOR HPTLC ANALYSIS OF PHARMACEUTICAL FORMULATION

Protocol No. 486

Formulation: Metformin hydrochloride, Gliclazide

Classification: Miscellaneous **Dosage form:** Tablets

Standard preparation: Prepare 50 mg/ml solution of metformin and 160 μg/ml solution of gliclazide, both in methanol. Further serial dilutions made with methanol for linearity profile. Apply 1–5 μl of each solution for chromatographic separation.

Sample preparation: An appropriate quantity of powdered sample equivalent to 30 mg of gliclazide suspended in 20 ml of methanol, sonicated for 15 min, diluted to 25 ml, filtered and the filtrate suitably diluted. Apply 3 μl of the resulting solution for assay.

Chromatographic equipments:

Sample applicator: Camag Linomat–V
Development chamber: Camag twin-trough glass chamber, 10 × 10 cm
Densitometric scanner: Camag TLC Scanner–III

Chromatographic conditions:

1. Stationary phase: Silica gel 60F_{254} pre-coated TLC plates, 10 × 10 cm (250 μm) – Merck, pre-washed with methanol, activated at 110°C for 5 min prior to use
2. Mobile phase (MP): 0.25% ammonium sulphate–methanol–ethyl acetate (10 : 2.5 : 2.5 v/v)
3. Standard/Sample application:
   Band length: 6 mm Volume applied: 1–5 μl Spacing: 5 mm
4. Chamber saturation: 30 min (MP)
5. RH (%): 60 ± 5
6. Temperature °C: 25 ± 2
7. Separation technique: Ascending
8. Quantity of mobile phase: 15 ml
8. Migration distance: 80 mm
9. Migration time: 18 min

Densitometric evaluation:

Wavelength: UV–236 nm (iso-absorption point)
Scanning mode: Reflectance/Absorbance
HRF: Metformin HCl—32; Gliclazide—73
Linearity: Metformin HCl—10–50 μg/band; Gliclazide—100–500 ng/band
Recovery (%): 99.58–100.74 for both the compounds

References: Shweta S. Havele and Sunil R. Dhaneshwar, *J. Liq. Chromatogr. and Related Technologies*, **34**, 966–980, 2011.

Comments: The method validated for accuracy, precision, linearity, LOD, LOQ, specificity and robustness.

HPTLC : High Performance Thin Layer Chromatography
HPTLC Densitogram

No. 487

Metformin hydrochloride

Glipizide

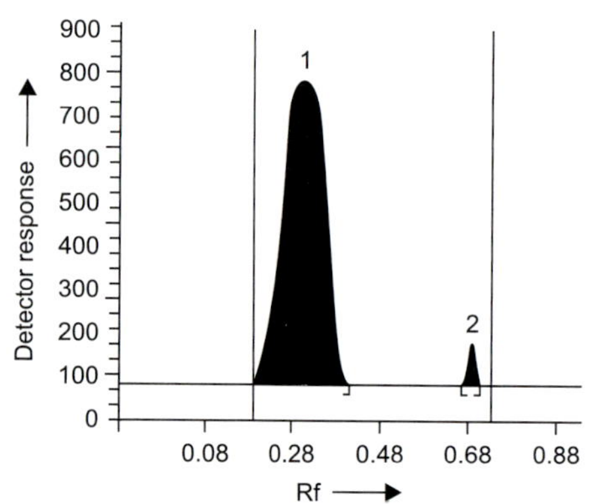

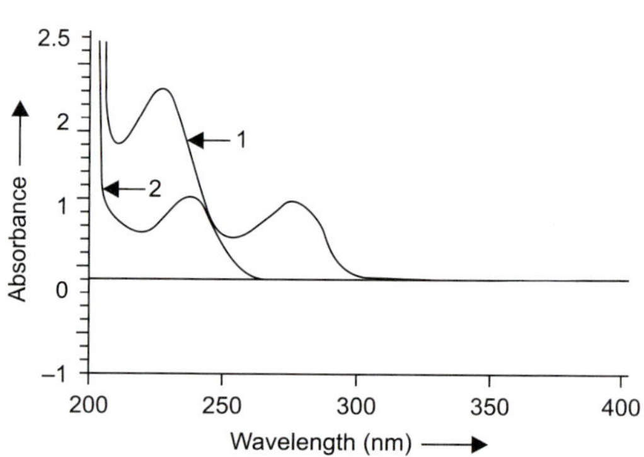

Overlaid UV-spectra of metformin HCl (1) and glipizide (2) for selection of suitable wavelength for densitometric scanning

Typical densitogram of the standard containing metformin HCl and glipizide. For detailed experimental and chromatographic conditions, refer to Protocol No. 487. Peaks identification: 1. Metformin HCl; 2. Glipizide.

PROTOCOL FOR HPTLC ANALYSIS OF PHARMACEUTICAL FORMULATION

Protocol No. 487

Formulation: Metformin hydrochloride, Glipizide

Classification: Miscellaneous **Dosage form:** Tablets

Standard preparation: Prepare solution of both the compounds separately in methanol to get 10 mg/ml of metformin HCl and 100 μg/ml of glipizide. Apply 1–5 μl of each solution for linearity profile.

Sample preparation: Powdered sample equivalent to 250 mg of metformin HCl and 2.5 mg of glipizide suspended in 20 ml of methanol, sonicated for 15 min, diluted to 25 ml and filtered through Whatman filter paper No. 41 and filtrate used for chromatographic separation and evaluation.

Chromatographic equipments:

Sample applicator: Camag Linomat–V

Development chamber: Camag twin-trough glass chamber, 10 × 10 cm

Denistometric scanner: Camag TLC Scanner–III

Chromatographic conditions:

1. Stationary phase: Silica gel $60F_{254}$ pre-coated HPTLC plates, 10 × 10 cm (200 μm) – Merck, pre-washed with methanol and activated at 80°C for 5 min prior to sample application
2. Mobile phase (MP): Ethylacetate–methanol–water–0.5% amm. sulphate (2.5 : 2.5 : 5 : 5 v/v)
3. Standard/Sample application:
   Band length: 6 mm Volume applied: 1–5 μl Spacing: 10 mm
4. Chamber saturation: 30 min (MP)
5. RH (%): 55 ± 5
6. Temperature °C: 25 ± 2
7. Separation technique: Ascending
8. Quantity of mobile phase: 15 ml
9. Migration distance: 80 mm
10. Migration time: 20 min

Densitometric evaluation:

Wavelength: UV–245 nm Scanning mode: Reflectance/Absorbance

HRF: Metformin HCl—31; Glipizide—70

Linearity (ng/band): Metformin HCl—1000–5000; Glipizide—100–500

Recovery (%): Metformin HCl—99.31–99.84; Glipizide—99.23–99.38

References: Shweta S Havel and Sunil R. Dhaneshwar, *Pelagia Research Library* (*Der Pharmacia Sinica*), **2(1)**, 40–8, 2011.

Comments: The method validated for accuracy, precision, linearity, LOD, LOQ, specificity and robustness.

HPTLC : High Performance Thin Layer Chromatography
HPTLC Densitogram

No. 488

Glimepride

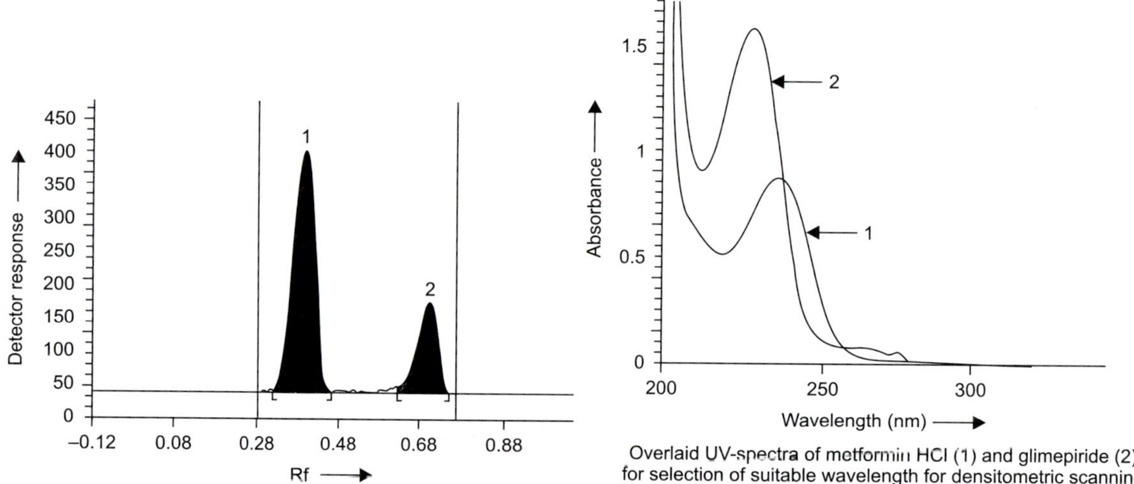

Overlaid UV-spectra of metformin HCl (1) and glimepiride (2) for selection of suitable wavelength for densitometric scanning

Typical densitogram of the standard containing metformin HCl and glimepiride. For detailed experimental and chromatographic conditions, refer to Protocol No. 488. Peaks identification: 1. Metformin HCl; 2. Glimepiride.

PROTOCOL FOR HPTLC ANALYSIS OF PHARMACEUTICAL FORMULATION

Protocol No. 488

Formulation: Metformin hydrochloride, Glimepiride

Classification: Miscellaneous **Dosage form:** Tablets

Standard preparation: Prepare 10 mg/ml solution of metformin HCl and 100 μg/ml solution of glimepiride, both in methanol. Further serial dilutions made with methanol for linearity studies. Apply 6–10 μl of each solution for chromatographic separation.

Sample preparation: Powdered sample equivalent to 1 mg of glimepiride suspended in 20 ml of methanol, sonicated for 15 min, diluted to 25 ml, filtered and the filtrate suitably diluted. Apply 8 μl of the resulting solution for assay.

Chromatographic equipments:

Sample applicator: Camag Linomat–V

Development chamber: Camag twin-trough glass chamber, 10 × 10 cm

Densitometric scanner: Camag TLC Scanner

Chromatographic conditions:

1. Stationary phase: Silica gel 60F_{254} pre-coated TLC plates, 10 × 10 cm (250 μm) – Merck, pre-washed with methanol, activated at 110°C for 5 min prior to use
2. Mobile phase (MP): 0.25% ammonium sulphate–methanol–ethyl acetate (10 : 2.5 : 2.5 v/v)
3. Standard/Sample application:
   Band length: 6 mm Volume applied: 6–10 μl Spacing: 5 mm
4. Chamber saturation: 30 min (MP)
5. RH (%): 60 ± 5
6. Temperature °C: 25 ± 2
7. Separation technique: Ascending
8. Quantity of mobile phase: 15 ml
8. Migration distance: 80 mm
9. Migration time: 18 min

Densitometric evaluation:

Wavelength: UV–236 nm (iso-absorption point)

Scanning mode: Reflectance/Absorbance

HRF: Metformin HCl—39; Glimepiride—69

Linearity: Metformin HCl—150–250 μg/band; Glimepiride—300–500 ng/band

Recovery (%): 99.23–99.84 for both the compounds

References: Jegnesh B. Patel et al., *Asian J. Chem.*, **18(4)**, 2875–2878, 2006

Comments: The method validated for accuracy, precision, linearity, LOD, LOQ, specificity, robustness and ruggedness.

HPTLC : High Performance Thin Layer Chromatography
HPTLC Densitogram

No. 489

Metformin hydrochloride

Nateglinide

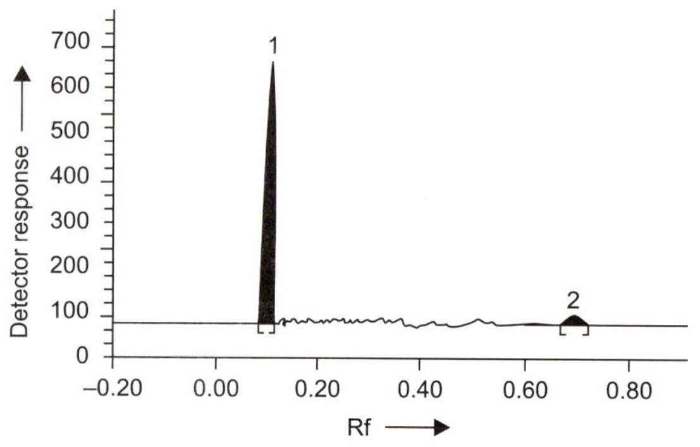

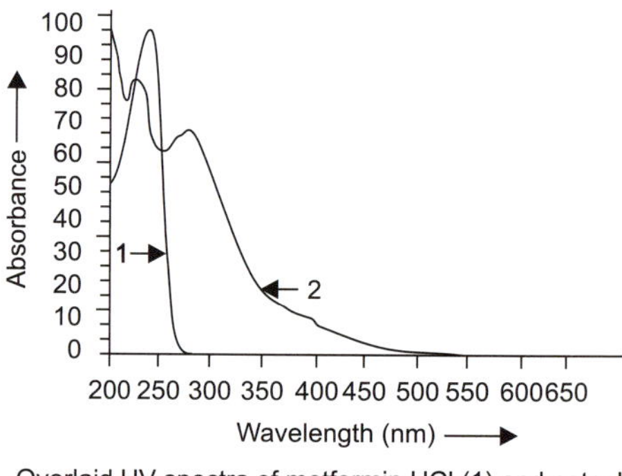

Overlaid UV-spectra of metformin HCl (1) and nateglinide (2) for selection of suitable wavelength for densitometric scanning

Typical densitogram of the sample containing metformin hydrochloride. For detailed experimental and chromatographic conditions, refer to Protocol No. 489. Peaks identification: 1. Metformin HCl; 2. Nateglinide.

PROTOCOL FOR HPTLC ANALYSIS OF PHARMACEUTICAL FORMULATION

Protocol No. 489

Formulation: Metformin hydrochloride, Nateglinide

Classification: Miscellaneous **Dosage form:** Tablets

Standard preparation: Prepare 1 mg/ml solution of each compound in methanol. Further serial dilutions made with methanol for linearity profile.

Sample preparation: Powdered sample equivalent to 100 mg of metformin hydrochloride suspended in 70 ml of methanol, sonicated for 30 min, diluted to 100 ml with methanol, filtered and further diluted suitably with methanol and used for chromatographic analysis.

Chromatographic equipments:

Sample applicator: Camag Linomat–V

Development chamber: Camag twin-trough glass chamber, 10 × 10 cm

Densitometric scanner: Camag TLC Scanner–III

Chromatographic conditions:

1. Stationary phase: Silica gel 60F_{254} pre-coated TLC plates, 10 × 10 cm (250 µm) – Merck
2. Mobile phase (MP): Chloroform–ethyl acetate–glacial acetic acid (4 : 6 : 0.1 v/v)
3. Standard/Sample application:
   Band length: 6 mm Volume applied: 10 µl Spacing: 10 mm
4. Chamber saturation: 20 min (MP)
5. RH (%): 55 ± 5
6. Temperature °C: 25 ± 2
7. Separation technique: Ascending
8. Quantity of mobile phase: 10 ml
8. Migration distance: 80 mm
9. Migration time: 15 min

Densitometric evaluation:

Wavelength: UV–216 nm Scanning mode: Reflectance/Absorbance

HRF: Metformin HCl—10; Nateglinide—70

Linearity (ng/band): Metformin HCl—500–3000; Nateglinide—600–2400

Recovery (%): 99.72–100.08 for both the compounds

References: A.B. Thomas et al., Personal communication.

Comments:

- The method validated for accuracy, precision, linearity, LOD, LOQ, specificity, robustness and ruggedness.
- The method is stability indicating (acid, base, oxidative, thermal, photolytic). The degradation products were separated from main compounds.

HPTLC : High Performance Thin Layer Chromatography
HPTLC Densitogram

No. 490

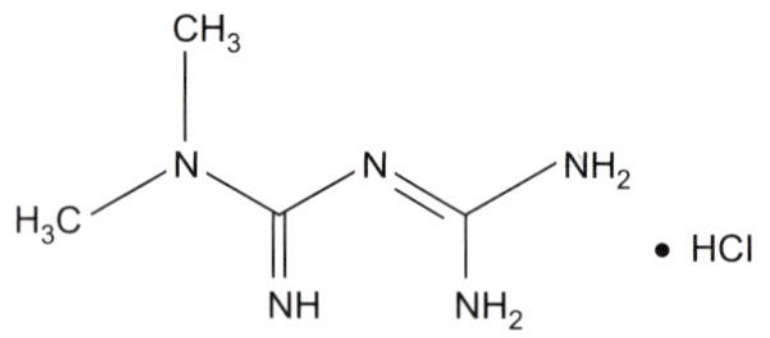

Metformin hydrochloride

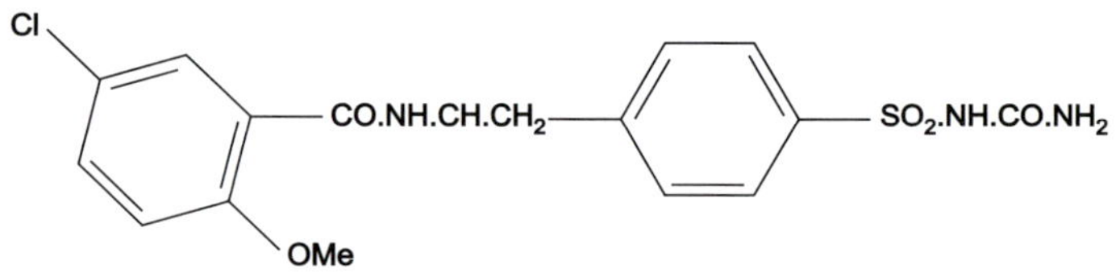

Glyburide

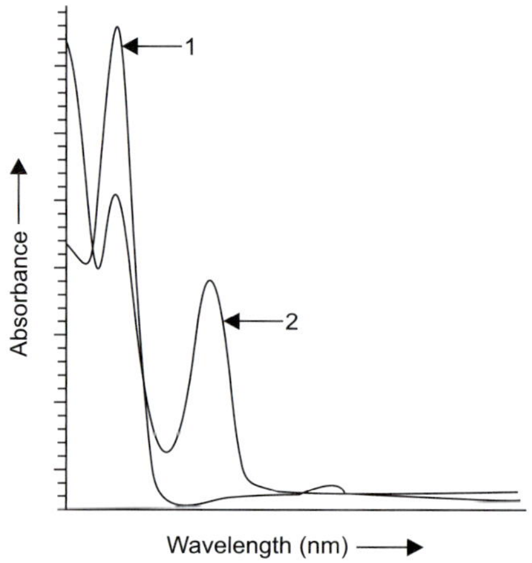

Overlaid UV-spectra of metformin HCl (1) and glyburide (2) for selection of suitable wavelength for densitometric scanning

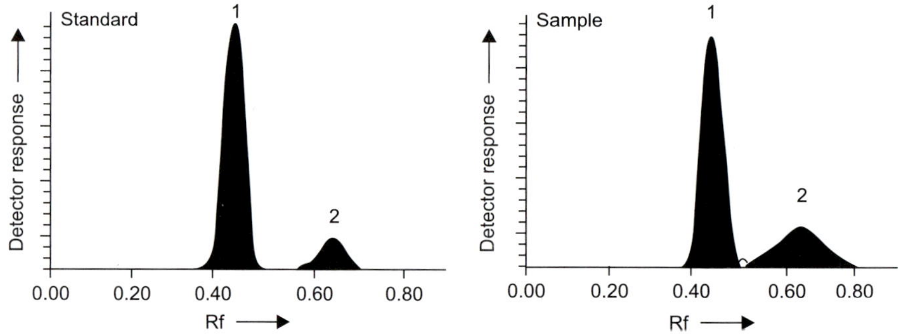

Typical densitogram of the standard and sample containing metformin HCl and glyburide. For detailed experimental and chromatographic conditions, refer to Protocol No. 490. Peaks identification: 1. Metformin HCl; 2. Glyburide.

PROTOCOL FOR HPTLC ANALYSIS OF PHARMACEUTICAL FORMULATION

Protocol No. 490

Formulation: Metformin hydrochloride, Glyburide

Classification: Miscellaneous **Dosage form:** Tablets

Standard preparation: Prepare solution of both the compounds separately in methanol. Further dilutions were made with methanol for linearity studies.

Sample preparation: Powdered sample equivalent to 500 mg of metformin HCl suspended in methanol, sonicated, suitably diluted with methanol, filtered and the filtrate used for chromatographic evaluation.

Chromatographic equipments:

Sample applicator: Camag Linomat–V

Development chamber: Camag horizontal chamber, 10 × 10 cm

Densitometric scanner: Camag TLC Scanner–III

Chromatographic conditions:

1. Stationary phase: Silica gel 60F_{254} pre-coated TLC plates, 10 × 10 cm (250 μm) – Merck
2. Mobile phase (MP): Water–methanol (2 : 1 v/v) containing 0.5% ammonium sulphate
3. Standard/Sample application:
   Band length: 4 mm Volume applied: 2 μl Spacing: 10 mm
4. Chamber saturation: —
5. RH (%): 55 ± 5
6. Temperature °C: 22 ± 2
7. Separation technique: Ascending
8. Quantity of mobile phase: 12 ml
8. Migration distance: 85 mm
9. Migration time: 25 min

Densitometric evaluation:

Wavelength: UV–237 nm Scanning mode: Reflectance/Absorbance

HRF: Metformin HCl—43; Glyburide—64

Linearity (ng/band): Metformin HCl—500–20000; Glyburide—50–2000

Recovery (%): Metformin HCl—95.16–103.19; Glyburide—91.10–108.31

References: A. Ghassempour, M. Ahmadi, S.N. Ebrahimi and H.Y. Aboul-Enein, *Chromatographia*, **64(1–2)**, 101–104, 2006.

Comments: The method validated for accuracy, precision, linearity, LOD, LOQ and selectivity.

HPTLC : High Performance Thin Layer Chromatography
HPTLC Densitogram

No. 491

• HCl

Metformin hydrochloride

• H_3PO_4 • H_2O

Sitagliptin phosphate monohydrate

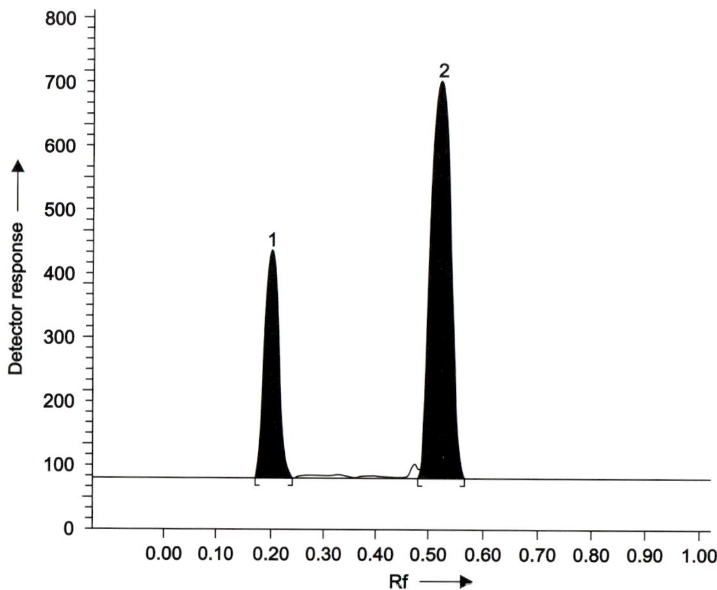

Typical densitogram of the standard containing metformin HCl and sitagliptin phosphate. For detailed experimental and chromatographic conditions, refer to Protocol No. 491. Peaks identification: 1. Sitagliptin phosphate; 2. Metformin HCl.

PROTOCOL FOR HPTLC ANALYSIS OF PHARMACEUTICAL FORMULATION

Protocol No. 491

Formulation: Metformin hydrochloride, Sitagliptin phosphate

Classification: Miscellaneous **Dosage form:** Tablets

Standard preparation: Both the drugs were initially dissolved in DMFO and further diluted with methanol to get final solutions to contain 10 μg/ml of sitagliptin and 100 μg/ml of metformin. Apply varying volumes of each solution for linearity profile.

Sample preparation: Powdered sample equivalent to 10 mg of sitagliptin suspended in 5 ml of methanol, shaken for 10 min, diluted to 10 ml with methanol, centrifuged for 5 min at 2000 rpm and 0.2 ml of supernatant diluted to 10 ml with methanol. Apply 2 μl for assay.

Chromatographic equipments:

Sample applicator: Camag Linomat–V

Development chamber: Camag twin-trough glass chamber, 10 × 10 cm

Densitometric scanner: Camag TLC Scanner–III

Chromatographic conditions:

1. Stationary phase: Silica gel 60F_{254} pre-coated HPTLC plates, 10 × 10 cm (200 μm) – Merck
2. Mobile phase (MP): Acetonitrile–methanol–glacial acetic acid (7 : 3 : 0.02 v/v)
3. Standard/Sample application:
   Band length: — Volume applied: 2 μl Spacing: —
4. Chamber saturation: 10 min (MP)
5. RH (%): 60 ± 5
6. Temperature °C: 20 ± 2
7. Separation technique: Ascending
8. Quantity of mobile phase: 10 ml
9. Migration distance: —
10. Migration time: —

Densitometric evaluation:

Wavelength: UV–216 nm Scanning mode: Reflectance/Absorbance

HRF: Sitagliptin—21; Metformin HCl—53

Linearity (ng/band): Metformin HCl—80–640; Sitagliptin—8–64

Recovery (%): 99.54–101.01 for both the drugs

References: D.S. Desai, P.S. Lohe, A.N. Maliye and S.G. Walode, Abstract No. F-266, 63rd IPC, 2011. Courtesy: Prof. S.G. Walode.

Comments:

- The method validated for accuracy, precision, linearity, LOD, LOQ, specificity, robustness and ruggedness.
- The method is stability indicating (acid, base, oxidative, thermal, photolytic). The degradation products were separated from main compounds.

HPTLC : High Performance Thin Layer Chromatography
HPTLC Densitogram

No. 492

Metformin hydrochloride

Pioglitazone

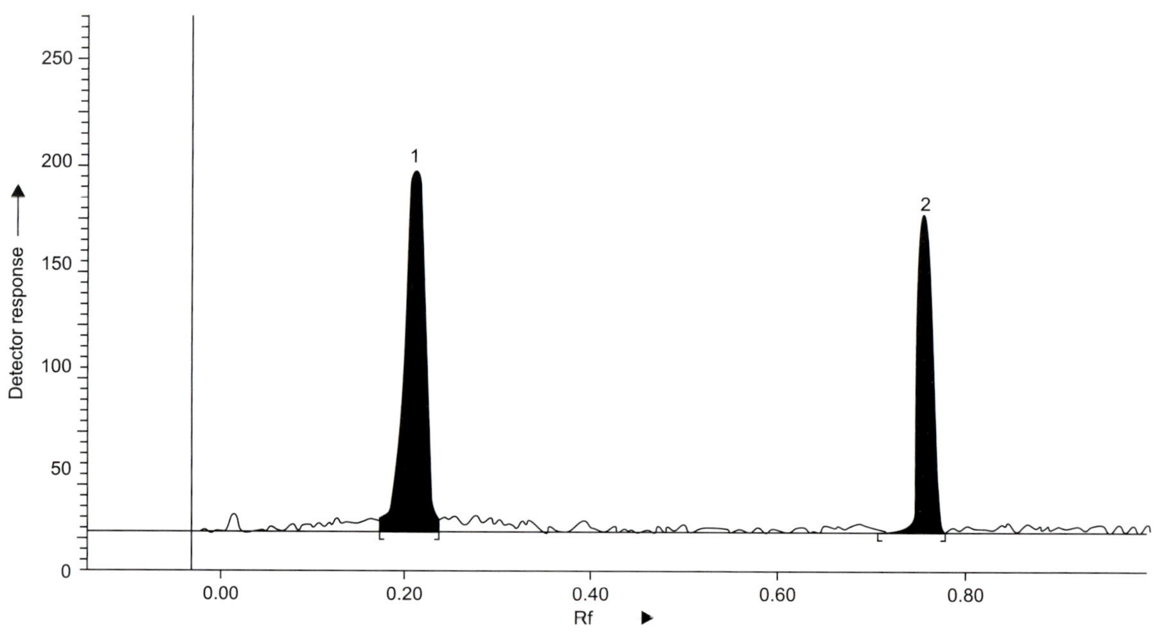

Typical densitogram of the standard containing metformin hydrochloride and pioglitazone hydrochloride. For detailed experimental and chromatographic conditions, refer to Protocol No. 492. Peaks identification: 1. Metformin HCl; 2. Pioglitazone.

PROTOCOL FOR HPTLC ANALYSIS OF PHARMACEUTICAL FORMULATION

Protocol No. 492

Formulation: Metformin hydrochloride, Pioglitazone

Classification: Miscellaneous **Dosage form:** Tablets

Standard preparation: Prepare solution of both the compounds separately in methanol to get 30 μg/ml of pioglitazone hydrochloride and 1000 μg/ml of metformin hydrochloride. Apply varying volumes of each solution for linearity profile.

Sample preparation: Weigh powdered sample equivalent to 500 mg of metformin hydrochloride, suspend in 80 ml of methanol, sonicate for 10 min, dilute to 100 ml with methanol, filter and dilute the filtrate to get 30 μg/ml of pioglitazone HCl and 1000 μg/ml of metformin HCl. Apply 5 μl for assay.

Chromatographic equipments:

Sample applicator: Camag Linomat–V

Development chamber: Camag twin-trough glass chamber, 10 × 10 cm

Denistometric scanner: Camag TLC Scanner–III

Chromatographic conditions:

1. Stationary phase: Silica gel $60F_{254}$ pre-coated HPTLC plates, 10 × 10 cm (200 μm) – Merck
2. Mobile phase (MP): Toluene–chloroform–5% amm. acetate in methanol (2.5 : 3.5 : 4 v/v)
3. Standard/Sample application:
   Band length: — Volume applied: 3–7 μl Spacing: —
4. Chamber saturation: 30 min (MP)
5. RH (%): —
6. Temperature °C: —
7. Separation technique: Ascending
8. Quantity of mobile phase: 10 ml
9. Migration distance: 80 mm
10. Migration time: 15 min

Densitometric evaluation:

Wavelength: UV-265 nm Scanning mode: Reflectance/Absorbance

HRF: Metformin HCl—20; Pioglitazone—76

Linearity (ng/band): Metformin HCl—3000–7000; Pioglitazone HCl—90–210

Recovery (%): Metformin HCl—98.29–102.62; Pioglitazone HCl—98.32–102.91

References: Tejas Vadher, Kashyap N. Thumar and Navin R. Sheth, Manuscript submitted for Dr. P.D. Sethi Award, 2011. Data courtesy, Prof. Kashyap.

Comments:

- The method validated for accuracy, precision, linearity, LOD, LOQ, specificity and robustness.
- Using RP–$18F_{254s}$ pre-coated plates as stationary phase and mixture of n-propanol–5% formic acid–25% ammonia (2 : 4 : 0.3 v/v) as MP, there was reversal of retention order; Pioglitazone—34; Metformin HCl—65 (K.M. Bhargav et al., Abstract No. F-346, 63rd IPC, 2011.

HPTLC : High Performance Thin Layer Chromatography
HPTLC Densitogram

No. 493

Metformin hydrochloride

Pioglitazone

Glimepride

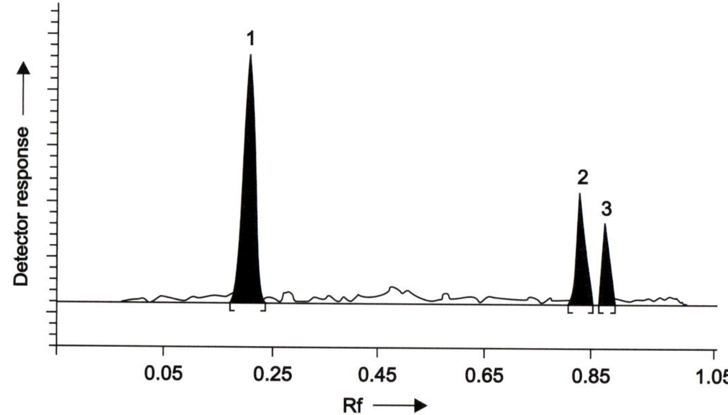

Typical densitogram of the sample containing metformin HCl, pioglitazone and glimepiride. For detailed experimental and chromatographic conditions, refer to Protocol No. 493. Peaks identification: 1. Metformin HCl; 2. Pioglitazone; 3. Glimepiride.

PROTOCOL FOR HPTLC ANALYSIS OF PHARMACEUTICAL FORMULATION

Protocol No. 493

Formulation: **Metformin hydrochloride, Pioglitazone, Glimepiride**

Classification: Miscellaneous **Dosage form:** Tablets

Standard preparation: Prepare 1.5, 10 and 0.5 mg/ml solutions of pioglitazone (Pio), metformin (Met) and glimepiride (Gli) in methanol. Further dilute with methanol to get 0.15, 5.0 and 0.02 mg/ml of Pio, Met and Gli respectively. Apply 1–10 μl of each solution for linearity profile.

Sample preparation: Powdered sample equivalent to 7.5 mg of pioglitazone suspended in 25 ml of methanol, sonicated for 30 min, cooled, diluted to 50 ml with methanol, filtered through Whatman grade-1 filter paper and filtrate used for chromatographic analysis.

Chromatographic equipments:

Sample applicator: Camag Linomat–V

Development chamber: Camag twin–trough glass chamber, 10 × 10 cm

Densitometric scanner: Camag TLC Scanner–III

Chromatographic conditions:

1. Stationary phase: Silica gel $60F_{254}$ pre-coated HPTLC plates, 10 × 10 cm (200 μm) – Merck, pre-washed with methanol, dried at 105°C for 60 min prior to use
2. Mobile phase (MP): Acetonitrile–methanol–n-propanol–1% ammonium acetate (7 : 2 : 1 : 1 v/v)
3. Standard/Sample application:
   Band length: 10 mm Volume applied: 8 μl Spacing: 10 mm
4. Chamber saturation: 10 min (MP)
5. RH (%): 55 ± 5
6. Temperature °C: 22 ± 2
7. Separation technique: Ascending
8. Quantity of mobile phase: 11 ml
9. Migration distance: 80 mm
10. Migration time: 20 min

Densitometric evaluation:

Wavelength: UV–240 nm Scanning mode: Reflectance/Absorbance

HRF: Metformin HCl—21; Pioglitazone—83; Glimepiride—88

Linearity (ng/band): Metformin—1000–40000; Pioglitazone—300–1200; Glimepiride—40–160

Recovery (%): Metformin—98.56–99.34; Pioglitazone—98.92–99.54; Glimepiride—98.65–99.67

References: Dipak Kale and Rajendra Kakde, *J. Planar Chromatogr.*, **24(4)**, 331–336, 2011.

Comments:

- The method validated for accuracy, precision, linearity, LOD, LOQ, specificity, robustness and ruggedness.
- The method is stability indicating (acid, base, oxidative, thermal, photolytic). The degradation products were separated from main compounds.

HPTLC : High Performance Thin Layer Chromatography
HPTLC Densitogram

No. 494

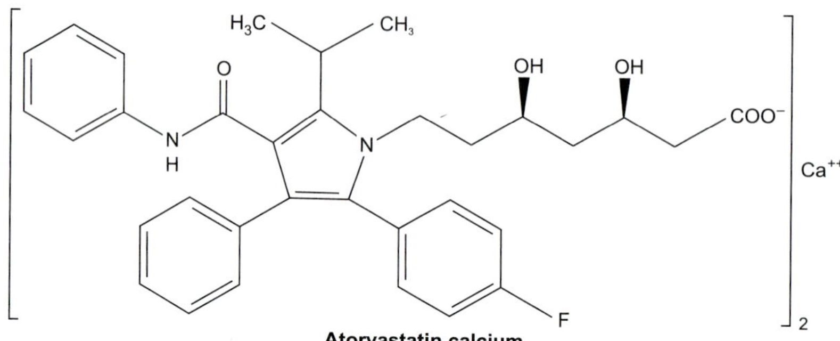

Atorvastatin calcium

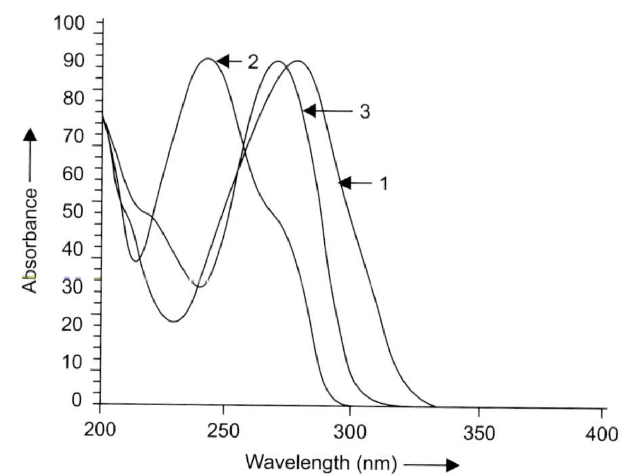

Overlaid UV-spectra of atorvastatin calcium (1), glimepiride (2) and metformin (3) for selection of suitable wavelength for densitometric scanning

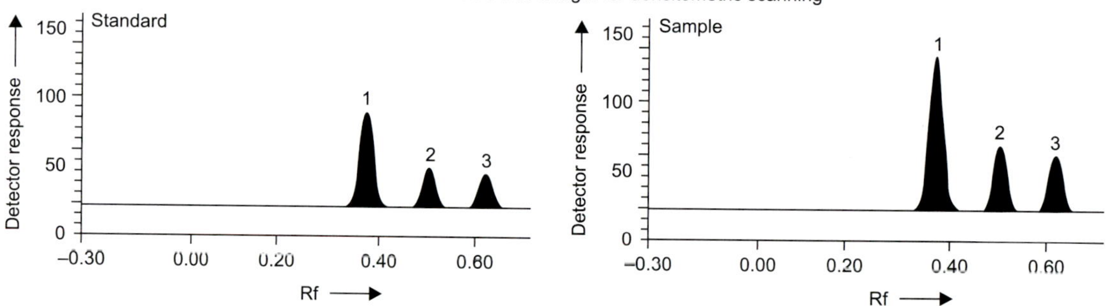

Typical densitogram of the sample and standard containing atorvastatin Ca^{++}, glimepiride and metformin. For detailed experimental and chromatographic conditions, refer to Protocol No. 494. Peaks identification: 1. Metformin; 2. Atorvastatin Ca^{++}; 3. Glimepiride.

PROTOCOL FOR HPTLC ANALYSIS OF PHARMACEUTICAL FORMULATION

Protocol No. 494

Formulation: Metformin, Glimepiride, Atorvastatin calcium

Classification: Miscellaneous **Dosage form:** Tablets

Standard preparation: Prepare 10 mg/ml solution of metformin, 100 μg/ml of glimepiride and 500 μg/ml of atorvastatin Ca^{++} in methanol. Further serial dilutions are made with methanol. Apply 5–10 μl of each solution for linearity profile.

Sample preparation: Suspend powdered sample equivalent to 1 mg of glimepiride in 20 ml of methanol, shake, dilute to 25 ml, filter and filtrate further diluted with methanol. Apply 5 μl of the resulting solution for assay.

Chromatographic equipments:

Sample applicator: Camag Linomat–V

Development chamber: Camag twin-trough glass chamber, 20 × 10 cm

Densitometric scanner: Camag TLC Scanner–III

Chromatographic conditions:

1. Stationary phase: Silica gel $60F_{254}$ pre-coated HPTLC plates, 20 × 10 cm (200 μm) – Merck
2. Mobile phase (MP): Methanol–water–1% ammonium sulphate (4.5 : 4.9 : 10.6 v/v)
3. Standard/Sample application:
   Band length: 6 mm Volume applied: 5 μl Spacing: 10 mm
4. Chamber saturation: 20 min (MP)
5. RH (%): 55 ± 5
6. Temperature °C: Ambient
7. Separation technique: Ascending
8. Quantity of mobile phase: 20 ml
9. Migration distance: 80 mm
10. Migration time: 15 min

Densitometric evaluation:

Wavelength: UV–245 nm Scanning mode: Reflectance/Absorbance

HRF: Metformin—33; Atorvastatin Ca^{++}—50; Glimepiride—65

Linearity (ng/band): Atorvastatin Ca^{++}—100–700; Metformin—100–1500; Glimepiride—20–140

Recovery (%): —

References: A. Manikanta Kumar, K.R. Alagawadi et al., Abstract No. F-286, 63rd IPC, 2011, Personal communication with the author.

Comments: The method validated for accuracy, precision, linearity, LOD, LOQ, specificity, robustness and ruggedness.

HPTLC : High Performance Thin Layer Chromatography
HPTLC Densitogram

No. 495

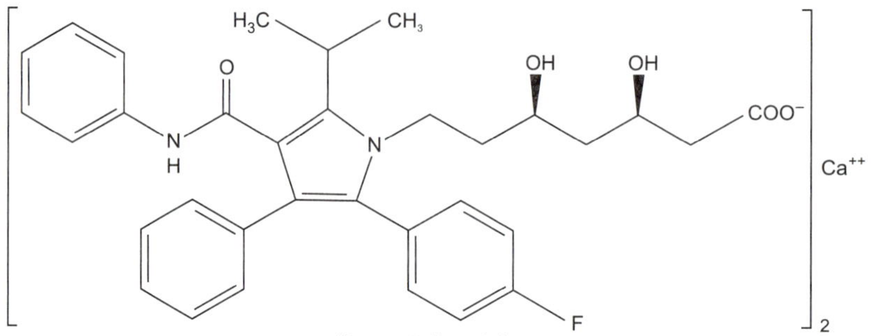

Atorvastatin calcium

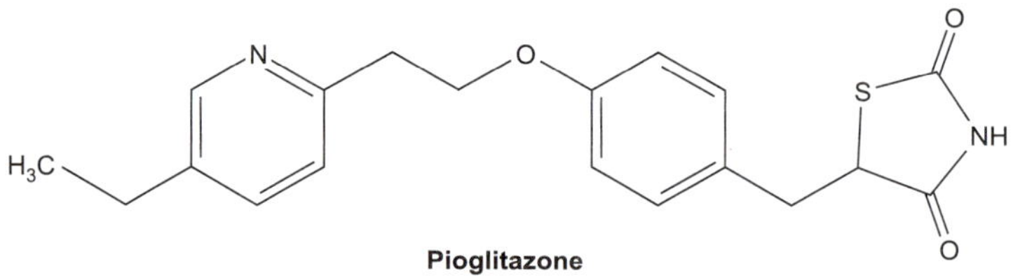

Pioglitazone

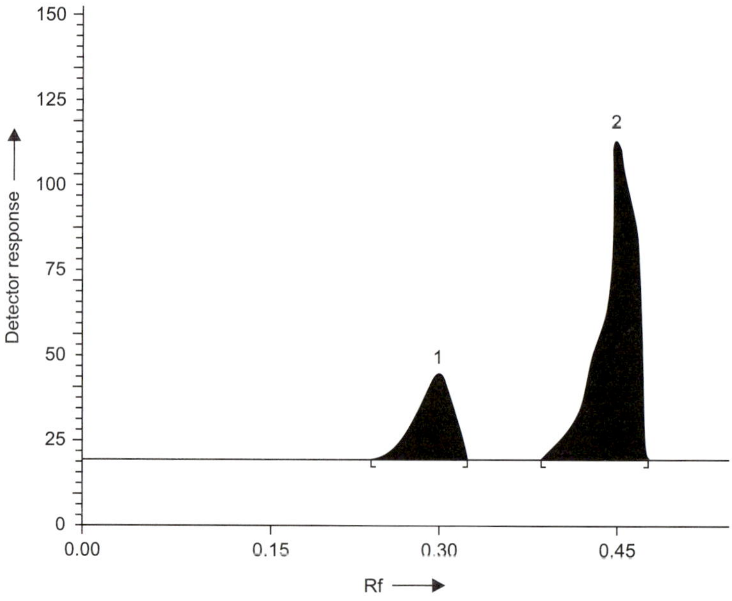

Typical densitogram of the standard containing atorvastatin calcium and pioglitazone. For detailed experimental and chromatographic conditions, refer to Protocol No. 495. Peaks identification: 1. Atorvastatin Ca^{++}; 2. Pioglitazone.

PROTOCOL FOR HPTLC ANALYSIS OF PHARMACEUTICAL FORMULATION

Protocol No. 495

Formulation: **Pioglitazone, Atorvastatin calcium**

Classification: Miscellaneous **Dosage form:** Tablets

Standard preparation: Prepare 100 μg/ml solution of each compound separately in methanol. Apply varying volumes of each solution for linearity profile.

Sample preparation: Powdered sample equivalent to 10 mg of atorvastatin calcium suspended in 70 ml of methanol, sonicated for 25 min, diluted to 100 ml. Filter and apply 4 μl of the filtrate for assay.

Chromatographic equipments:

Sample applicator: Camag Linomat–V

Development chamber: Camag twin-trough glass chamber, 10 × 10 cm

Denistometric scanner: Camag TLC Scanner–III

Chromatographic conditions:

1. Stationary phase: Silica gel 60F_{254} pre-coated TLC plates, 10 × 10 cm (250 μm) – Merck, pre-washed with methanol, activated at 95°C for 30 min prior to use
2. Mobile phase (MP): Chloroform–methanol–toluene (6 : 3 : 4 v/v)
3. Standard/Sample application:
   Band length: 9 mm Volume applied: 2–10 μl Spacing: 10 mm
4. Chamber saturation: 20 min (MP)
5. RH (%): 55 ± 5
6. Temperature °C: Ambient
7. Separation technique: Ascending
8. Quantity of mobile phase: 13 ml
9. Migration distance: —
10. Migration time: —

Densitometric evaluation:

Wavelength: UV–259 nm Scanning mode: Reflectance/Absorbance

HRF: Atorvastatin Ca^{++}—30; Pioglitazone—45

Linearity: 100–400 ng/band for both the compounds

Recovery (%): Atorvastatin Ca^{++}—98.93–100.05, Pioglitazone—99.93–100.05

References: M.C. Sharma, Smita Sharma and D.V. Kohli, *Annals Biol. Res.*, **1(1)**, 124–129, 2010.

Comments: The method was validated for accuracy, precision, linearity, LOD and LOQ.

HPTLC : High Performance Thin Layer Chromatography
HPTLC Densitogram

No. 496

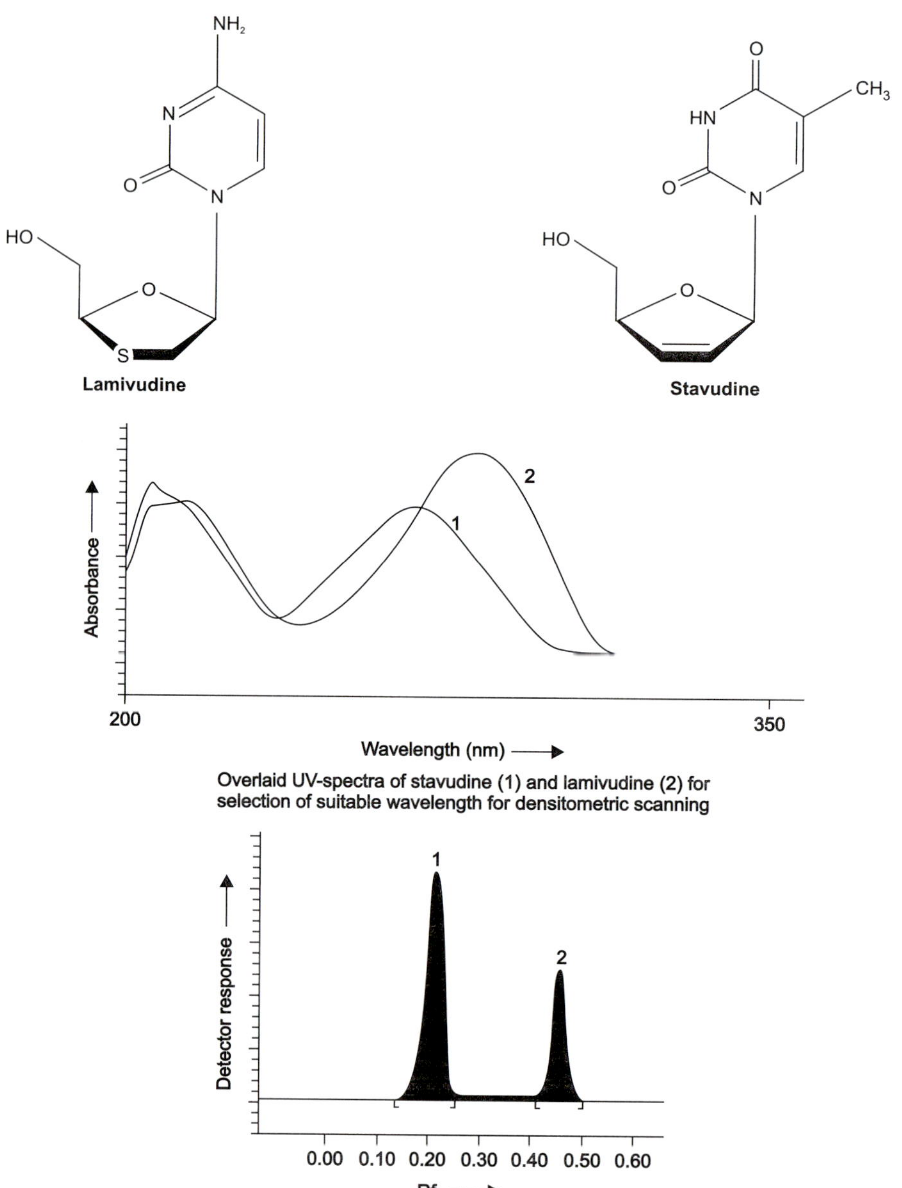

Typical densitogram of the sample containing lamivudine and stavudine. For detailed experimental and chromatographic conditions, refer to Protocol No. 496. Peaks identification: 1. Lamivudine; 2. Stavudine.

PROTOCOL FOR HPTLC ANALYSIS OF PHARMACEUTICAL FORMULATION

Protocol No. 496

Formulation: Lamivudine, Stavudine

Classification: Miscellaneous **Dosage form:** Tablets

Standard preparation: Prepare standard solution of each compound in methanol to get 1 mg/ml of lamivudine and 0.2 mg/ml of stavudine. Further serial dilutions made with methanol for linearity studies. Apply 5 μl of each solution.

Sample preparation: Powdered sample equivalent to 10 mg of stavudine suspended in methanol, sonicated for 10 min, diluted and filtered. The filtrate suitably diluted and used for chromatographic evaluation. Apply 5 μl of the resulting solution.

Chromatographic equipments:

Sample applicator: Camag Linomat–IV

Development chamber: Camag twin-trough glass chamber, 10 × 10 cm

Densitometric scanner: Camag TLC Scanner–III

Chromatographic conditions:

1. Stationary phase: Silica gel $60F_{254}$ pre-coated HPTLC plates, 10 × 10 cm (200 μm) – Merck
2. Mobile phase (MP): Toluene–n-hexane–tetrahydrofuran (7 : 1.5 : 1.5 v/v)
3. Standard/Sample application:
   Band length: 4 mm Volume applied: 5 μl Spacing: 4 mm
4. Chamber saturation: 20 min (MP)
5. RH (%): 55 ± 5
6. Temperature °C: 22 ± 2
7. Separation technique: Ascending
8. Quantity of mobile phase: 10 ml
8. Migration distance: 80 mm
9. Migration time: 20 min

Densitometric evaluation:

Wavelength: UV–253 nm Scanning mode: Reflectance/Absorbance

HRF: Lamivudine—20; Stavudine—45

Linearity (ng/band): Lamivudine—25–75; Stavudine—5–20

Recovery (%): 98.8–100.2 for both the drugs

References: S.B. Wankhede, K.R. Gupta and S.G. Wadodkar, *Indian J. Pharm Sci.*, **67(1)**, 96–97, 2005.

Comments:

- The method validated for accuracy, precision, linearity, LOD, LOQ, specificity, robustness and ruggedness.
- The method is stability indicating (acid, base, oxidative, thermal, photolytic). The degradation products were separated from main compounds.

HPTLC : High Performance Thin Layer Chromatography
HPTLC Densitogram

No. 497

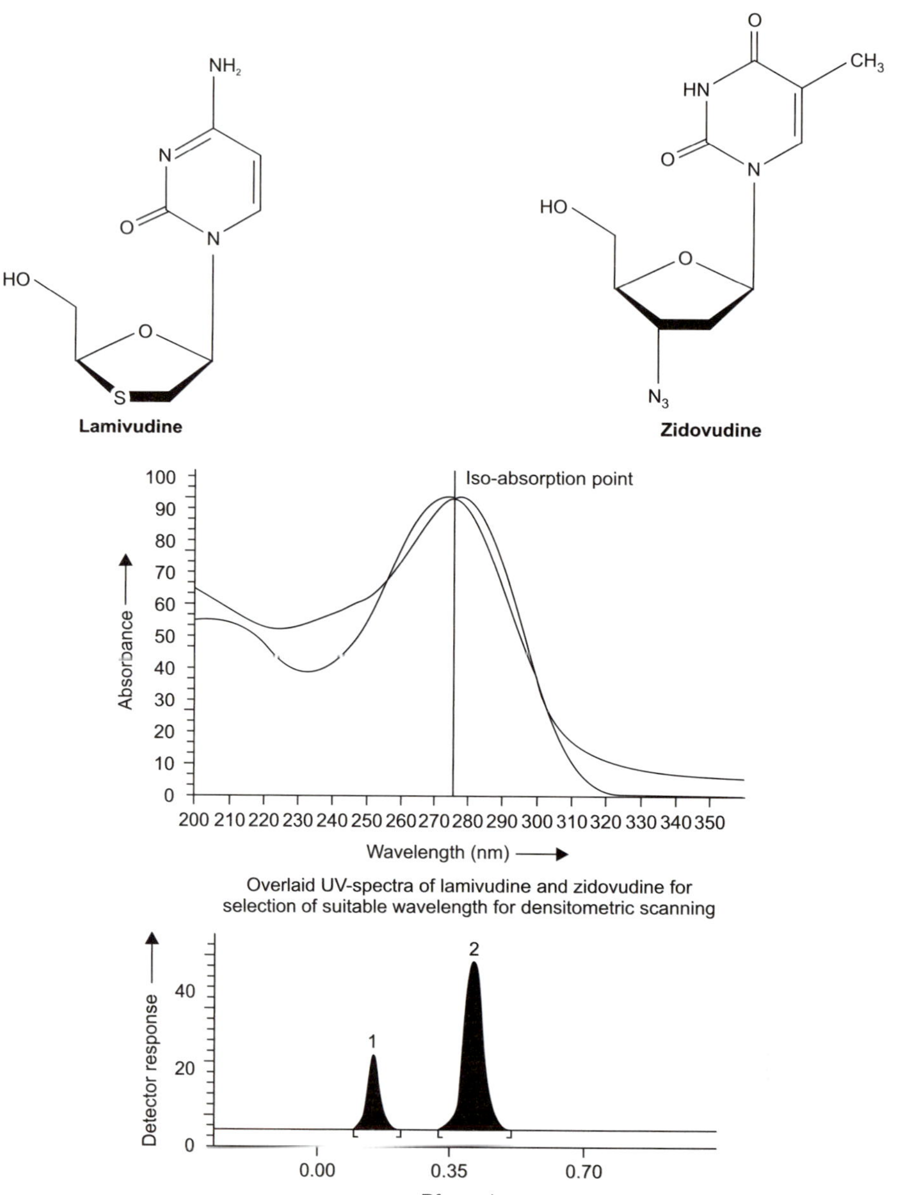

Typical densitogram of the sample containing lamivudine and zidovudine. For detailed experimental and chromatographic conditions, refer to Protocol No. 497. Peaks identification: 1. Lamivudine; 2. Zidovudine.

PROTOCOL FOR HPTLC ANALYSIS OF PHARMACEUTICAL FORMULATION

Protocol No. 497

Formulation: Lamivudine, Zidovudine

Classification: Miscellaneous **Dosage form:** Tablets

Standard preparation: Prepare solution of both the compounds separately in methanol to get 500 μg/ml (lamivudine) and 1000 μg/ml (zidovudine). Further dilutions made with methanol to get 500 ng/ml and apply different volumes for linearity profile.

Sample preparation: Powdered sample equivalent to 500 mg of lamivudine suspended in methanol, sonicated for 5 min, diluted and filtered. The filtrate suitably diluted to get 500 ng/μl of both the substances and used for chromatographic separation.

Chromatographic equipments:

Sample applicator: Camag Linomat–IV
Development chamber: Camag twin-trough glass chamber, 10 × 10 cm
Densitometric scanner: Camag TLC Scanner–III

Chromatographic conditions:

1. Stationary phase: Silica gel $60F_{254}$ pre-coated TLC plates, 10 × 10 cm (250 μm) – Merck
2. Mobile phase (MP): Toluene–methanol–n-hexane (7 : 1.5 : 1.0 v/v)
3. Standard/Sample application:
   Band length: 4 mm Volume applied: 5 μl Spacing: 5 mm
4. Chamber saturation: 10 min (MP)
5. RH (%): 55 ± 5
6. Temperature °C: 25 ± 5
7. Separation technique: Ascending
8. Quantity of mobile phase: 19 ml
8. Migration distance: 70 mm
9. Migration time: 15 min

Densitometric evaluation:

Wavelength: UV–275 nm (iso-absorption point)
Scanning mode: Reflectance/Absorbance
HRF: Lamivudine—13; Zidovudine—40
Linearity (ng/band): Lamivudine—20–250; Zidovudine—50–500
Recovery (%): 99.43–100.01 for both the compounds

References: Sagar B. Wankhede, K.R. Gupta, M.R. Tajne and Sudhir G. Wadodkar, *Asian J. Chem.*, **18(4)**, 2669–2672, 2006.

Comments:

- The method validated for accuracy, precision, linearity, LOD, LOQ, specificity, robustness and ruggedness.
- The method is stability indicating (acid, base, oxidative, thermal, photolytic). The degradation products were separated from main compounds.

HPTLC : High Performance Thin Layer Chromatography
HPTLC Densitogram

No. 498

NH_2 / N / O / N / HO / O / S

Lamivudine

O / CH_3 / HN / O / N / HO / O / N_3

Zidovudine

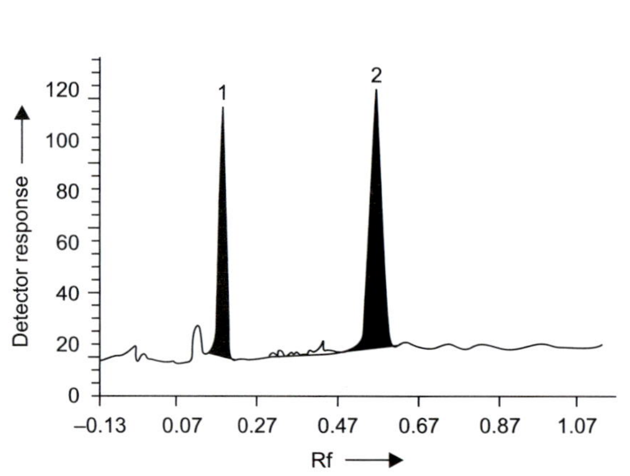

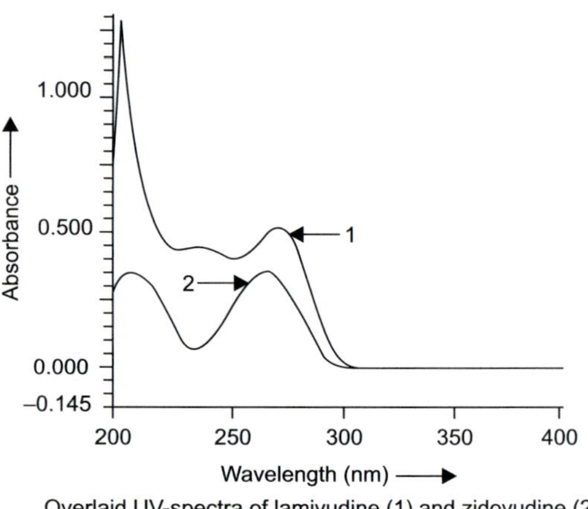

Overlaid UV-spectra of lamivudine (1) and zidovudine (2) for selection of suitable wavelength for densitometric scanning

Typical densitogram of the standard containing lamivudine and zidovudine. For detailed experimental and chromatographic conditions, refer to Protocol No. 498. Peaks identification: 1. Lamivudine; 2. Zidovudine.

PROTOCOL FOR HPTLC ANALYSIS OF PHARMACEUTICAL FORMULATION

Protocol No. 498

Formulation: Lamivudine, Zidovudine

Classification: Miscellaneous **Dosage form:** Tablets

Standard preparation: Prepare solution of both the drugs in methanol to get 2.25 mg/ml of lamivudine and zidovudine. Further dilutions were made to get 50, 80, 100, 120 and 150% of the claim. Apply 5 µl of each solution for linearity profile.

Sample preparation: Powdered composite sample was weighed accurately, suspended in methanol, suitably diluted with methanol and used for chromatographic assay.

Chromatographic equipments:

Sample applicator: Camag Linomat–V

Development chamber: Camag twin-trough glass chamber, 20 × 10 cm

Densitometric scanner: Camag TLC Scanner–III

Chromatographic conditions:

1. Stationary phase: Silica gel $60F_{254}$ pre-coated HPTLC plates, 20 × 10 cm (200 µm) – Merck
2. Mobile phase (MP): Ethyl acetate–toluene–methanol (12 : 5 : 3 v/v)
3. Standard/Sample application:
   Band length: 8 mm Volume applied: 5 µl Spacing: 10 mm
4. Chamber saturation: 20 min (MP)
5. RH (%): 55 ± 5
6. Temperature °C: 25 ± 2
7. Separation technique: Ascending
8. Quantity of mobile phase: 20 ml
8. Migration distance: 70 mm
9. Migration time: 15 min

Densitometric evaluation:

Wavelength: UV–289 nm Scanning mode: Reflectance/Absorbance

HRF: Lamivudine—19; Zidovudine—57

Linearity: —

Recovery (%): 99.90–103.61 for both the drugs

References: Eliangiringa Kaale and Peter Risha, Eike Reich and Thomas P. Layloff, *J. AOAC International*, **93(6)**, 1836–42, 2010.

Comments: This is based on inter-laboratory collaboration studies by the authors as per ICH guidelines for validation of methods.

HPTLC : High Performance Thin Layer Chromatography
HPTLC Densitogram

No. 499

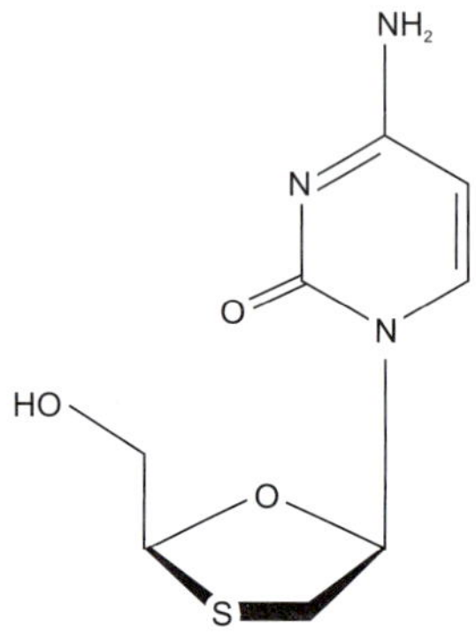

NH2
N
O
N
HO
O
S
Lamivudine

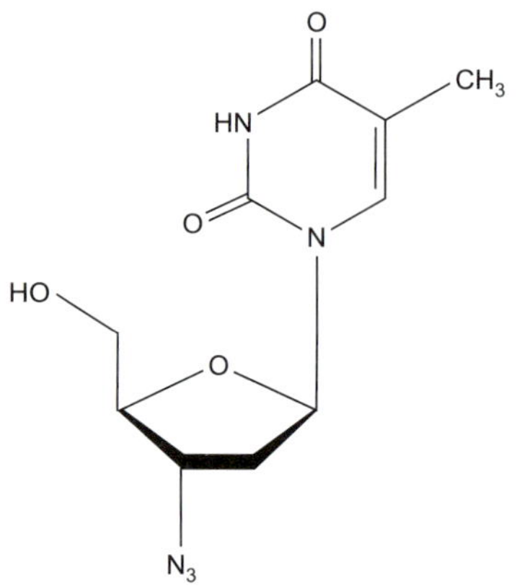

O
CH3
HN
O
N
HO
O
N3
Zidovudine

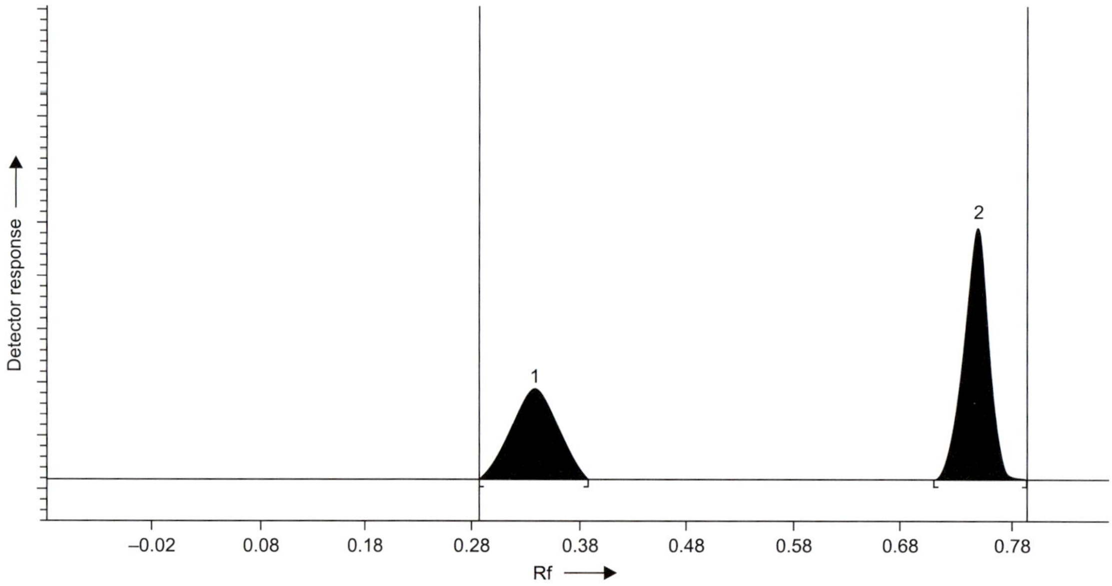

Detector response ⟶
1
2
–0.02 0.08 0.18 0.28 0.38 0.48 0.58 0.68 0.78
Rf ⟶

Typical densitogram of the sample containing lamivudine and zidovudine. For detailed experimental and chromatographic conditions, refer to Protocol No. 499. Peaks identification: 1. Lamivudine; 2. Zidovudine.

PROTOCOL FOR HPTLC ANALYSIS OF PHARMACEUTICAL FORMULATION

Protocol No. 499

Formulation: Lamivudine, Zidovudine

Classification: Miscellaneous **Dosage form:** Tablets

Standard preparation: Prepare solution of both the compounds separately in the solvent to get 30 μg/ml (lamivudine) and 60 μg/ml zidovudine. Carry out further serial dilutions and apply 4 μl of each solution.

Solvent: Acetone–methanol (1 : 1 v/v).

Sample preparation: The powdered sample suspended in solvent, sonicated, diluted and filtered. The filtrate suitably diluted with solvent. Apply 4 μl for assay.

Chromatographic equipments:

Sample applicator: Camag Linomat–IV

Development chamber: Camag twin-trough glass chamber, 10 × 10 cm

Densitometric scanner: Camag TLC Scanner–III

Chromatographic conditions:

1. Stationary phase: Silica gel $60F_{254}$ pre-coated HPTLC plates, 10 × 10 cm (200 μm) – Merck
2. Mobile phase (MP): Acetone–toluene–methanol (4 : 4 : 2 v/v)
3. Standard/Sample application:
   Band length: 5 mm Volume applied: 4 μl Spacing: 5 mm
4. Chamber saturation: 20 min (MP)
5. RH (%): 55 ± 5
6. Temperature °C: 22 ± 2
7. Separation technique: Ascending
8. Quantity of mobile phase: 10 ml
8. Migration distance: 80 mm
9. Migration time: 20 min

Densitometric evaluation:

Wavelength: UV–267 nm and 272 nm Scanning mode: Reflectance/Absorbance

HRF: Lamivudine—34; Zidovudine—74

Linearity (ng/band): Lamivudine—10–210; Zidovudine—30–420

Recovery (%): 99.46–100.36 for both the drugs

References: P.K. Saini, R.M. Singh, S.C. Mathur, G.N. Singh, S. Tuteja and U.K. Singh, *Indian Drugs*, **47(5)**, 42–45, 2010.

Comments: The method validated for accuracy, precision, linearity, LOD, LOQ, specificity, robustness and ruggedness.

HPTLC : High Performance Thin Layer Chromatography
HPTLC Densitogram

No. 500

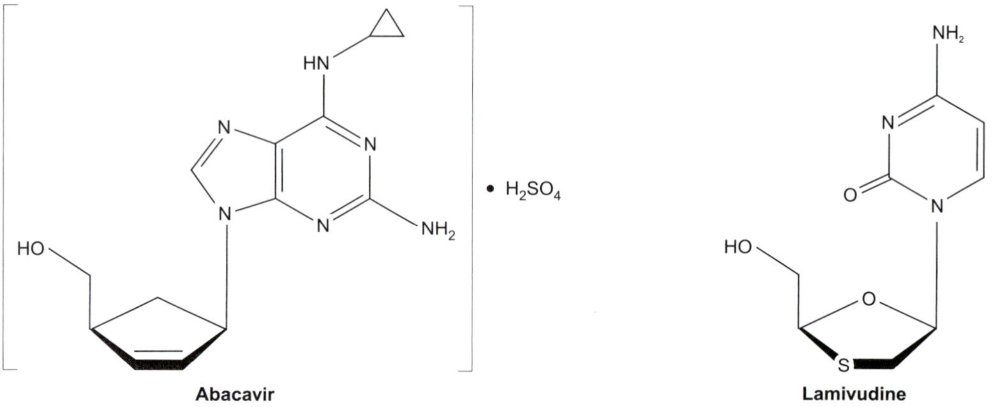

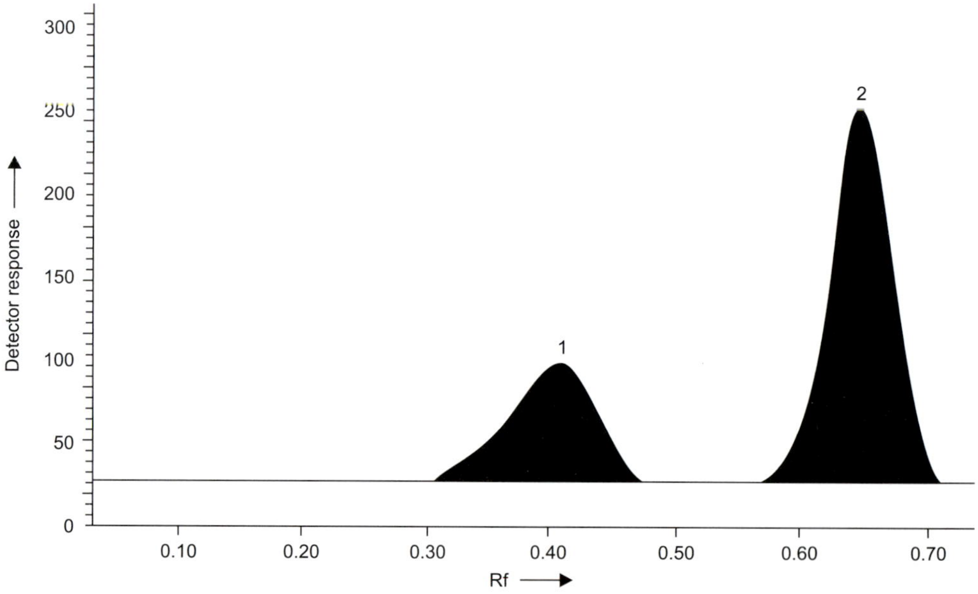

• H_2SO_4

Abacavir

Lamivudine

Typical densitogram of the sample containing abacavir sulphate and lamivudine. For detailed experimental and chromatographic conditions, refer to Protocol No. 500. Peaks identification: 1. Lamivudine; 2. Abacavir sulphate.

PROTOCOL FOR HPTLC ANALYSIS OF PHARMACEUTICAL FORMULATION

Protocol No. 500

Formulation: Lamivudine, Abacavir sulphate

Classification: Miscellaneous **Dosage form:** Tablets

Standard preparation: Prepare solution of both the compounds in methanol to get 1.2 mg/ml of abacavir sulphate and 0.6 mg/ml of lamivudine. Further dilutions were made with methanol for linearity studies.

Sample preparation: Powdered sample equivalent to 120 mg of abacavir sulphate or 60 mg of lamivudine suspended in methanol, sonicated for 30 min, diluted to 100 ml with methanol. Filtered and 2 ml of filtrate diluted to 10 ml with methanol, centrifuged and supernatant used for analysis.

Chromatographic equipments:

Sample applicator: Camag Linomat–IV
Development chamber: Camag twin-trough glass chamber, 10 × 10 cm
Densitometric scanner: Camag TLC Scanner–III

Chromatographic conditions:

1. Stationary phase: Silica gel 60F_{254} pre-coated HPTLC plates, 10 × 10 cm (200 µm) – Merck, pre-washed with methanol and activated (60°C) for 5 min prior to use
2. Mobile phase (MP): Methanol–acetone–n-butylacetate (1 : 1 : 2 v/v)
3. Standard/Sample application:
   Band length: 5 mm Volume applied: 3 µl Spacing: 5 mm
4. Chamber saturation: 20 min (MP)
5. RH (%): 60 ± 5
6. Temperature °C: 25 ± 2
7. Separation technique: Ascending
8. Quantity of mobile phase: 12 ml
8. Migration distance: 60 mm
9. Migration time: 20 min

Densitometric evaluation:

Wavelength: UV–284 nm Scanning mode: Reflectance/Absorbance
HRF: Lamivudine—40; Abacavir sulphate—65
Linearity (ng/band): Abacavir sulphate—240–1200; Lamivudine—120–600
Recovery (%): Abacavir sulphate—99.42–100.66; Lamivudine—99.54–101.4

References: P.K. Saini, C.L. Jain, R.M. Singh, S.C. Madhur, G.N. Singh and M. Naslam, *J. Pharm. Research*, **8(4)**, 187–191, 2009.

Comments:

- The method validated for accuracy, precision, linearity, LOD, LOQ, specificity, robustness and ruggedness.
- The method is stability indicating (acid, base, oxidative, thermal, photolytic). The degradation products were separated from main compounds.

HPTLC : High Performance Thin Layer Chromatography
HPTLC Densitogram

No. 501

Tenofovir

Lamivudine

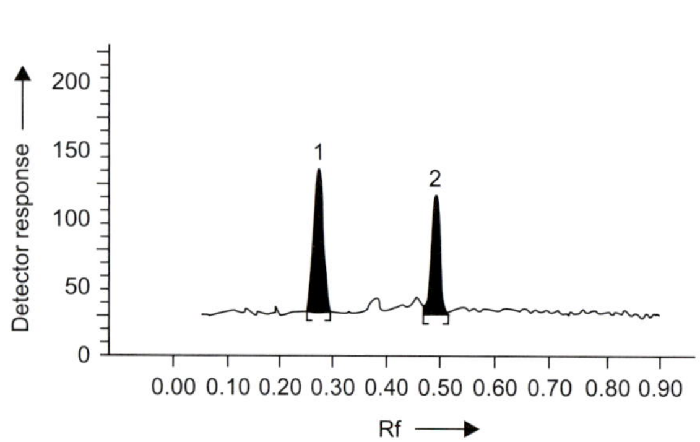

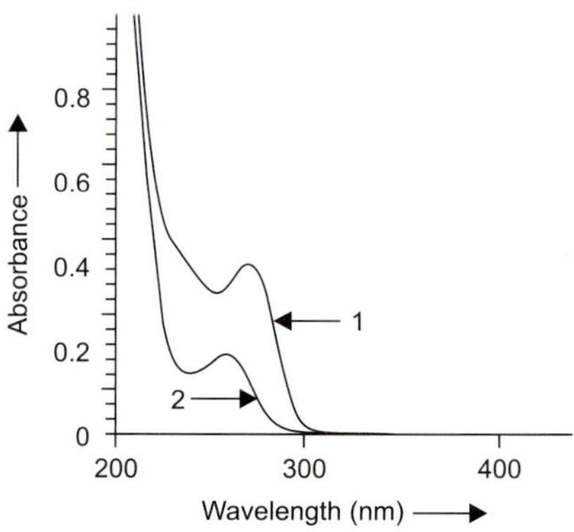

Overlaid UV-spectra of lamivudine (1) and tenofovir (2) for selection of suitable wavelength for densitometric scanning

Typical densitogram of the sample containing lamivudine and tenofovir. For detailed experimental and chromatographic conditions, refer to Protocol No. 501. Peaks identification: 1. Lamivudine; 2. Tenofovir disoproxil fumarate.

PROTOCOL FOR HPTLC ANALYSIS OF PHARMACEUTICAL FORMULATION

Protocol No. 501

Formulation: Lamivudine, Tenofovir disoproxil fumarate

Classification: Miscellaneous **Dosage form:** Tablets

Standard preparation: Prepare 3 mg/ml solution of each compound in methanol. Further serial dilutions made for linearity studies. Apply 10 µl of each solution for chromatographic separation.

Sample preparation: Appropriate quantity of powdered sample suspended in methanol, sonicated, diluted and filtered. Further dilutions suitably made with methanol for chromatographic evaluation.

Chromatographic equipments:

Sample applicator: Camag Linomat–IV

Development chamber: Camag twin-trough glass chamber, 20 × 10 cm

Densitometric scanner: Camag TLC Scanner–III

Chromatographic conditions:

1. Stationary phase: Silica gel $60F_{254}$ pre-coated TLC plates, 20 × 10 cm (250 µm) – Merck, pre-washed with methanol and activated at 110°C for 5 min prior to use
2. Mobile phase (MP): Chloroform–methanol–toluene (8 : 2 : 2 v/v)
3. Standard/Sample application:
   Band length: 6 mm Volume applied: 10 µl Spacing: 6 mm
4. Chamber saturation: 30 min (MP)
5. RH (%): 60 ± 5
6. Temperature °C: 25 ± 2
7. Separation technique: Ascending
8. Quantity of mobile phase: 24 ml
8. Migration distance: 80 mm
9. Migration time: 20 min

Densitometric evaluation:

Wavelength: UV–265 nm Scanning mode: Reflectance/Absorbance

HRF: Lamivudine—27; Tenofovir—51

Linearity (ng/band): 60–210 for both the drugs

Recovery (%): 99.37–100.93 for both the compounds

References: P. Chandra, A.S. Rathore, L. Sathiyanarayanan and K.R. Mahadik, *J. Chil. Chem Soc.*, **56(2)**, 701–705, 2011.

Comments: The method validated for accuracy, precision, linearity, LOD, LOQ, specificity, and robustness.

HPTLC : High Performance Thin Layer Chromatography
HPTLC Densitogram

No. 502

Stavudine

Nevirapine

Overlaid UV-spectra of lamivudine (1), nevirapine (2) and stavudine (3) for selection of suitable wavelength for densitometric scanning

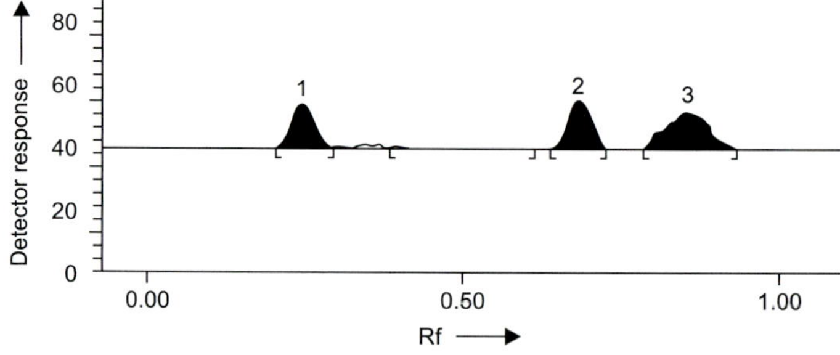

Typical densitogram of the sample containing lamivudine, stavudine and nevirapine. For detailed experimental and chromatographic conditions, refer to Protocol No. 502. Peaks identification: 1. Stavudine; 2. Lamivudine; 3. Nevirapine.

PROTOCOL FOR HPTLC ANALYSIS OF PHARMACEUTICAL FORMULATION

Protocol No. 502

Formulation: Lamivudine, Stavudine, Nevirapine
Classification: Miscellaneous **Dosage form:** Tablets
Standard preparation: Prepare standard solution of each compound in MP to get final concentrations in the range of 10–50 μg/ml (Stavudine) 50–300 μg/ml (Lamivudine), 60–400 μg/ml (Nevirapine). Apply 10 μl of each solution for linearity profile.
Sample preparation: Accurately weighed quantity of powdered sample suspended in MP, sonicated for 10 min, diluted and filtered. The filtrate suitably diluted with MP to get concentration within linearity range. Apply 10 μl of each solution for linearity profile.
Chromatographic equipments:
Sample applicator: Camag Linomat–IV
Development chamber: Camag twin-trough glass chamber, 10 × 10 cm
Densitometric scanner: Camag TLC Scanner–II
Chromatographic conditions:
1. Stationary phase: Silica gel $60F_{254}$ pre-coated TLC plates, 10 × 10 cm (250 μm) – Merck
2. Mobile phase (MP): Chloroform–methanol (9 : 1 v/v)
3. Standard/Sample application:
   Band length: 4 mm Volume applied: 10 μl Spacing: 4 mm
4. Chamber saturation: 20 min (MP)
5. RH (%): 55 ± 5
6. Temperature °C: 22 ± 2
7. Separation technique: Ascending
8. Quantity of mobile phase: 10 ml
8. Migration distance: 70 mm
9. Migration time: 15 min

Densitometric evaluation:
Wavelength: UV–265 nm Scanning mode: Reflectance/Absorbance
HRF: Stavudine—25; Lamivudine—65; Nevirapine—85
Linearity (ng/band): Stavudine—10–60; Lamivudine—50–500; Nevirapine—60–400
Recovery (%): 99.16–101.99 for all the three compounds
References: Sockalingam Anbazhagan, Narayanareddy Indumathy, Pitchaimuthu Shanmugapandiyan, Seshaiah Krishnan Sridhar, *J. Pharm. Biomed. Anal.*, **39**, 801–804, 2005.
Comments:
- The method validated for accuracy, precision, linearity, LOD, LOQ, specificity, robustness and ruggedness.
- The method is stability indicating (acid, base, oxidative, thermal, photolytic). The degradation products were separated from main compounds.

HPTLC : High Performance Thin Layer Chromatography
HPTLC Densitogram

No. 503

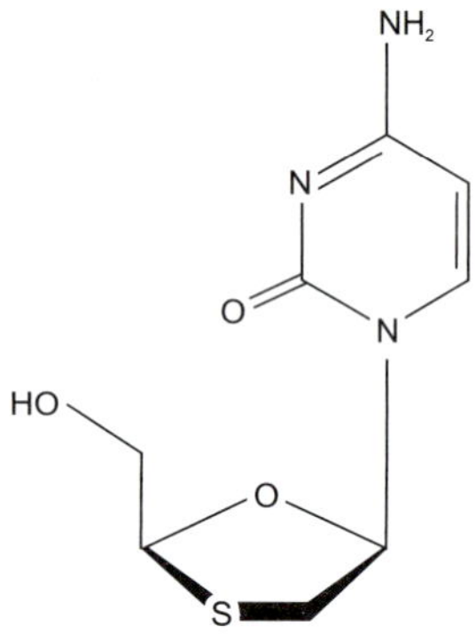

NH2

O

CH3

N

HN

H3C

O

HN

O

N

O

N

HO

HO

N

N

N

O

O

S

Lamivudine

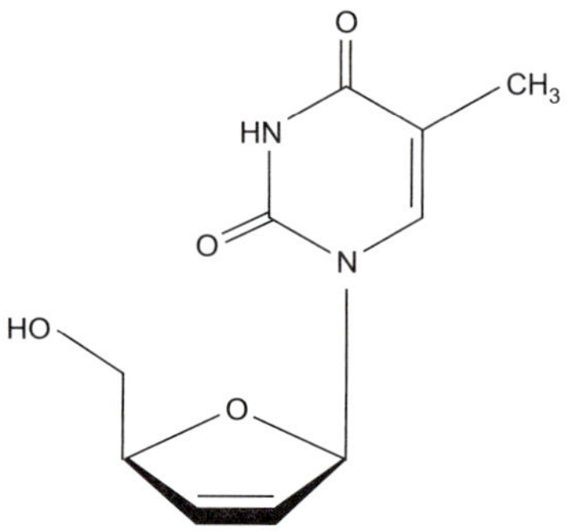

Stavudine

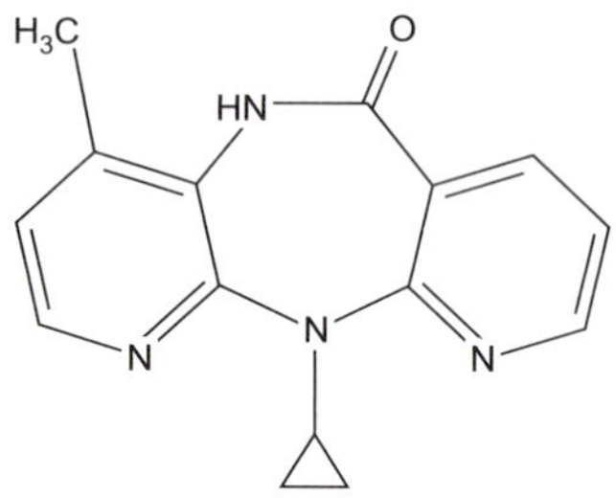

Nevirapine

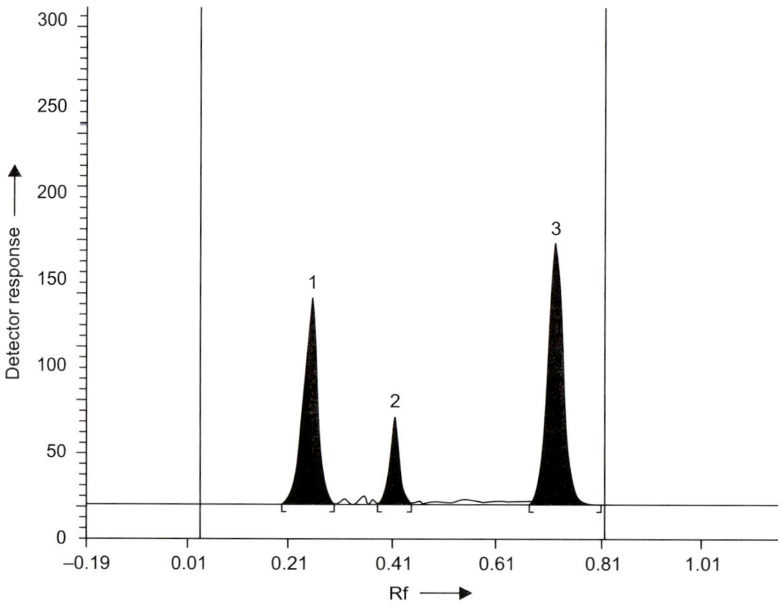

300

250

200

Detector response

150

100

50

0

–0.19 0.01 0.21 0.41 0.61 0.81 1.01

Rf

1

2

3

Typical densitogram of the sample containing lamivudine, stavudine and nevirapine. For detailed experimental and chromatographic conditions, refer to Protocol No. 503. Peaks identification: 1. Lamivudine; 2. Stavudine; 3. Nevirapine.

PROTOCOL FOR HPTLC ANALYSIS OF PHARMACEUTICAL FORMULATION

Protocol No. 503

Formulation: Lamivudine, Stavudine, Nevirapine

Classification: Miscellaneous **Dosage form:** Tablets

Standard preparation: Prepare 5 mg/ml solution of each compound separately in methanol. Further dilute to get 524 μg/ml (lamivudine), 480 μg/ml (stavudine) and 520 μg/ml (nevirapine). Further serial dilutions made for linearity profile. Apply 2 μl of each solution.

Sample preparation: Powdered sample equivalent to 50 mg of lamivudine suspended in 15 ml of methanol, sonicated for 10 min, diluted to 25 ml with methanol and filtered. Dilute 5 ml of the filtrate to 100 ml with methanol for lamivudine and 5 ml and 2 ml to 25 ml with methanol for stavudine and nevirapine respectively and use the final solution for spotting.

Chromatographic equipments:

Sample applicator: Camag Linomat–V

Development chamber: Camag twin-trough glass chamber, 20 × 20 cm

Densitometric scanner: Camag TLC Scanner–III

Chromatographic conditions:

1. Stationary phase: Silica gel $60F_{254}$ pre-coated HPTLC plates, 10 × 20 cm (200 μm) – Merck
2. Mobile phase (MP): Ethyl acetate–methanol–toluene–25% ammonia (12 : 6 : 12 : 1 v/v)
3. Standard/Sample application:
   Band length: 6 mm Volume applied: 2 μl Spacing: 10 mm
4. Chamber saturation: 20 min (MP)
5. RH (%): 55 ± 5
6. Temperature °C: 20 ± 2
7. Separation technique: Ascending
8. Quantity of mobile phase: 31 ml
8. Migration distance: 70 mm
9. Migration time: 15 min

Densitometric evaluation:

Wavelength: UV–254 nm Scanning mode: Reflectance/Absorbance

HRF: Lamivudine—24; Stavudine—42; Nevirapine—69

Linearity (ng/band): Lamivudine—41.9–209; Stavudine—38.4–192; Nevirapine—41.6–208

Recovery (%): 96.41–101.63 for all the three compounds

References: D.H. Shewiyo, E. Kaale, C. Ugullam, M.N. Sigonda, P.G. Risha, B. Dejaegher, J. Smeyers-Verbeke and Y. Vander Heyden, *J. Pharm. Biomed. Anal.*, **54(3)**, 445–450, 2011.

Comments: The method validated for accuracy, precision, linearity, LOD, LOQ, specificity, robustness and ruggedness.

HPTLC : High Performance Thin Layer Chromatography
HPTLC Densitogram

No. 504

Emtricitabine **Tenofovir**

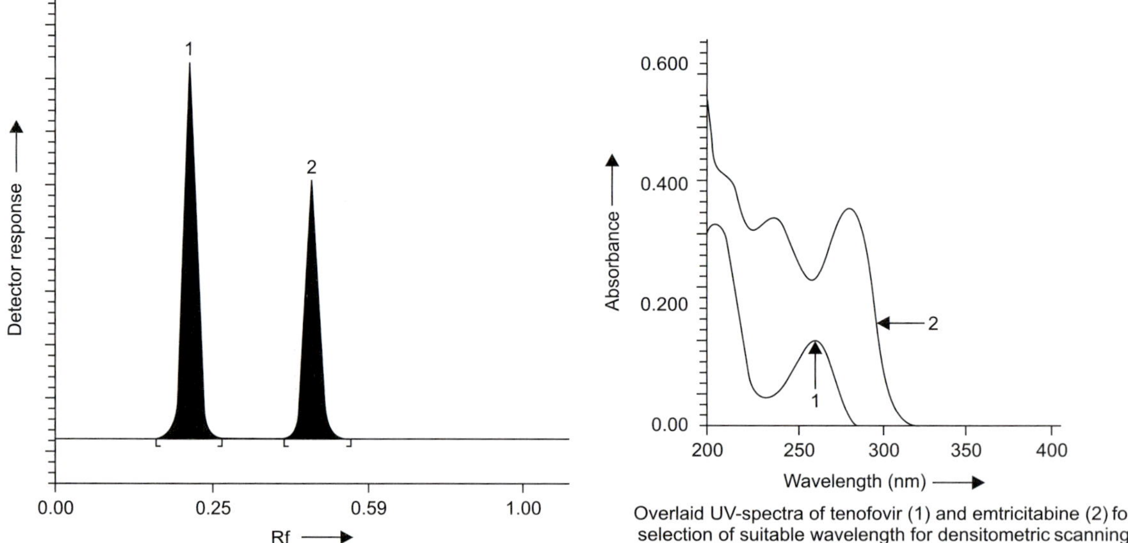

Overlaid UV-spectra of tenofovir (1) and emtricitabine (2) for selection of suitable wavelength for densitometric scanning

Typical densitogram of the sample containing tenofovir and emtricitabine. For detailed experimental and chromatographic conditions, refer to Protocol No. 504. Peaks identification: 1. Emtricitabine; 2. Tenofovir.

PROTOCOL FOR HPTLC ANALYSIS OF PHARMACEUTICAL FORMULATION

Protocol No. 504

Formulation: Tenofovir, Emtricitabine

Classification: Miscellaneous **Dosage form:** Tablets

Standard preparation: Prepare solution of each compound separately in methanol to get final concentration of 100 ng/μl. Apply 2–10 μl of each solution for linearity studies.

Sample preparation: Powdered sample equivalent to 10 mg of tenofovir suspended in methanol, sonicated for 15 min, diluted and filtered. The filtrate suitably diluted with methanol. Apply 5 μl for chromatographic analysis.

Chromatographic equipments:

Sample applicator: Camag Linomat–V

Development chamber: Camag twin-trough glass chamber, 10 × 10 cm

Densitometric scanner: Camag TLC Scanner–III

Chromatographic conditions:

1. Stationary phase: Silica gel $60F_{254}$ pre-coated TLC plates, 10 × 10 cm (250 μm) – Merck, pre-washed with methanol, dried at 50°C for 5 min prior to use
2. Mobile phase (MP): Chloroform–methanol (9 : 1 v/v)
3. Standard/Sample application:
   Band length: 5 mm Volume applied: 2–10 μl Spacing: 5 mm
4. Chamber saturation: 30 min (MP)
5. RH (%): 55 ± 5
6. Temperature °C: 22 ± 2
7. Separation technique: Ascending
8. Quantity of mobile phase: 10 ml
8. Migration distance: 80 mm
9. Migration time: 20 min

Densitometric evaluation:

Wavelength: UV–265 nm Scanning mode: Reflectance/Absorbance

HRF: Emtricitabine—18; Tenofovir—48

Linearity (ng/band): Tenofovir—200–1000; Emtricitabine—200–1000

Recovery (%): 99.07–100.08 for both the compounds

References: Maithilee Joshi, A.P. Nikalje, M. Shahed and M. Dehghan, *Ind. J. Pharm. Sci.*, **71(1)**, 95–97, 2009.

Comments: The method validated for accuracy, precision, linearity, LOD, LOQ, specificity, robustness and ruggedness.

HPTLC : High Performance Thin Layer Chromatography
HPTLC Densitogram

No. 505

Emtricitabine

Tenofovir

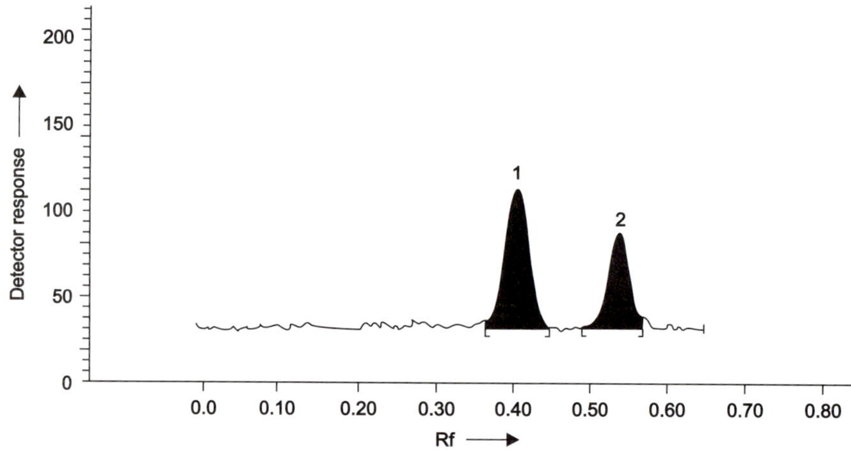

Typical densitogram of the standard containing tenofovir and emtricitabine. For detailed experimental and chromatographic conditions, refer to Protocol No. 505. Peaks identification: 1. Emtricitabine; 2. Tenofovir.

PROTOCOL FOR HPTLC ANALYSIS OF PHARMACEUTICAL FORMULATION

Protocol No. 505

Formulation: Tenofovir, Emtricitabine

Classification: Miscellaneous **Dosage form:** Tablets

Standard preparation: Prepare solution of both the substances in methanol to get 120 μg/ml of tenofovir and 80 μg/ml of emtricitabine. Apply varying volumes of each solution for linearity profile.

Sample preparation: Powdered sample equivalent to 300 mg of tenofovir suspended in 70 ml of methanol, sonicated, diluted to 100 ml with methanol. The solution was further diluted to get 120 ng/μl of tenofovir and 80 ng/μl of emtricitabine. Apply 4 μl for assay.

Chromatographic equipments:

Sample applicator: Camag Linomat–V

Development chamber: Camag twin-trough glass chamber, 20 × 10 cm

Densitometric scanner: Camag TLC Scanner–III

Chromatographic conditions:

1. Stationary phase: Silica gel 60F_{254} pre-coated HPTLC plates, 20 × 10 cm (200 μm) – Merck, pre-washed with methanol and activated at 115°C for 10 min prior to use
2. Mobile phase (MP): Toluene–methanol–ethyl acetate–glacial acetic acid (4 : 2 : 5 : 0.1 v/v)
3. Standard/Sample application:
   Band length: 6 mm Volume applied: 4 μl Spacing: 5 mm
4. Chamber saturation: 20 min (MP)
5. RH (%): 60 ± 5
6. Temperature °C: Ambient
7. Separation technique: Ascending
8. Quantity of mobile phase: 22 ml
8. Migration distance: 80 mm
9. Migration time: 20 min

Densitometric evaluation:

Wavelength: UV–270 nm Scanning mode: Reflectance/Absorbance

HRF: Emtricitabine—40; Tenofovir—52

Linearity (ng/band): Tenofovir—120–600; Emtricitabine—80–560

Recovery (%): 99.54–99.87 for both the compounds

References: Janhavi R. Rao, Shweta A. Gondkar and Savita S. Yadav, *Int. J. Pharm. Tech. Research*, **3(3)**, 1430–1434, 2011.

Comments: The method validated for accuracy, precision, linearity, LOD, LOQ, specificity, robustness and ruggedness.

HPTLC : High Performance Thin Layer Chromatography
HPTLC Densitogram

No. 506

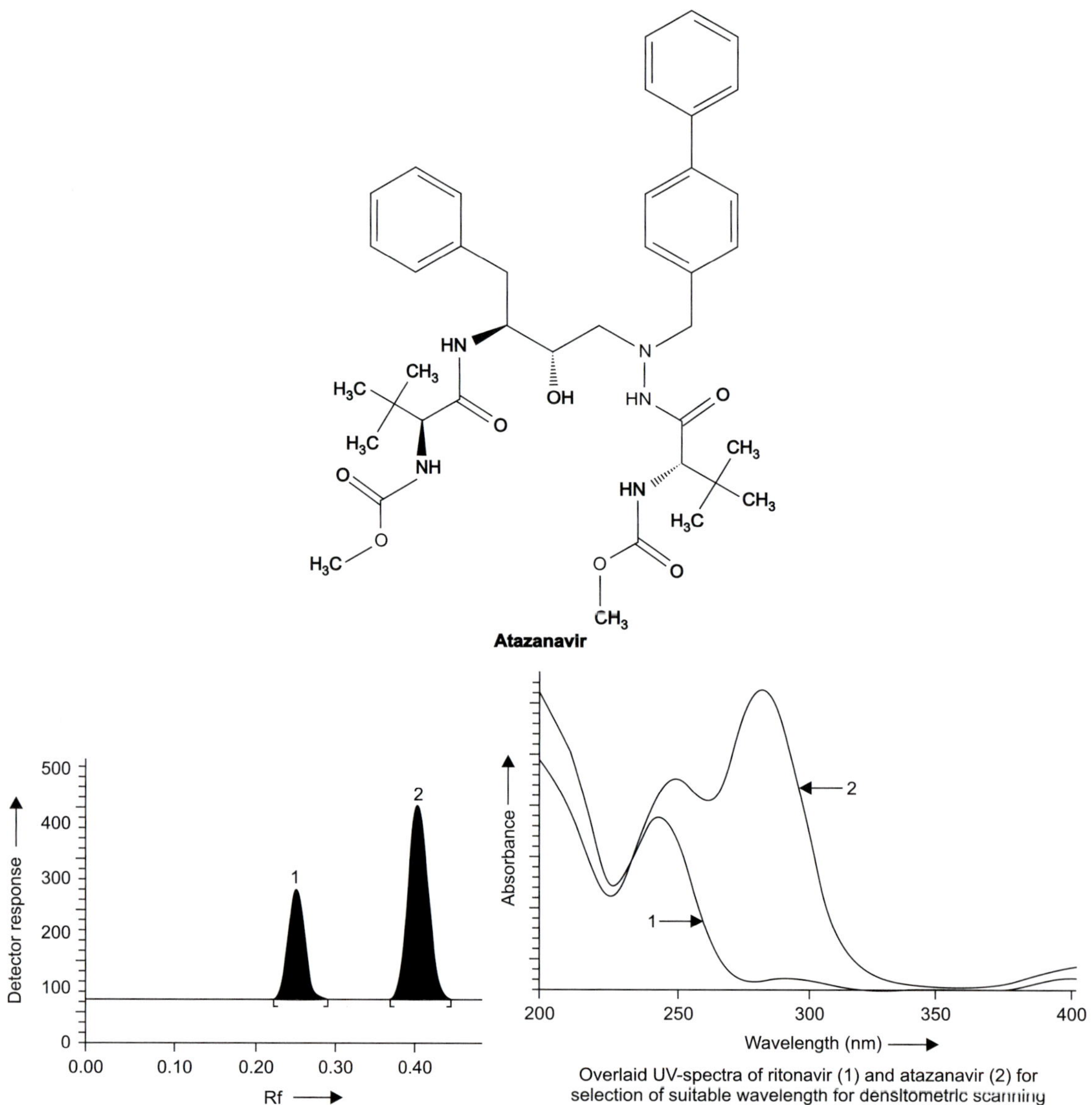

Overlaid UV-spectra of ritonavir (1) and atazanavir (2) for selection of suitable wavelength for densitometric scanning

Typical densitogram of the standard containing ritonavir and atazanavir. For detailed experimental and chromatographic conditions, refer to Protocol No. 506. Peaks identification: 1. Ritonavir; 2. Atazanavir.

PROTOCOL FOR HPTLC ANALYSIS OF PHARMACEUTICAL FORMULATION

Protocol No. 506

Formulation: Ritonavir, Atazanavir

Classification: Miscellaneous **Dosage form:** Tablets

Standard preparation: Prepare 500 μg/ml solution of each compound separately in methanol. Apply varying volumes for linearity studies.

Sample preparation: Powdered sample equivalent to 5 mg of ritonavir suspended in methanol, sonicated, diluted suitably and 2 μl applied for assay.

Chromatographic equipments:

Sample applicator: Camag Linomat–V

Development chamber: Camag twin-trough glass chamber, 10 × 10 cm

Densitometric scanner: Camag TLC Scanner–III

Chromatographic conditions:

1. Stationary phase: Silica gel 60F_{254} pre-coated TLC plates, 10 × 10 cm (250 μm) – Merck
2. Mobile phase (MP): Toluene–ethyl acetate–methanol (6 : 4.5 : 0.6 v/v)
3. Standard/Sample application:
   Band length: 6 mm Volume applied: 1–8 μl; 2–16 μl
   Spacing: 10 mm
4. Chamber saturation: 15 min (MP)
5. RH (%): 55 ± 5
6. Temperature °C: Ambient
7. Separation technique: Ascending
8. Quantity of mobile phase: 11 ml
8. Migration distance: 90 mm
9. Migration time: 15 min

Densitometric evaluation:

Wavelength: UV–240 nm Scanning mode: Reflectance/Absorbance

HRF: Ritonavir—25; Atazanavir—41

Linearity (ng/band): Ritonavir—500–4000; Atazanavir—1000–8000

Recovery (%): 99.59–100.40 for both the compounds

References: Santosh V. Gandhi, Personal communication (in press).

Comments: The method validated for accuracy, precision, linearity, LOD, LOQ, specificity, robustness and ruggedness.

HPTLC : High Performance Thin Layer Chromatography
HPTLC Densitogram

No. 507

Ritonavir

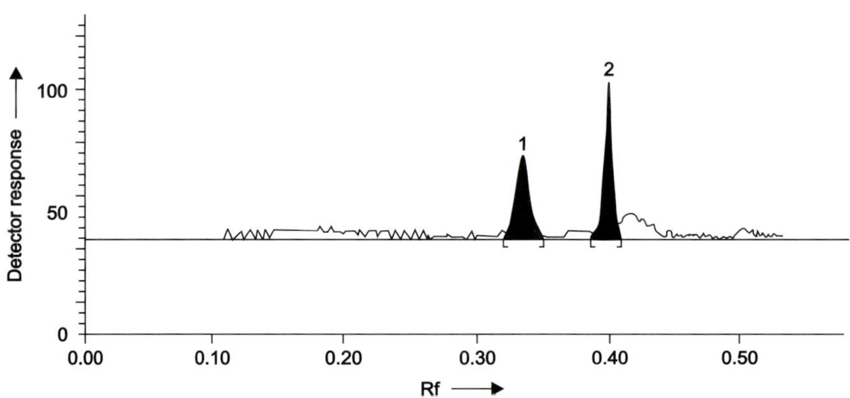

Typical densitogram of the standard containing lopinavir and ritonavir. For detailed experimental and chromatographic conditions, refer to Protocol No. 507. Peaks identification: 1. Ritonavir; 2. Lopinavir.

PROTOCOL FOR HPTLC ANALYSIS OF PHARMACEUTICAL FORMULATION

Protocol No. 507

Formulation: Ritonavir, Lopinavir

Classification: Miscellaneous **Dosage form:** Capsules

Standard preparation: Prepare 2.5 mg/ml solution of lopinavir (L) and 1 mg/ml solution of ritonavir (R), both in methanol. Mix 26.6 ml of solution L and 16.65 ml of solution R and dilute to 50 ml with methanol. Apply varying volumes for linearity studies.

Sample preparation: An appropriate quantity of the sample was accurately weighed, suspended in methanol, sonicated, suitably diluted to obtain concentration within linearity range. Apply 10 μl for chromatographic evaluation.

Chromatographic equipments:

Sample applicator: Camag Linomat–IV

Development chamber: Camag twin-trough glass chamber, 10 × 10 cm

Densitometric scanner: Camag TLC Scanner–II

Chromatographic conditions:

1. Stationary phase: Silica gel $60F_{254}$ pre-coated HPTLC plates, 10 × 10 cm (200 μm) – Merck, pre-washed with methanol, dried at 105°C for 2 hrs prior to use
2. Mobile phase (MP): Toluene–ethyl acetate–methanol–glacial acetic acid (7 : 2 : 0.5 : 0.5 v/v)
3. Standard/Sample application:
   Band length: 10 mm Volume applied: 10 μl Spacing: 10 mm
4. Chamber saturation: 15 min (MP)
5. RH (%): 55 ± 5
6. Temperature °C: 22 ± 2
7. Separation technique: Ascending
8. Quantity of mobile phase: 10 ml
8. Migration distance: 85 mm
9. Migration time: 30 min

Densitometric evaluation:

Wavelength: UV–263 nm Scanning mode: Reflectance/Absorbance

HRF: Ritonavir—32; Lopinavir—39

Linearity (ng/band): Lopinavir—6.67–20.0; Ritonavir—1.67–5.0

Recovery (%): Lopinavir—98.58–101.49; Ritonavir—96.45–102.14

References: A.V. Sulebhavikar, U.D. Pawar, K.V. Mangoankar and N.D. Prabhu-Navelkar, *E.J. Chem.*, **5(4)**, 706–712, 2008.

Comments: The method validated for accuracy, precision, linearity, LOD and LOQ.

HPTLC : High Performance Thin Layer Chromatography
HPTLC Densitogram

No. 508

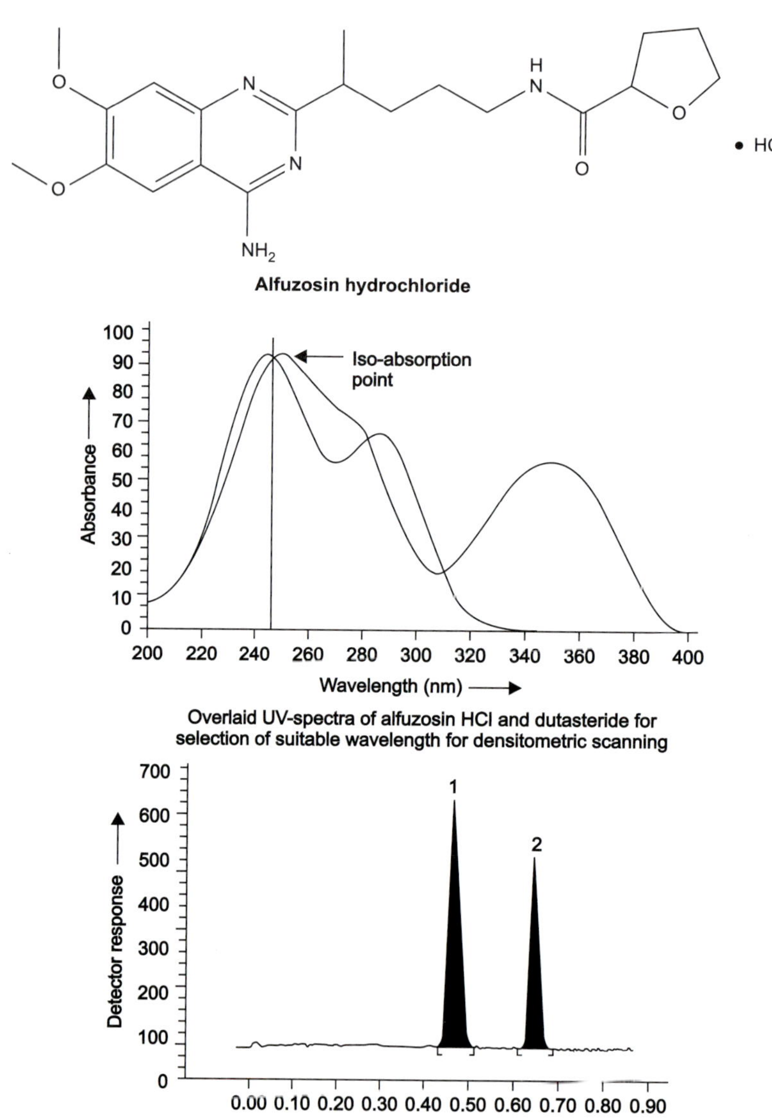

Typical densitogram of the standard containing alfuzosin and dutasteride. For detailed experimental and chromatographic conditions, refer to Protocol No. 508. Peaks identification: 1. Alfuzosin HCl; 2. Dutasteride.

PROTOCOL FOR HPTLC ANALYSIS OF PHARMACEUTICAL FORMULATION

Protocol No. 508

Formulation: **Alfuzosin hydrochloride, Dutasteride**

Classification: Miscellaneous **Dosage form:** Tablets

Standard preparation: Prepare 1 mg/ml solution of each compound in methanol. Further serial dilutions are made for linearity studies by applying 1 μl of each solution.

Sample preparation: Powdered sample equivalent to 10 mg of alfuzosin and 0.5 mg of dutasteride suspended in 20 ml of methanol, sonicated for 10 min, diluted to 25 ml with methanol, centrifuged at 7000 rpm and 22 μl of supernatant applied for chromatographic analysis.

Chromatographic equipments:

Sample applicator: Camag Linomat–V

Development chamber: Camag twin–trough glass chamber, 20 × 10 cm

Densitometric scanner: Camag TLC Scanner–III

Chromatographic conditions:

1. Stationary phase: Silica gel 60F_{254} pre-coated HPTLC plates, 20 × 10 cm (200 μm), pre-washed with methanol, activated at 110°C for 5 min prior to use
2. Mobile phase (MP): Toluene–methanol–dichloromethane–triethylamine (6 : 1 : 1 : 0.6 v/v)
3. Standard/Sample application:
   Band length: 6 mm Volume applied: 22 μl Spacing: 6 mm
4. Chamber saturation: 30 min (MP)
5. RH (%): 60 ± 5
6. Temperature °C: 25 ± 2
7. Separation technique: Ascending
8. Quantity of mobile phase: 17 ml
8. Migration distance: 80 mm
9. Migration time: 20 min

Densitometric evaluation:

Wavelength: UV–247 nm (iso-absorption point)

Scanning mode: Reflectance/Absorbance

HRF: Alfuzosin hydrochloride—46; Dutasteride—65

Linearity (ng/band): Alfuzosin HCl—300–600; Dutasteride—500–1000

Recovery (%): 99.29–100.55 for both the compounds

References: Shivprasad S. Deshmukh, Vaishali V. Musale, Vidhya K. Bhusari and Sunil S. Dhaneshwar, *J. Planar Chromatogr.*, **24(3)**, 218–221, 2011.

Comments: The method validated for accuracy, precision, linearity, LOD, LOQ, specificity, robustness and ruggedness.

HPTLC : High Performance Thin Layer Chromatography
HPTLC Densitogram

No. 509

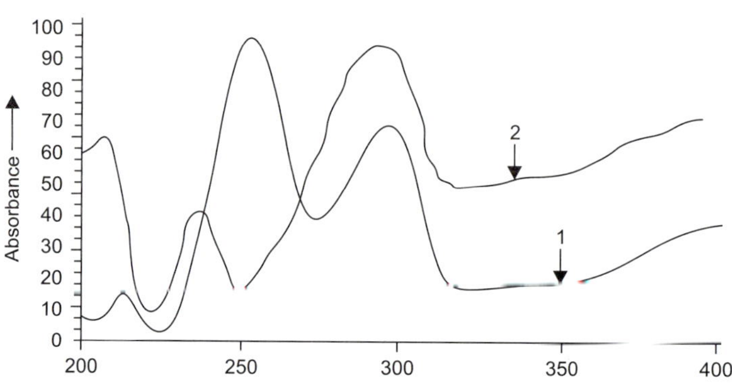

Tamsulosin hydrochloride

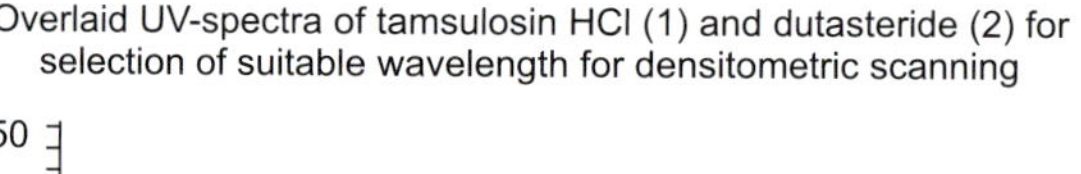

Overlaid UV-spectra of tamsulosin HCl (1) and dutasteride (2) for selection of suitable wavelength for densitometric scanning

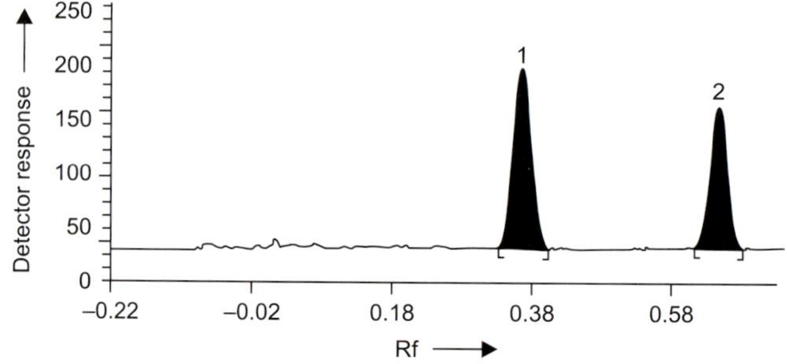

Typical densitogram of the sample containing tamsulosin HCl and dutasteride. For detailed experimental and chromatographic conditions, refer to Protocol No. 509. Peaks identification: 1. Tamsulosin HCl; 2. Dutasteride.

PROTOCOL FOR HPTLC ANALYSIS OF PHARMACEUTICAL FORMULATION

Protocol No. 509

Formulation: Tamsulosin hydrochloride, Dutasteride

Classification: Miscellaneous **Dosage form:** Tablets

Standard preparation: Prepare 1 mg/ml solution of each compound in methanol. Further dilutions are made with methanol to get 100 μg/ml. Apply varying volumes for linearity profile.

Sample preparation: Powdered sample equivalent to 8 mg of tamsulosin HCl and 10 mg of dutasteride suspended in 80 ml of methanol, sonicated for 15 min, diluted and filtered. Carry out further dilutions to get 8 μg/ml of tamsulosin HCl and 10 μg/ml of dutasteride and use for analysis.

Chromatographic equipments:

Sample applicator: Camag Linomat–V

Development chamber: Camag twin–trough glass chamber, 10 × 10 cm

Densitometric scanner: Camag TLC Scanner–III

Chromatographic conditions:

1. Stationary phase: Silica gel $60F_{254}$ pre-coated HPTLC plates, 10 × 10 cm (200 μm) – Merck
2. Mobile phase (MP): Toluene–methanol–triethylamine (9 : 1.5 : 1 v/v)
3. Standard/Sample application:
   Band length: 6 mm Volume applied: 1–10 μl Spacing: 10 mm
4. Chamber saturation: 30 min (MP)
5. RH (%): 55 ± 5
6. Temperature °C: Ambient
7. Separation technique: Ascending
8. Quantity of mobile phase: 11.5 ml
8. Migration distance: 85 mm
9. Migration time: 18 min

Densitometric evaluation:

Wavelength: UV–280 nm Scanning mode: Reflectance/Absorbance

HRF: Tamsulosin HCl—36; Dutasteride—65

Linearity (ng/band): 200–2000 for both the compounds

Recovery (%): 99.10–100.20 for both the compounds

References: D.B. Patel and N.J. Patel, *Acta Chromatographica*, **22(3)**, 419–431, 2010.

Comments: The method validated for accuracy, precision, linearity, LOD, LOQ, specificity and robustness.

HPTLC : High Performance Thin Layer Chromatography
HPTLC Densitogram

No. 510

Tamsulosin hydrochloride

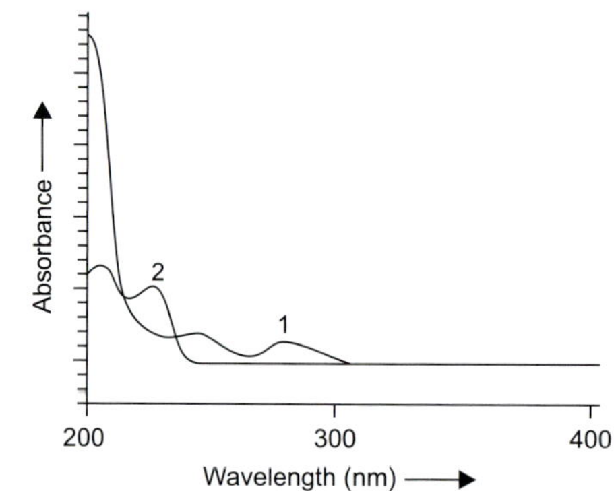

Overlaid UV-spectra of finasteride (1) and tamsulosin HCl (2)
for selection of suitable wavelength for densitometric scanning

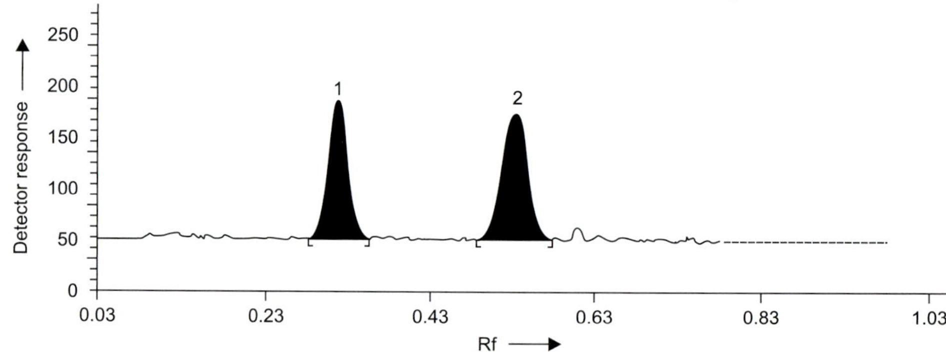

Typical densitogram of the sample containing tamsulosin hydrochloride and finasteride. For detailed experimental and chromatographic conditions, refer to Protocol No. 510. Peaks identification: 1. Tamsulosin HCl; 2. Finasteride.

PROTOCOL FOR HPTLC ANALYSIS OF PHARMACEUTICAL FORMULATION

Protocol No. 510

Formulation: Tamsulosin hydrochloride, Finasteride

Classification: Miscellaneous **Dosage form:** Tablets

Standard preparation: Prepare 1 mg/ml solution of each compound in methanol. From this take 1 ml of TAM and 2.5 ml of FN solutions and dilute to 10 ml with methanol. Apply 1, 2, 4, 8, 12, 16, 20 μl for linearity studies.

Sample preparation: Powdered sample equivalent to 1 mg of TAM or 12.5 mg of FN suspended in 80 ml of methanol, sonicated for 15 min, dilute to 100 ml, filtered and used for analysis.

Chromatographic equipments:

Sample applicator: Camag Linomat–V with 100 μl syringe

Development chamber: Camag twin–trough glass chamber, 10 × 10 cm

Densitometric scanner: Camag TLC Scanner–III

Chromatographic conditions:

1. Stationary phase: Silica gel $60F_{254}$ pre-coated HPTLC plates, 10 × 10 cm (250 μm) – Merck
2. Mobile phase (MP): (i) Toluene–methanol–triethylamine (9 : 1.5 : 0.1 v/v); (ii) Toluene–1,4-dioxane–25% ammonia (4.5 : 5.5 : 0.1 v/v)
3. Standard/Sample application:
   Band length: 6 mm Volume applied: 1–20 μl Spacing: 10 mm
4. Chamber saturation: 30 min (MP)
5. RH (%): 55 ± 5
6. Temperature °C: 22 ± 2
7. Separation technique: Ascending
8. Quantity of mobile phase: 10.5 ml
8. Migration distance: 85 mm
9. Migration time: 50 min

Densitometric evaluation:

Wavelength: UV–270 nm or 282 nm Scanning mode: Reflectance/Absorbance

HRF: Tamsulosin HCl—36, 45; Finasteride—54; 68

Linearity (ng/band): Tamsulosin HCl—100–2000; Finasteride—250–5000

Recovery (%): 99.63–100.64 for both the compounds

References: Susheel John Verghese, Leela Madhuri Pola, K.R. Ramesh Krishnan and T.K. Ravi, Abstract No. F-278; 61st IPC, 2009. Personal communication, Prof. T.K. Ravi.

Comments: The method validated for accuracy, precision, linearity, LOD, LOQ, specificity, robustness and ruggedness.

HPTLC : High Performance Thin Layer Chromatography
HPTLC Densitogram

No. 511

Tamsulosin hydrochloride

Finasteride

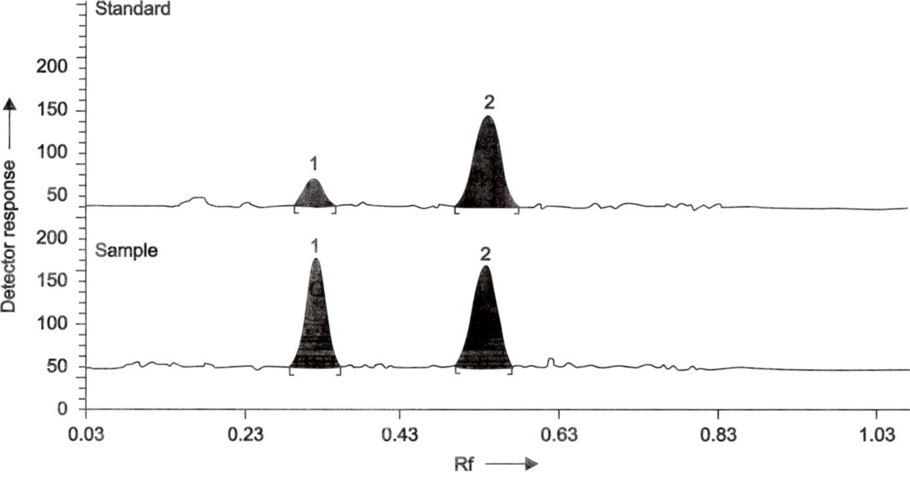

Typical densitogram of the standard and sample containing tamsulosin HCl and finasteride. For detailed experimental and chromatographic conditions, refer to Protocol No. 511. Peaks identification: 1. Tamsulosin HCl; 2. Finasteride.

PROTOCOL FOR HPTLC ANALYSIS OF PHARMACEUTICAL FORMULATION

Protocol No. 511

Formulation: Tamsulosin hydrochloride, Finasteride

Classification: Miscellaneous **Dosage form:** Tablets

Standard preparation: Prepare 1 mg/ml solution of each compound in methanol. Further dilute to get 100 μg/ml of tamsulosin hydrochloride and 250 μg/ml of finasteride. Apply varying volumes of each solution for linearity profile.

Sample preparation: Dissolve powdered sample equivalent to 1 mg of tamsulosin, suspend in 80 ml of methanol, sonicate for 15 min, dilute to 100 ml, filter and use the filtrate for chromatographic evaluation.

Chromatographic equipments:

Sample applicator: Camag Linomat–V

Development chamber: Camag twin–trough glass chamber, 10 × 10 cm

Densitometric scanner: Camag TLC Scanner–III

Chromatographic conditions:

1. Stationary phase: Silica gel $60F_{254}$ pre-coated HPTLC plates, 10 × 10 cm (200 μm) – Merck
2. Mobile phase (MP): Toluene–methanol–triethylamine (9 : 1.5 : 1 v/v)
3. Standard/Sample application:
   Band length: 5 mm Volume applied: 1–20 μl Spacing: 10 mm
4. Chamber saturation: 30 min (MP)
5. RH (%): 55 ± 5
6. Temperature °C: 25 ± 2
7. Separation technique: Ascending
8. Quantity of mobile phase: 11 ml
8. Migration distance: 85 mm
9. Migration time: 20 min

Densitometric evaluation:

Wavelength: UV–270 Scanning mode: Reflectance/Absorbance

HRF: Tamsulosin HCl—33; Finasteride—53

Linearity (ng/band): Tamsulosin HCl—100–2000; Finasteride—250–5000

Recovery (%): 99.80–100.00 for both the compounds

References: Dipti B. Patel and Nathubhai J. Patel, *Acta Pharm.*, **60**, 197–205, 2010.

Comments:

- The method validated for accuracy, precision, linearity, LOD and LOQ.
- The sample was also analysed by RP-HPLC and results were comparable by both the methods.

HPTLC : High Performance Thin Layer Chromatography
HPTLC Densitogram

No. 512

Finasteride

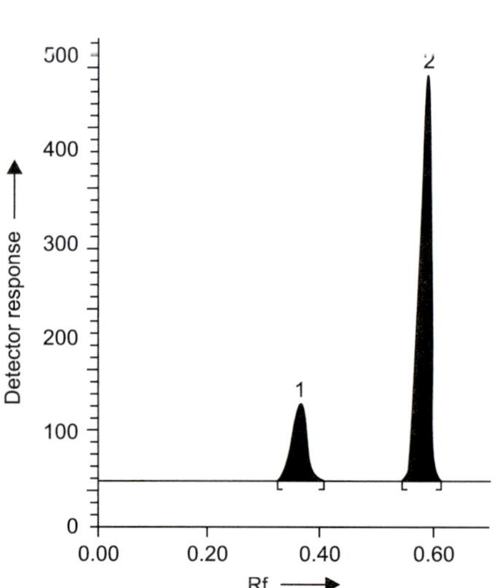

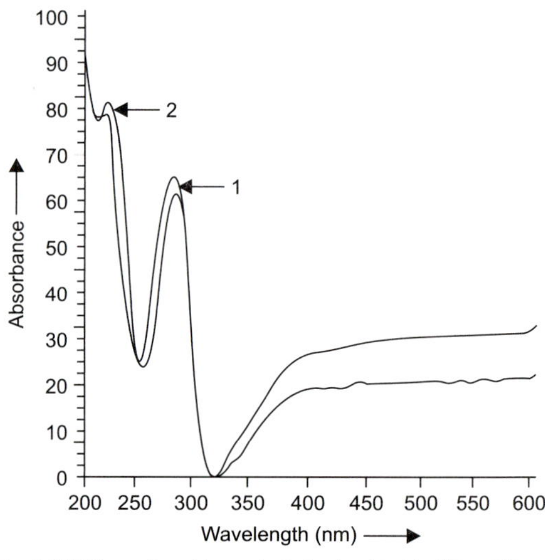

Overlaid UV-spectra of tamsulosin hydrochloride (1) and finasteride (2) for selection of suitable wavelength for densitometric scanning

Typical densitogram of the sample containing tamsulosin HCl and finasteride. For detailed experimental and chromatographic conditions, refer to Protocol No. 512. Peaks identification: 1. Tamsulosin HCl; 2. Finasteride.

PROTOCOL FOR HPTLC ANALYSIS OF PHARMACEUTICAL FORMULATION

Protocol No. 512

Formulation: Tamsulosin hydrochloride, Finasteride

Classification: Miscellaneous **Dosage form:** Tablets

Standard preparation: Prepare solution of both the compounds in methanol to get 1 mg/ml of tamsulosin and 5 mg/ml of finasteride. Dilute 2 ml of each solution to 10 ml with methanol and apply varying volumes for linearity profile.

Sample preparation: Powdered sample equivalent to 4 mg of tamsulosin suspended in 15 ml of methanol, sonicated for 10 min, diluted to 25 ml, filtered and the filtrate used for chromatographic evaluation.

Chromatographic equipments:

Sample applicator: Camag Linomat–V

Development chamber: Camag twin–trough glass chamber, 20 × 10 cm

Densitometric scanner: Camag TLC Scanner–III

Chromatographic conditions:

1. Stationary phase: Silica gel $60F_{254}$ pre-coated HPTLC plates, 20 × 10 cm (200 μm) – Merck
2. Mobile phase (MP): Toluene–n-propanol–triethylamine (3 : 1.5 : 0.2 v/v)
3. Standard/Sample application:
   Band length: 6 mm Volume applied: 1–6 μl Spacing: 15 mm
4. Chamber saturation: —
5. RH (%): 60 ± 5
6. Temperature °C: 25 ± 2
7. Separation technique: Ascending
8. Quantity of mobile phase: 23 ml
8. Migration distance: 80 mm
9. Migration time: 20 min

Densitometric evaluation:

Wavelength: UV–260 nm Scanning mode: Reflectance/Absorbance

HRF: Tamsulosin HCl—35; Finasteride—56

Linearity (ng/band): Tamsulosin HCl—200–1200; Finasteride—1000–6000

Recovery (%): 99.75–99.77 for both the compounds

References: Sanjay B. Bari, Pritam S. Jain, Abdul R. Bakshi and Sanjay B. Surana, *J. Analytical and Bioanalytical Techniques*, **2(2)**, 1–4, 2011.

Comments: The method validated for accuracy, precision, linearity, LOD, LOQ, specificity, robustness and ruggedness.

HPTLC : High Performance Thin Layer Chromatography
HPTLC Densitogram

No. 513

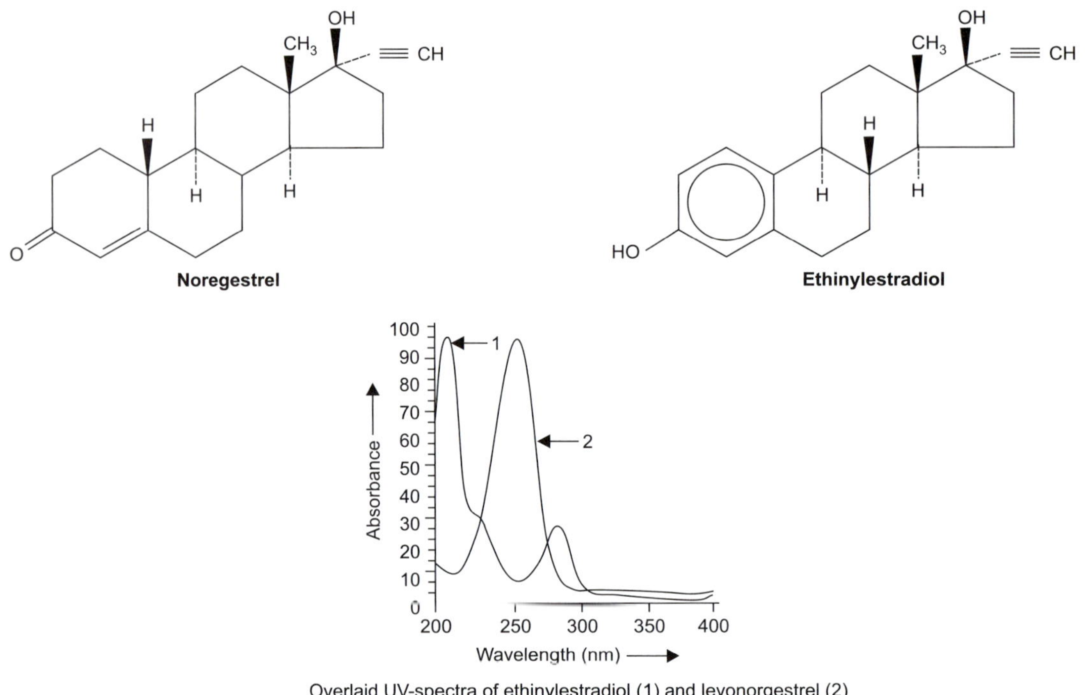

Overlaid UV-spectra of ethinylestradiol (1) and levonorgestrel (2) for selection of suitable wavelength for densitometric scanning

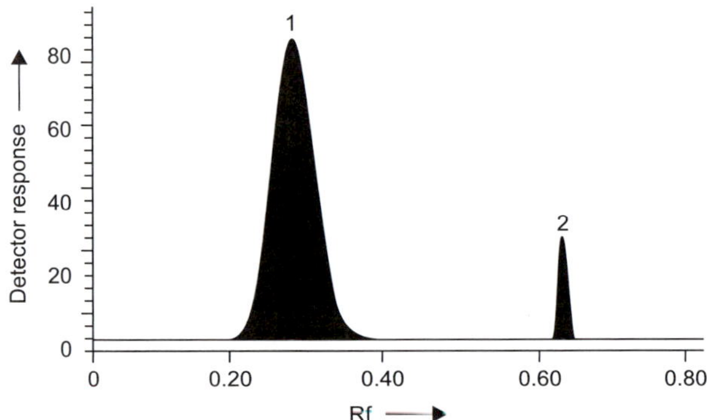

Typical densitogram of the sample containing norgestrel and ethinylestradiol. For detailed experimental and chromatographic conditions, refer to Protocol No. 513. Peaks identification: 1. Norgestrel; 2. Ethinylestradiol.

PROTOCOL FOR HPTLC ANALYSIS OF PHARMACEUTICAL FORMULATION

Protocol No. 513

Formulation: **dl-Norgestrel, Ethinylestradiol**

Classification: Miscellaneous **Dosage form:** Tablets

Standard preparation: Prepare solution of each compound separately in methanol to get 150 ng/μl (dl-norgestrel) and 15 ng/μl of ethinyloestradiol. Apply 1 μl for analysis.

Sample preparation: Powdered sample equivalent to 1 tablet extracted with methanol to make 10 ml, centrifuge and use clear solution for analysis. Apply 1 μl for chromatographic separation and analysis.

Chromatographic equipments:

Sample applicator: Camag Linomat–V
Development chamber: Camag twin-trough glass chamber, 10 × 10 cm
Densitometric scanner: Camag TLC Scanner–III

Chromatographic conditions:

1. Stationary phase: Silica gel $60F_{254}$ pre-coated HPTLC plates, 10 × 10 cm (200 μm) – Merck, pre-washed with methanol dried at 105°C for 5 min prior to use
2. Mobile phase (MP): Chloroform–methanol (9.6 : 0.4 v/v)
3. Standard/Sample application:
   Band length: 5 mm Volume applied: 1 μl Spacing: 5 mm
4. Chamber saturation: 30 min (MP)
5. RH (%): 55 ± 5
6. Temperature °C: 20 ± 2
7. Separation technique: Ascending
8. Quantity of mobile phase: 10 ml
8. Migration distance: 55 mm 9. Migration time: 22 min

Densitometric evaluation:

Wavelength: UV–240 nm, 366 nm Scanning mode: Reflectance/Absorbance
HRF: dl-Norgestrel—30; Ethinylestradiol—62
Linearity (ng/band): dl-Norgestrel—200–1000; Ethinylestradiol—10–100
Recovery (%): Norgestrel—98–105; Ethinylestradiol—95–110

References: —

Comments:

- The method was developed and optimized at CIPL, Ghaziabad.
- After development, the plate was scanned at 240 nm under reflectance mode for norgestrel. The plate was then sprayed with 20% methanolic sulphuric acid (v/v) and heated at 110°C for 3 min in an oven with non-perforated shelf, cooled and scanned at 366 nm under fluorescence mode for ethinylestradiol.
- The method was routinely used in the laboratory. More than 5000 samples were analysed with good reproducibility.

HPTLC : High Performance Thin Layer Chromatography
HPTLC Densitogram

No. 514

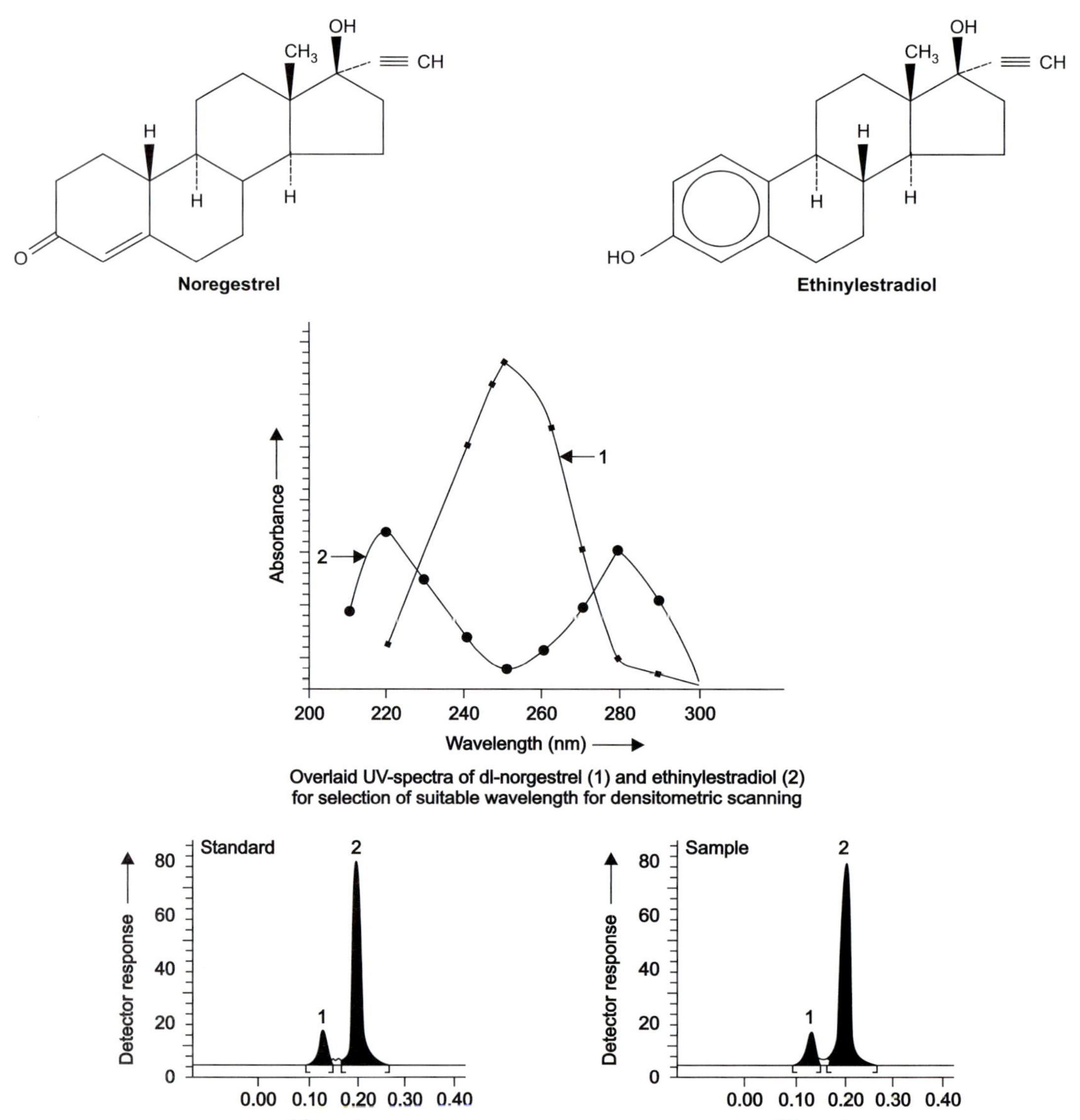

Overlaid UV-spectra of dl-norgestrel (1) and ethinylestradiol (2) for selection of suitable wavelength for densitometric scanning

Typical densitogram of the sample and the standard containing dl-norgestrel and ethinylestradiol. For detailed experimental and chromatographic conditions, refer to Protocol No. 514. Peaks identification: 1. Ethinylestradiol; 2. dl-Norgestrel.

PROTOCOL FOR HPTLC ANALYSIS OF PHARMACEUTICAL FORMULATION

Protocol No. 514

Formulation: dl–Norgestrel, Ethinylestradiol

Classification: Miscellaneous **Dosage form:** Tablets

Standard preparation: Prepare solution of both the compounds separately in methanol to get 300 μg/ml (dl-norgestrel) and 30 μg/ml (ethinylestradiol). Further dilutions made with methanol for application and analysis.

Sample preparation: Powdered sample equivalent to 300 mg of dl-norgestrel suspended in methanol, sonicated for 20 min, centrifuged and clear supernatant suitably diluted. Apply 1 μl for chromatographic separation and assay.

Chromatographic equipments:

Sample applicator: Camag Linomat–IV

Development chamber: Rectangular flat bottom glass chamber, 20 × 20 cm

Densitometric scanner: Shimadzu CS 910 Dual wavelength TLC scanner

Chromatographic conditions:

1. Stationary phase: Silica gel $60F_{254}$ pre-coated TLC plates, 10 × 10 cm (250 μm) – Merck, pre-washed with methanol, dried for 60 min prior to use
2. Mobile phase (MP): n-hexane–chloroform–carbon tetrachloride–ethanol (7 : 18 : 22 : 1 v/v)
3. Standard/Sample application:
   Band length: 3 mm Volume applied: 1 μl Spacing: 5 mm
4. Chamber saturation: 10 min (MP)
5. RH (%): 55 ± 5
6. Temperature °C: 25 ± 1
7. Separation technique: Ascending
8. Quantity of mobile phase: 45 ml
8. Migration distance: 50 mm
9. Migration time: 2 × 15 min

Densitometric evaluation:

Wavelength: UV–220 nm Scanning mode: Reflectance/Absorbance

HRF: Ethinylestradiol—12; dl–Norgestrel—22

Linearity (ng/band): Ethinylestradiol—10–100; dl-Norgestrel—100–500

Recovery (%): 98.75–101.25 for both the drugs

References: J.A. Berndt, C.F. Poole, *J. Planar Chromatogr.*, **1**, 173–177, 1988.

Comments: Although λ_{max} of dl-norgestrel is about 250 nm but considering that ethinylestradiol is minor compound, UV–220 nm was selected for densitometric scanning.

HPTLC : High Performance Thin Layer Chromatography
HPTLC Densitogram

No. 515

Levonorgestrel

Ethinylestradiol

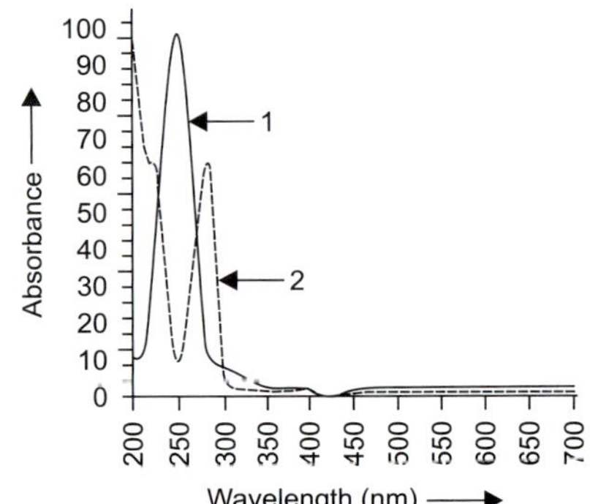

Overlaid UV-spectra of levonorgestrel (1) and ethinylestradiol (2) for selection of suitable wavelength for densitometric scanning

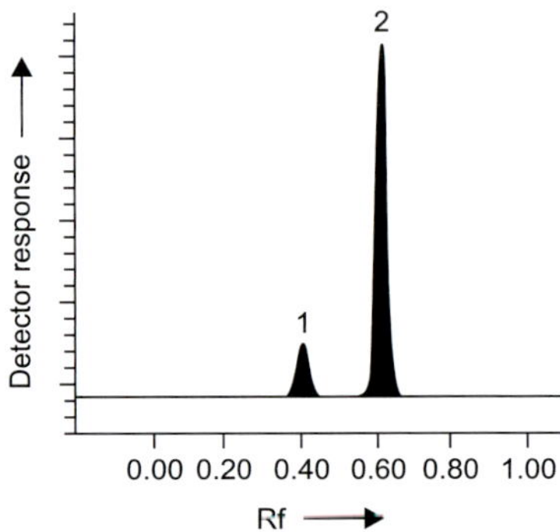

Typical densitogram of the sample containing levonorgestrel and ethinylestradiol. For detailed experimental and chromatographic conditions, refer to Protocol No. 515. Peaks identification: 1. Levonorgestrel; 2. Ethinylestradiol.

PROTOCOL FOR HPTLC ANALYSIS OF PHARMACEUTICAL FORMULATION

Protocol No. 515

Formulation: Levonorgestrel, Ethinylestradiol

Classification: Miscellaneous **Dosage form:** Tablets

Standard preparation: Stock solution of both the compounds were prepared separately in methanol. Further serial dilutions made with methanol to get different concentrations, i.e. 100–400 μg/ml (levonorgestrel) and 20–80 μg/ml (ethinyl-estradiol). Apply 2 μl of each solution for linearity profile.

Sample preparation: Powdered sample equivalent to 15 mg of levonorgestrel suspended in diethylether, sonicated for 15 min, filtered and diluted. Organic phase evaporated to dryness and the residue taken up in methanol. Apply 2 μl for chromatographic evaluation.

Chromatographic equipments:

Sample applicator: Camag Linomat–IV

Development chamber: Rectangular flat bottom glass chamber, 10 × 10 cm

Densitometric scanner: Camag TLC Scanner–III

Chromatographic conditions:

1. Stationary phase: Silica gel $60F_{254}$ pre-coated TLC plates, 10 × 10 cm (250 μm) – Merck
2. Mobile phase (MP): n-hexane–chloroform–methanol (3 : 9 : 0.75 v/v)
3. Standard/Sample application:
   Band length: 6 mm Volume applied: 2 μl Spacing: 5 mm
4. Chamber saturation: 15 min (MP)
5. RH (%): 55 ± 5
6. Temperature °C: 25 ± 4
7. Separation technique: Ascending
8. Quantity of mobile phase: 12 ml
8. Migration distance: 60 mm
9. Migration time: 15 min

Densitometric evaluation:

Wavelength: UV–225 nm Scanning mode: Reflectance/Absorbance

HRF: Ethinylestradiol—43; Levonorgestrel—65

Linearity (ng/band): Levonorgestrel—200–800; Ethinylestradiol—40–160

Recovery (%): 98.5–101.0 for both the drugs

References: Ali Reza Fakhan, Afshin Rajabi Khorrami and Mojtaba Shamsipur, *Analytica Chimica Acta*, **572**, 237–242, 2006

Comments:

- The method validated for accuracy, precision, linearity, LOD, LOQ, specificity, robustness and ruggedness.
- The method is stability indicating (acid, base, oxidative, thermal, photolytic). The degradation products were separated from main compounds.

HPTLC : High Performance Thin Layer Chromatography
HPTLC Densitogram

No. 516

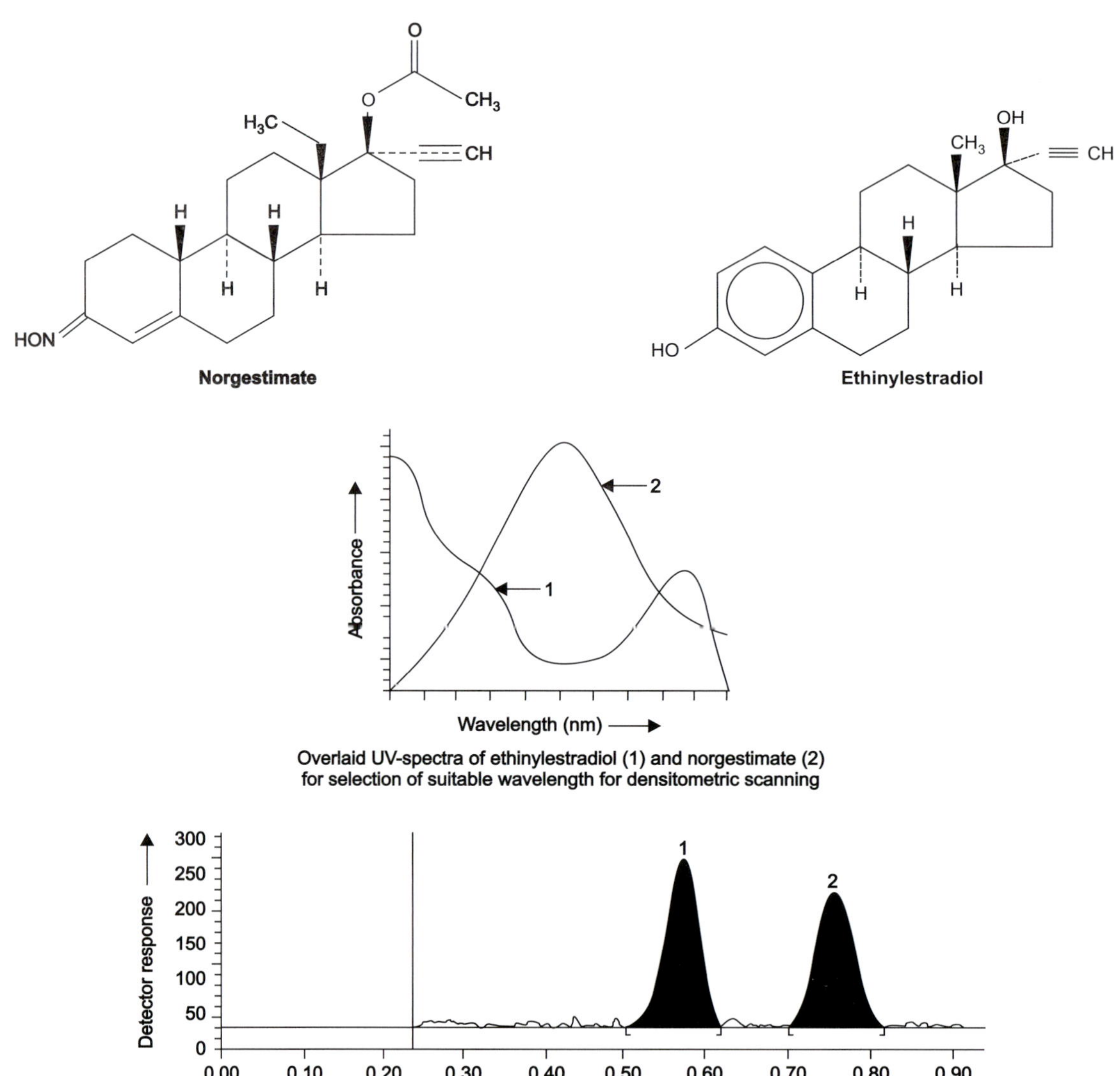

Overlaid UV-spectra of ethinylestradiol (1) and norgestimate (2) for selection of suitable wavelength for densitometric scanning

Typical densitogram of the standard containing ethinylestradiol and norgestimate. For detailed experimental and chromatographic conditions, refer to Protocol No. 516. Peaks identification: 1. Ethinylestradiol; 2. Norgestimate.

PROTOCOL FOR HPTLC ANALYSIS OF PHARMACEUTICAL FORMULATION

Protocol No. 516

Formulation: Ethinylestradiol, Norgestimate

Classification: Miscellaneous **Dosage form:** Tablets

Standard preparation: Prepare 500 μg/ml solution of norgestimate and 100 μg/ml of ethinylestradiol, both in methanol. Apply varying volumes for linearity studies.

Sample preparation: For norgestimate, weigh sample equivalent to 1 mg, suspend in 5 ml of methanol, sonicate, dilute to 10 ml, filter and apply 20 μl for assay. For ethinylestradiol, sample equivalent to 0.2 mg suspended in methanol, sonicated, diluted to 10 ml, filtered and 20 μl applied for assay.

Chromatographic equipments:

Sample applicator: Camag Linomat–V

Development chamber: Camag twin–trough glass chamber, 10 × 10 cm

Densitometric scanner: Camag TLC Scanner–III

Chromatographic conditions:

1. Stationary phase: Silica gel 60F_{254} pre-coated TLC plates, 10 × 10 cm (250 μm) – Merck, pre-washed with methanol, activated at 110°C (5 min) prior to use
2. Mobile phase (MP): Benzene–ethyl acetate–triethylamine (7 : 2 : 1 v/v)
3. Standard/Sample application:
   Band length: 6 mm Volume applied: 2–10 μl Spacing: 5 mm
4. Chamber saturation: 20 min (MP)
5. RH (%): 55 ± 5
6. Temperature °C: Ambient
7. Separation technique: Ascending
8. Quantity of mobile phase: 10 ml
8. Migration distance: 90 mm
9. Migration time: 20 min

Densitometric evaluation:

Wavelength: UV–280 nm Scanning mode: Reflectance/Absorbance

HRF: Ethinylestradiol—58; Norgestimate—77

Linearity (ng/band): Ethinylestradiol—200–1000; Norgestimate—1000–5000

Recovery (%): 99.40–99.80 for both the compounds

References: P.B. Deshpande, S.V. Gandhi, A.V. Patel, V.A. Khandelwal, U.V. Bhasvar and B.P. Pawaskar, *Res. J. Pharm and Tech.*, **4(4)**, 582–584, 2011.

Comments: The method validated for accuracy, precision, linearity, LOD, LOQ and robustness.

HPTLC : High Performance Thin Layer Chromatography
HPTLC Densitogram

No. 517

Drospirenone

Ethinylestradiol

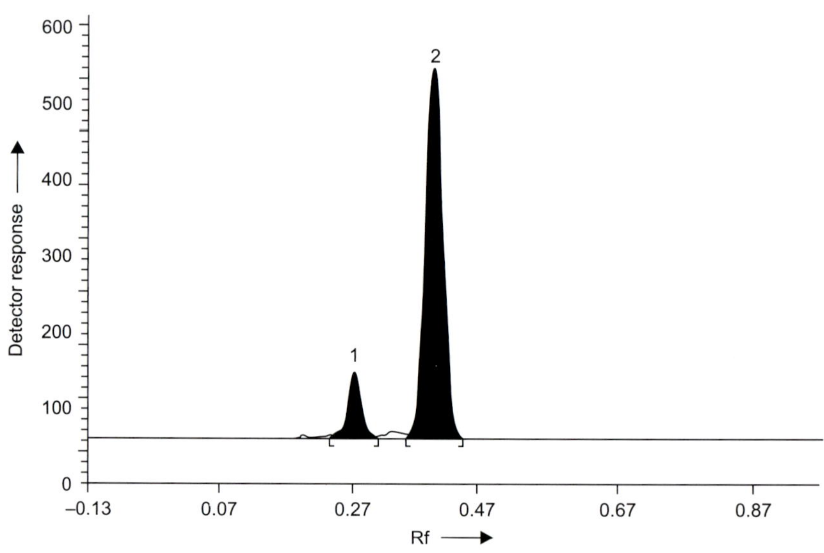

Typical densitogram of the standard containing ethinylestradiol and drospirenone. For detailed experimental and chromatographic conditions, refer to Protocol No. 517. Peaks identification: 1. Ethinylestradiol; 2. Drospirenone.

PROTOCOL FOR HPTLC ANALYSIS OF PHARMACEUTICAL FORMULATION

Protocol No. 517

Formulation: **Ethinylestradiol, Drospirenone**

Classification: Miscellaneous **Dosage form:** Tablets

Standard preparation: Prepare 1 mg/ml solution of each compound in methanol. Further serial dilutions of each solution made with methanol. Apply 10 μl of each solution for linearity profile.

Sample preparation: Powdered sample equivalent to 1 mg of ethinylestradiol suspended in methanol, sonicated for 15 min, diluted to 10 ml with methanol. Filtered and the filtrate suitably diluted to get 200 μg/ml solution of ethinylestradiol. Apply 10 μl for chromatographic separation and assay.

Chromatographic equipments:

Sample applicator: Camag Linomat–V

Development chamber: Camag twin–trough glass chamber, 20 × 10 cm

Densitometric scanner: Camag TLC Scanner–III

Chromatographic conditions:

1. Stationary phase: Silica gel $60F_{254}$ pre-coated TLC plates, 20 × 10 cm (250 μm) – Merck, pre-washed with methanol, activated at 110°C for 5 min prior to use
2. Mobile phase (MP): Toluene–methanol–25% ammonia (8 : 2 : 0.1 v/v)
3. Standard/Sample application:
   Band length: 6 mm Volume applied: 10 μl Spacing: 10 mm
4. Chamber saturation: 30 min (MP)
5. RH (%): 60 ± 5
6. Temperature °C: 25 ± 2
7. Separation technique: Ascending
8. Quantity of mobile phase: 20 ml
8. Migration distance: 80 mm
9. Migration time: 20 min

Densitometric evaluation:

Wavelength: UV–280 nm Scanning mode: Reflectance/Absorbance

HRF: Ethinylestradiol—29; Drospirenone—42

Linearity (ng/band): Ethinylestradiol—150–400; Drospirenone—30–80

Recovery (%): 98.30–99.75 for both the compounds

References: Vidya K. Bhusari and Sunil R. Dhaneshwar, Abstract No. 260, 63rd IPC, 2011, Personal correspondence with Prof. S. Dhaneshwar.

Comments: The method validated for accuracy, precision, linearity, LOD, LOQ, specificity and robustness as per ICH guidelines.

HPTLC : High Performance Thin Layer Chromatography
HPTLC Densitogram

No. 518

Icariin

Cyproterone

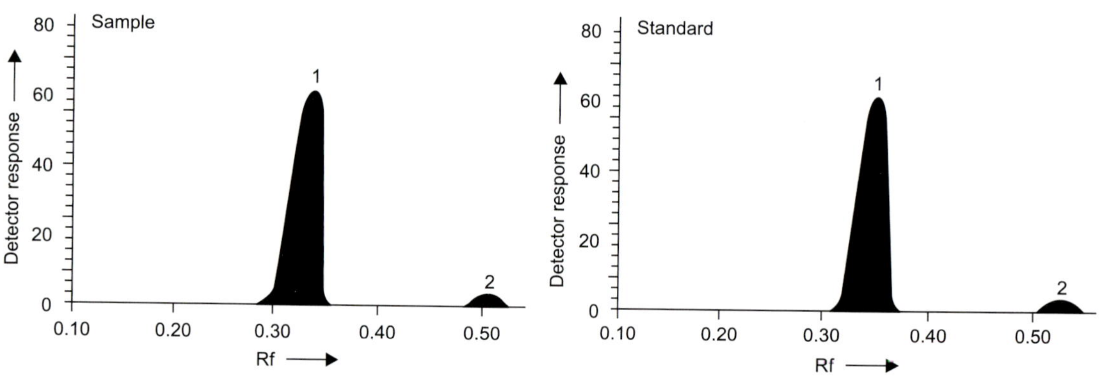

Typical densitogram of the sample and the standard containing cyproterone acetate and ethinylestradiol. For detailed experimental and chromatographic conditions, refer to Protocol No. 518. Peaks identification: 1. Cyproterone acetate; 2. Ethinylestradiol.

PROTOCOL FOR HPTLC ANALYSIS OF PHARMACEUTICAL FORMULATION

Protocol No. 518

Formulation: Ethinylestradiol, Cyproterone acetate

Classification: Miscellaneous **Dosage form:** Tablets

Standard preparation: Prepare 1 mg/ml solution of cyproterone acetate (CA) in solvent. Further prepare serial dilutions so that application of 1 μl of each solution covers the range of 250–4000 ng/band. For ethinylestradiol (EE) prepare 1 mg/ml solution in solvent. Further dilute to cover linearity range of 100–500 ng/band.

Sample preparation: Powdered sample equivalent to 10 mg of CA suspended in solvent, sonicated for 10 min, filtered and diluted suitably to get 1000 ng/μl. Apply 1 μl of CA solution and 5 μl of EE solution for assay.

Solvent: Chloroform–methanol (1 : 1 v/v).

Chromatographic equipments:

Sample applicator: Camag Nanomat–III

Development chamber: Camag twin-trough glass chamber, 10 × 20 cm

Densitometric scanner: Camag TLC Scanner–II

Chromatographic conditions:

1. Stationary phase: Silica gel 60F_{254} pre-coated HPTLC plates, 10 × 20 cm (200 μm) – Merck
2. Mobile phase (MP): Cyclohexane–ethyl acetate (6 : 4 v/v)
3. Standard/Sample application:
   Band length: 5 mm Volume applied: 1 μl, 5 μl Spacing: 10 mm
4. Chamber saturation: 15 min (MP)
5. RH (%): —
6. Temperature °C: 24 ± 1
7. Separation technique: Ascending
8. Quantity of mobile phase: 20 ml
8. Migration distance: 80 mm
9. Migration time: 20 min

Densitometric evaluation:

Wavelength: UV–221 (ethinylestradiol); 284 nm (cyproterone acetate)

Scanning mode: Reflectance/Absorbance

HRF: Cyproterone acetate—34; Ethinylestradiol—52

Linearity (ng/band): Cyproterone acetate—250–4000; Ethinylestradiol—100–500

Recovery (%): Cyproterone acetate—97.81–102.31; Ethinylestradiol—98.90–100.51

References: Katarina Pavič, Olivera čudina, Danica Agbaba and Soté Vladimirov, *J. Planar Chromatogr.*, **16(1)**, 45–47, 2003.

Comments: The method validated for accuracy, precision, linearity, LOD, LOQ, specificity, robustness and ruggedness.

HPTLC : High Performance Thin Layer Chromatography
HPTLC Densitogram

No. 519

Results obtained from analysis of ten tablets by three methods			
No.	Content [%] by HPTLC	Content [%] by HPLC (BP)	Content [%] by UV (IP)
1	96.22	96.01	96.09
2	100.40	99.21	100.65
3	99.71	98.72	100.07
4	97.42	96.69	97.90
5	96.55	95.92	97.03
6	98.44	99.71	99.01
7	102.68	101.19	102.49
8	100.42	100.37	100.65
9	96.85	95.96	96.50
10	97.46	100.04	97.63
Average	98.62	98.38	98.80
RSD (%)	2.1	2.0	2.1

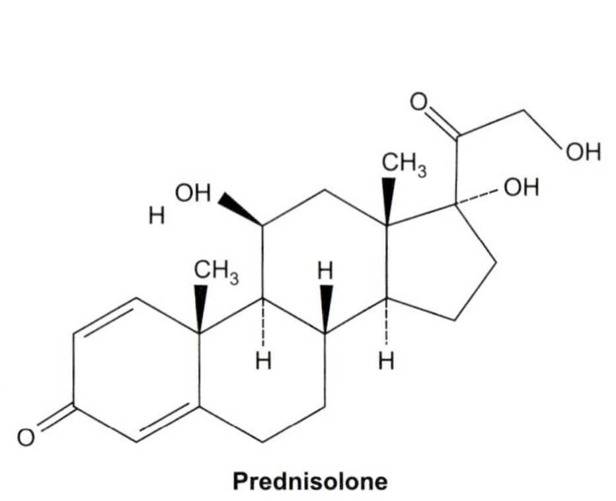

Prednisolone

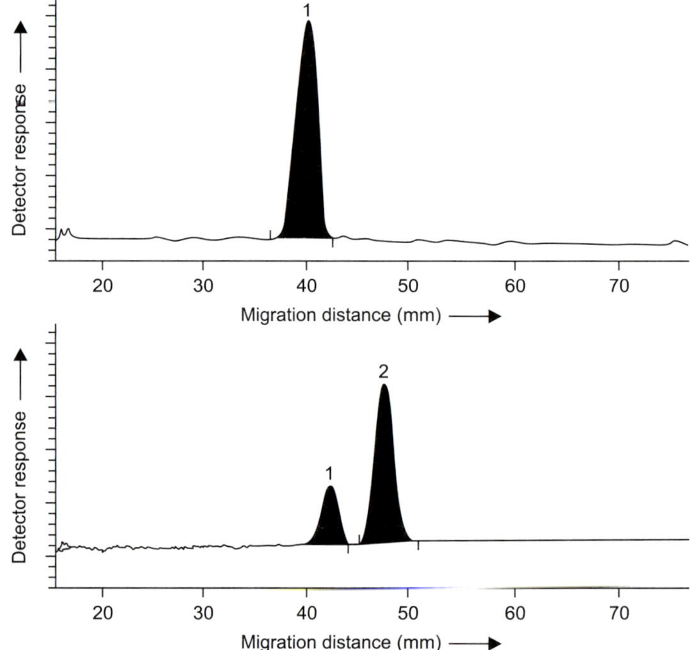

Typical densitograms of the standard (prednisolone) along with hydrocortisone (related substance). For detailed experimental and chromatographic conditions, refer to Protocol No. 519. Peaks identification: 1. Prednisolone; 2. Hydrocortisone.

PROTOCOL FOR HPTLC ANALYSIS OF PHARMACEUTICAL FORMULATION

Protocol No. 519

Formulation: Prednisolone, Hydrocortisone (related substance)

Classification: Miscellaneous **Dosage form:** Tablets

Standard preparation: Prepare 1 mg/ml solution of the substance in methanol. Further dilute with methanol to get 500 μg/ml. Apply varying volumes for linearity profile.

Sample preparation: Powdered sample equivalent to 5 mg suspended in 5–8 ml of methanol, sonicated for 15 min, dilute to 10 ml to get 0.5 μg/ml. Apply 10 μl (5 μg) for chromatographic separation and analysis.

Chromatographic equipments:

Sample applicator: Desaga AS–30

Plate-coater: Camag twin-trough glass chamber, 20 × 20 cm

Densitometric scanner: Desaga CD–60

Chromatographic conditions:

1. Stationary phase: Silica gel $60F_{254}$ pre-coated HPTLC plates, 20 × 20 cm (200 μm) – Merck, pre-washed with methanol before use
2. Mobile phase (MP): Chloroform–methanol (9.5 : 0.5 v/v)
3. Standard/Sample application:
   Band length: 5 mm Volume applied: 10 μl Spacing: 5 mm
4. Chamber saturation: 30 min (MP)
5. RH (%): 55 ± 5
6. Temperature °C: 22 ± 2
7. Separation technique: Ascending
8. Quantity of mobile phase: 20 ml
8. Migration distance: 75 mm
9. Migration time: 20 min

Densitometric evaluation:

Wavelength: UV–250 nm Scanning mode: Reflectance/Absorbance

HRF: See densitogram

Linearity: 2–10 μg/band

Recovery (%): 98.3–101.3 for both the compounds

References: Astha Mehta and Anil Thaker, *J. Planar Chromatogr.*, **23(3)**, 208–211, 2010.

Comments:

- The method is suitable for assay and content uniformity.
- The results by HPTLC are comparable with compendial methods (UV and HPLC).

HPTLC : High Performance Thin Layer Chromatography
HPTLC Densitogram

No. 520

HO OH R_1 R_2 O H

$R_1 = R_2 = OCH_3$, Curcumin
$R_1 = OCH_3$, $R_2 = H$, Demethoxycurcumin
$R_1 = R_2 = H$, Bis-Demethoxycurcumin

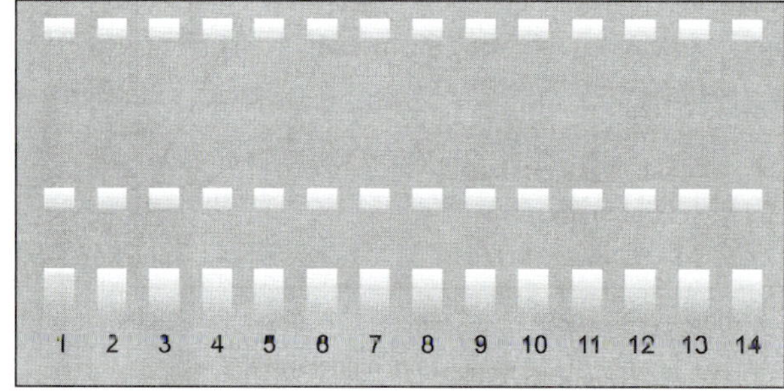

TLC profile of Curcuma longa when examined under 366 nm;
Tracks 1–5 of standard curcumin, demethoxycurcumin and bis-demethoxycurcumin;
Tracks 6–14 of sample of Curcuma longa collected from different geographical zones

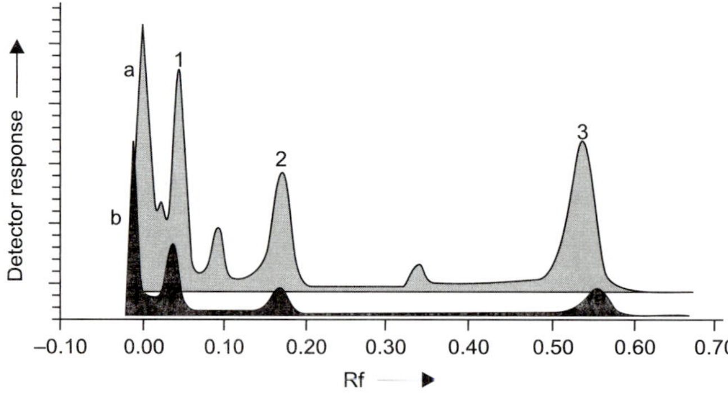

Typical densitograms of the sample (b) and standard (a). For detailed experimental and chromatographic conditions, refer to Protocol No. 520. Peaks identification: 1. Bis-Demethoxycurcumin; 2. Demethoxycurcumin; 3. Curcumin.

PROTOCOL FOR HPTLC ANALYSIS OF PHARMACEUTICAL FORMULATION

Protocol No. 520

Formulation: Curcuminoids (Curcumin, Demethoxycurcumin, Bis-Demethoxy-curcumin)

Classification: Miscellaneous **Dosage form:** Raw material

Standard preparation: Prepare 50 μg/ml solution of each curcuminoid in methanol. Apply varying concentrations of each in the range of 100–100 ng and carry out the chromatographic analysis.

Sample preparation: Extract 100 mg of curcuma longa, finely powdered with acetone (3 × 10 ml), concentrate under vacuum, dissolve in methanol to produce 5 ml and use for HPTLC analysis.

Chromatographic equipments:

Sample applicator: Camag Linomat–IV

Plate-coater: Camag glass chamber, 20 × 20 cm

Densitometric scanner: Camag TLC Scanner–III

Chromatographic conditions:

1. Stationary phase: Silica gel $60F_{254}$ pre-coated HPTLC plates, 20 × 20 cm (200 μm) – Merck
2. Mobile phase (MP): Chloroform–methanol (9.8 : 0.2 v/v)
3. Standard/Sample application:
   Band length: 6 mm Volume applied: 2–10 μl Spacing: 10 mm
4. Chamber saturation: 30 min (MP)
5. RH (%): 37.5 ± 2.5
6. Temperature °C: 25 ± 1
7. Separation technique: Ascending
8. Quantity of mobile phase: 20 ml
8. Migration distance: 80 mm
9. Migration time: 25 min

Densitometric evaluation:

Wavelength: UV–366 nm Scanning mode: Reflectance/Fluorescence

HRF: See densitogram

Linearity: 100–1000 ng/band for all the three curcuminoids

Recovery (%): Curcumin—98.75–100.73; Demethoxycurcumin—95.37–98.57; bis-Demethoxycurcumin—97.78–101.18

References: Vijaylata Pathania, Ajay Prakash Gupta and Bikram Singh, *J. Liq. Chromatogr. and Related Tech.*, **29**, 877–87, 2006.

Comments: The method validated for accuracy, precision, linearity, LOD, LOQ, specificity, robustness and ruggedness.

HPTLC : High Performance Thin Layer Chromatography
HPTLC Densitogram

No. 521

Curcuminoid content in extract (% w/w) of samples*				
Samples	**C**	**DMC**	**BDMC**	**Total content of curcuminoids**
m_1	0.99 ± 0.13	0.53 ± 0.07	0.49 ± 0.03	2.01 ± 0.23
m_2	0.79 ± 0.07	0.35 ± 0.06	0.34 ± 0.09	1.48 ± 0.22
m_3	0.70 ± 0.12	0.38 ± 0.10	0.30 ± 0.02	1.38 ± 0.24
m_4	0.61 ± 0.06	0.36 ± 0.08	0.26 ± 0.05	1.23 ± 0.19
m_5	0.23 ± 0.02	0.16 ± 0.01	0.13 ± 0.01	0.52 ± 0.04

*Expressed as mean values (n = 3) ± SD.

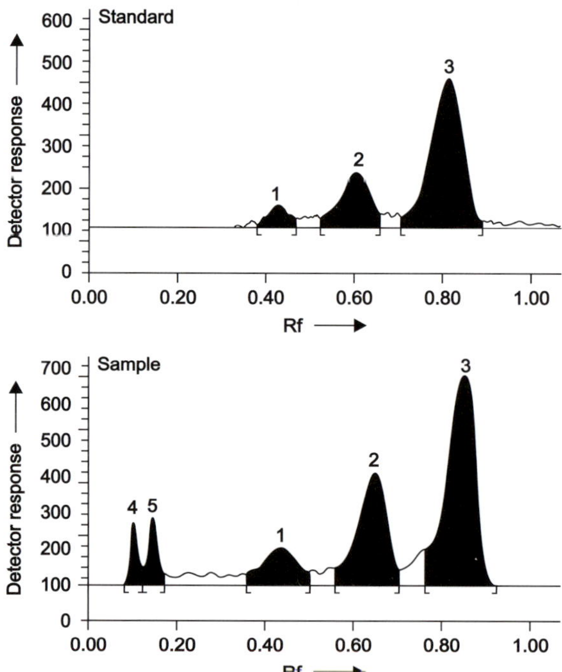

Typical densitograms of the sample and standard containing curcumin, demethoxycurcumin and bis-demethoxycurcumin. For detailed experimental and chromatographic conditions, refer to Protocol No. 521. Peaks identification: 1. bis-Demethoxycurcumin; 2. Demethoxycurcumin; 3. Curcumin; 4. Not identified; 5. Not identified.

PROTOCOL FOR HPTLC ANALYSIS OF PHARMACEUTICAL FORMULATION

Protocol No. 521

Formulation: Curcuminoids (Curcumin, Demethoxycurcumin, Bis-Demethoxy-curcumin)

Classification: Miscellaneous **Dosage form:** Raw material

Standard preparation: Prepare 1 mg/ml solution of each curcumin in methanol. Further serial dilutions are made with methanol to get 25–250 ng/ml. Apply 4 μl of each for linearity profile.

Sample preparation: 1 g of powdered sample extracted with methanol (20 ml × 3) for 15 min, filtered, total extract concentrated at 50°C under reduced pressure and the residue dissolved in 1 ml of methanol and the resulting solution used for HPTLC analysis.

Chromatographic equipments:

Sample applicator: Camag Linomat–V
Plate-coater: Camag glass chamber, 20 × 10 cm
Densitometric scanner: Camag TLC Scanner–III

Chromatographic conditions:

1. Stationary phase: Silica gel $60F_{254}$ pre-coated HPTLC plates, 20 × 10 cm (200 μm) – Merck
2. Mobile phase (MP): Chloroform–methanol (9.6 : 0.4 v/v)
3. Standard/Sample application:
   Band length: 6 mm Volume applied: 4 μl Spacing: 11 mm
4. Chamber saturation: 30 min (MP)
5. RH (%): 50 ± 5
6. Temperature °C: 25 ± 5
7. Separation technique: Ascending
8. Quantity of mobile phase: 20 ml
8. Migration distance: 70 mm
9. Migration time: 20 min

Densitometric evaluation:

Wavelength: UV–Vis—425 nm Scanning mode: Reflectance/Absorbance
HRF: See densitogram
Linearity: 100–1000 ng/band for all the three curcuminoids
Recovery (%): 96–98 for all the three curcuminoids

References: M. Paramasiram, Rajlakshmi and Hemanta Banerjee, *Current Science*, **95(11)**, 1529–1531, 2008.

Comments:

- Several commercially available samples of curcumin were analysed by the proposed methanol. The contents of curcuminoids varied from 0.5–2% w/w, curcumin being the major component.
- The method validated for accuracy, precision, linearity, LOD and LOQ.

HPTLC : High Performance Thin Layer Chromatography
HPTLC Densitogram

No. 522

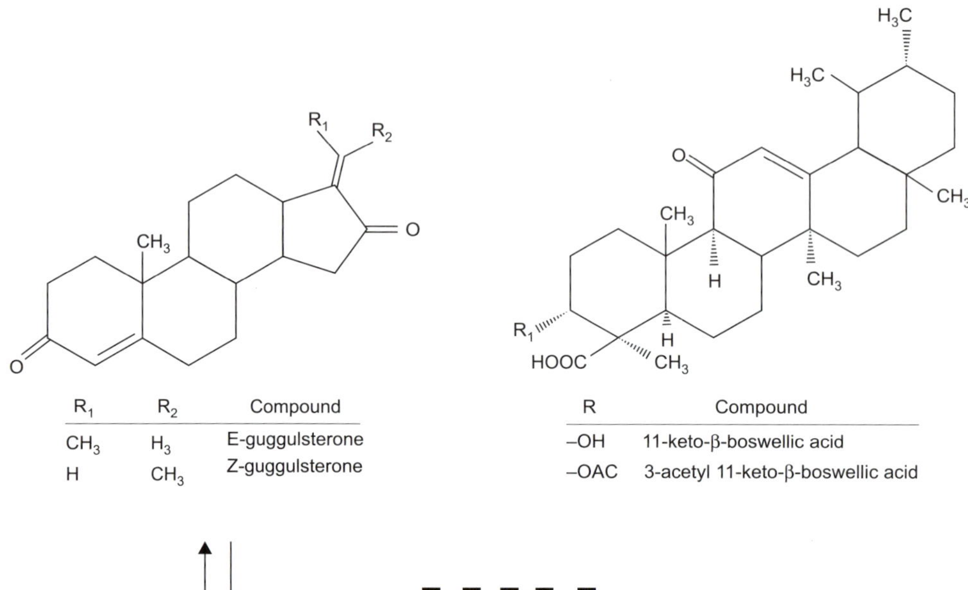

R_1	R_2	Compound
CH_3	H_3	E-guggulsterone
H	CH_3	Z-guggulsterone

R	Compound
–OH	11-keto-β-boswellic acid
–OAC	3-acetyl 11-keto-β-boswellic acid

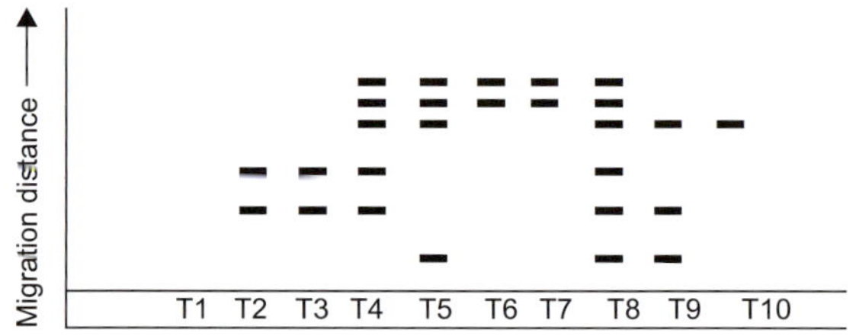

Photo documentation of plate at 254 nm. T1, blank; T2, 11-KBA and A-11-KBA standards; T3, shallaki extract; T4 and T8, formulation; T5, shallaki placebo; T6, EG and ZG standards; T7, guggul extract; T9, guggul placebo; T10, plain placebo

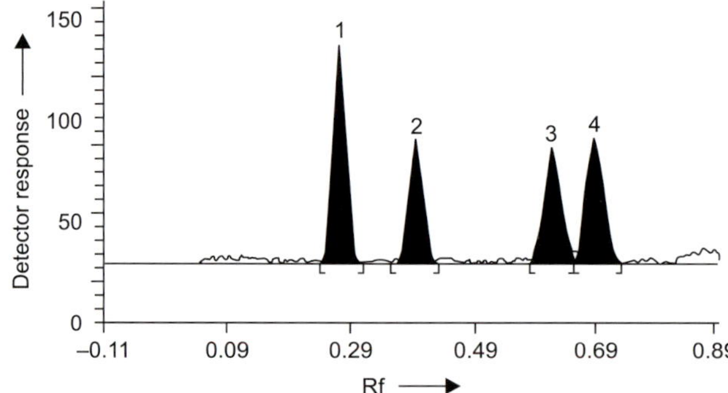

Typical densitograms of the standard containing EG, ZG, 11-KBA, 3-A-11-KBA. For detailed experimental and chromatographic conditions, refer to Protocol No. 522. Peaks identification: 1. 11-KBA; 2. 3-A-11-KBA; 3. EG; 4. ZG.

PROTOCOL FOR HPTLC ANALYSIS OF PHARMACEUTICAL FORMULATION

Protocol No. 522

Formulation: E-Guggulsterone, Z-Guggulsterone, 11-Keto-β-Boswellic acid, 3-Acetyl-11-Keto-β-Boswellic acid

Classification: Miscellaneous **Dosage form:** Capsules

Standard preparation: Prepare solution of each compound separately in methanol to get 100 μg/ml of EG and ZG and 250 μg/ml of 11-KBA and 3-A-11-KBA. Further dilutions made to get 10 μg/ml of EG and ZG and 50 μg/ml of 11-KBA and 3-A-11-KBA. Apply varying volumes of each solution for linearity profile.

Sample preparation: Accurately weighed amount equivalent to one capsule suspended in 70 ml of methanol, sonicated for 30 min, diluted to 100 ml with methanol, filtered through Whatman No. 41 filter paper and the resultant solution used for chromatographic analysis.

Chromatographic equipments:

Sample applicator: Camag Linomat–V

Plate-coater: Camag twin-trough glass chamber, 20 × 10 cm

Densitometric scanner: Camag TLC Scanner–III

Chromatographic conditions:

1. Stationary phase: Silica gel 60F_{254} pre-coated HPTLC plates, 20 × 10 cm (200 μm) – Merck, pre-washed with methanol, dried prior to use.
2. Mobile phase (MP): n-hexane–chloroform–ethyl acetate–methanol (10 : 3 : 3 : 1 v/v)
3. Standard/Sample application:
   Band length: 6 mm Volume applied: 1–10 μl Spacing: 6 mm
4. Chamber saturation: 15 min (MP)
5. RH (%): 60 ± 5
6. Temperature °C: 25 ± 2
7. Separation technique: Ascending
8. Quantity of mobile phase: 17 ml
8. Migration distance: 80 mm
9. Migration time: 20 min

Densitometric evaluation:

Wavelength: UV–254 nm Scanning mode: Reflectance/Absorbance

HRF: 11-KBA—28; 3-A-11-KBA—39; EG—61; ZG—68

Linearity (ng/band): 11-KBA and 3-A-11-KBA—50–450; EG and ZG—10–90

Recovery (%): EG—96.73–97.22; ZG—97.45–97.53; 11-KBA—97.06–98.05; 3-A-11-KBA—97.01–97.64.

References: Nitin N. Shelke, Vinod Kumar V. Kuber, Shrinivas G. Bhope and Ramachandra B. Jadhav, *J. Planar Chromatogr.*, **24(3)**, 242–247, 2011.

Comments: The method validated for accuracy, precision, linearity, LOD, LOQ, specificity, robustness and ruggedness.

HPTLC : High Performance Thin Layer Chromatography
HPTLC Densitogram

No. 523

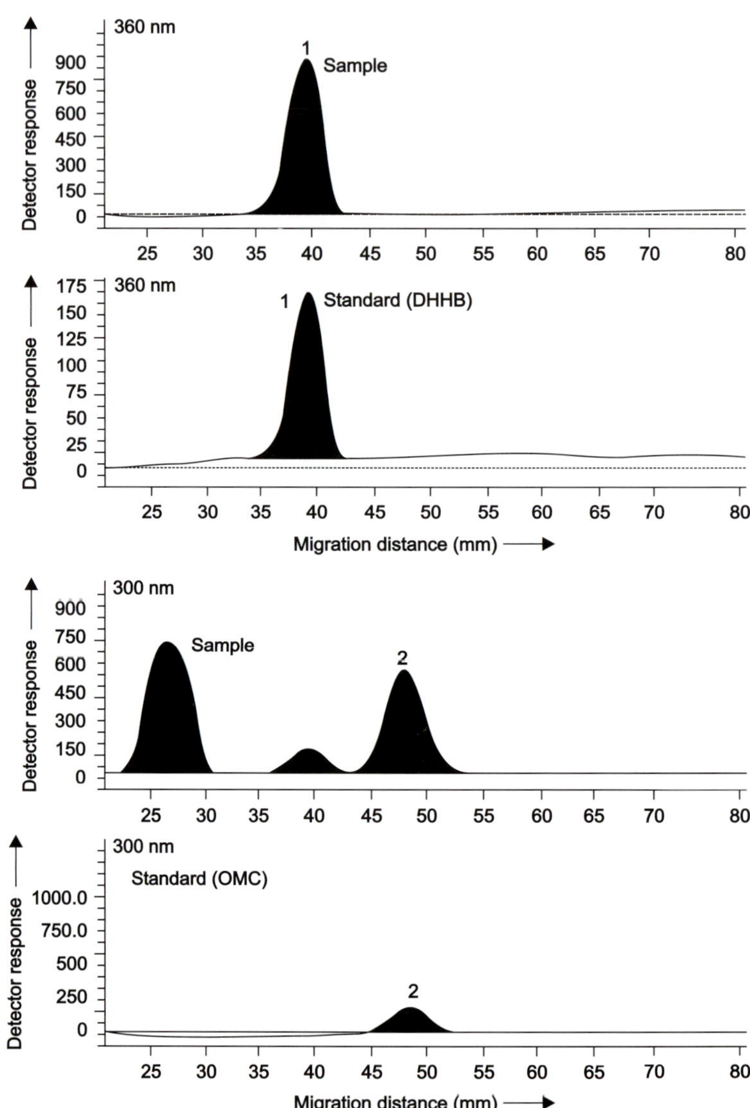

Typical densitograms of the sample and the standard containing OMC and DHHB. For detailed experimental and chromatographic conditions, refer to Protocol No. 523. Peaks identification: 1. DHHB; 2. OMC.

PROTOCOL FOR HPTLC ANALYSIS OF PHARMACEUTICAL FORMULATION

Protocol No. 523

Formulation: Diethylamine hydroxybenzoyl hexylbenzoate (DHHB), Octyl methoxycinnamate (OMC)

Classification: Miscellaneous **Dosage form:** Lotion

Standard preparation: Prepare 5 mg/ml solution of each compound separately in methanol. Further dilutions made to get 200 μg/ml. Apply 1–10 μl for chromatographic separation and linearity profile.

Sample preparation: 1000 mg of the suncare lotion suspended in 70 ml of methanol, shaken for 60 min, diluted to 100 ml. Apply 4 μl for assay of DHHB and 1 μl for assay of OMC and carry out the chromatographic separation and analysis.

Chromatographic equipments:

Sample applicator: Hamilton 10 μl TLC microsyringe

Plate-coater: Flat bottom glass vertical chamber

Densitometric scanner: Desaga CD 60 densitometer

Chromatographic conditions:

1. Stationary phase: Silica gel $60F_{254}$ pre-coated TLC plates, 20 × 10 cm (250 μm) – Merck
2. Mobile phase (MP): Cyclohexane–diethylether–acetone (15 : 1 : 2 v/v)
3. Standard/Sample application:
   Band length: 5 mm Volume applied: 1–10 μl Spacing: 10 mm
4. Chamber saturation: 20 min (MP)
5. RH (%): 55 ± 5
6. Temperature °C: 20 ± 1
7. Separation technique: Ascending
8. Quantity of mobile phase: 18 ml
8. Migration distance: 80 mm
9. Migration time: 20 min

Densitometric evaluation:

Wavelength: OMC (300 nm); DHHB (360 mm)

Scanning mode: Reflectance/Absorbance

HRF: See densitogram

Linearity: 200–2000 ng/band for both the compounds

Recovery (%): DHHB—97.8–101.9; OMC—99.1–102.7

References: Anna W. Sobanako and Elzbieta Bizezinska, *J. Planar Chromatogr.*, **24(3)**, 227, 231, 2011.

Comments: The method validated for accuracy, precision, linearity, LOD and LOQ.

HPTLC : High Performance Thin Layer Chromatography
HPTLC Densitogram

No. 524

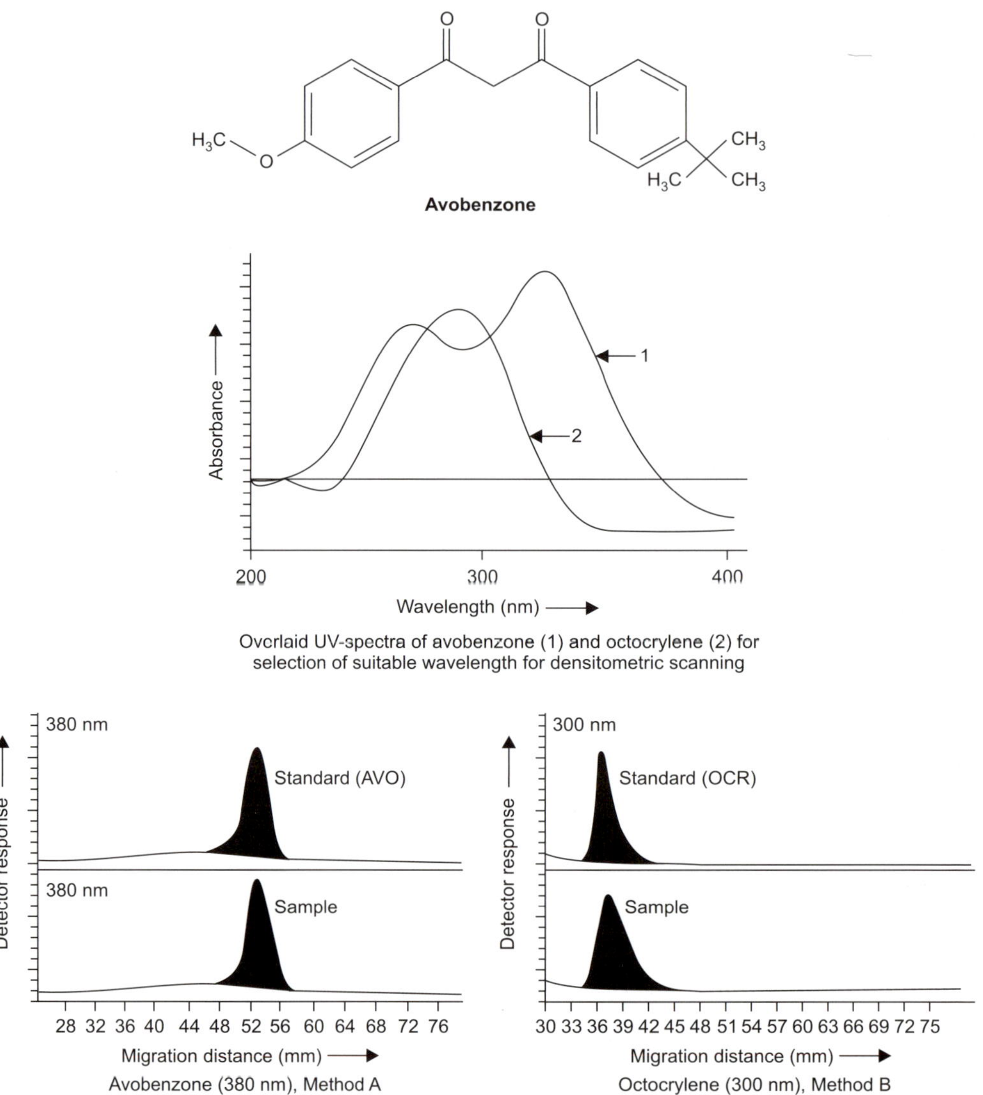

Overlaid UV-spectra of avobenzone (1) and octocrylene (2) for selection of suitable wavelength for densitometric scanning

Avobenzone (380 nm), Method A

Octocrylene (300 nm), Method B

Typical densitograms of the sample and the standard containing avobenzone and octocrylene. For detailed experimental and chromatographic conditions, refer to Protocol No. 524. Peaks identification: See densitograms above.

PROTOCOL FOR HPTLC ANALYSIS OF PHARMACEUTICAL FORMULATION

Protocol No. 524

Formulation: Avobenzone, Octocrylene

Classification: Miscellaneous **Dosage form:** Lotion

Standard preparation: Prepare 5 mg/ml solution of each compound separately in methanol. Further dilutions made with methanol to get 200 μg/ml. Apply varying volumes (1–10 μl) for linearity profile.

Sample preparation: 1000 mg of the suncare lotion suspended in 70 ml of methanol, shaken for 60 min, diluted to 100 ml. Apply 4 μl for assay of avobenzone and 1 μl for assay of octocrylene and carry out the chromatographic separation and analysis.

Chromatographic equipments:

Sample applicator: 10 μl TLC microsyringe

Plate-coater: Vertical flat bottom chromatographic chamber, lined with filter paper

Densitometric scanner: Desaga CD for densitometer

Chromatographic conditions:

1. Stationary phase: Silica gel $60F_{254}$ pre-coated TLC plates, 10 × 10 cm (250 μm) – Merck
2. Mobile phase (MP): (A) Cyclohexane–diethylether (1 : 1 v/v) (avobenzone); (B) Cyclohexane–piperidine (15 : 1 v/v) (octocrylene)
3. Standard/Sample application:
   Band length: 5 mm Volume applied: 1–10 μl Spacing: 10 mm
4. Chamber saturation: 20 min (MP)
5. RH (%): 55 ± 5
6. Temperature °C: 20 ± 1
7. Separation technique: Ascending
8. Quantity of mobile phase: 16 ml
8. Migration distance: 80 mm
9. Migration time: 20 min

Densitometric evaluation:

Wavelength: Avobenzone (380 nm); Octocrylene (300 nm)

Scanning mode: Reflectance/Absorbance

HRF: See densitograms

Linearity: 200–1800 ng/band for both the compounds

Recovery (%): 98.80–102.7 for both the compounds

References: Anna W. Sobanake and Elzbieta Bizezinska, *J. Planar Chromatogr.*, **24(2)**, 154–159, 2011.

Comments: The method validated for accuracy, precision, linearity, LOD and LOQ.

HPTLC : High Performance Thin Layer Chromatography
HPTLC Densitogram

No. 525

Vitamin B_2

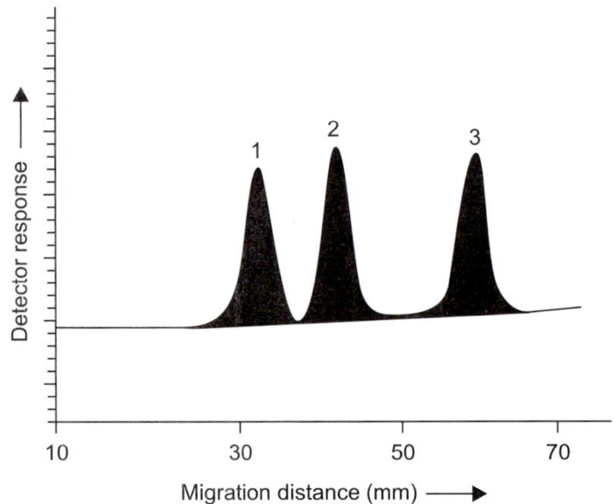

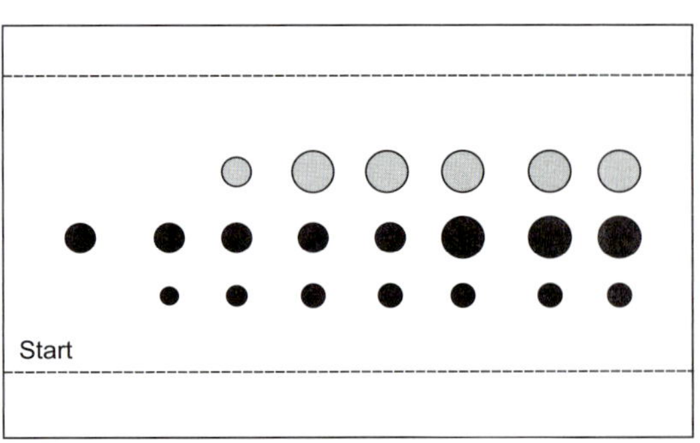

TLC profile of vitamins B_1, B_6 and B_{12} applying 5–40 µg/band

Typical densitogram of the standard containing vitamins B_1, B_6 and B_{12}. For detailed experimental and chromatographic conditions, refer to Protocol No. 525. Peaks identification: 1. Vitamin B_{12}; 2. Vitamin B_1; 3. Vitamin B_6.

PROTOCOL FOR HPTLC ANALYSIS OF PHARMACEUTICAL FORMULATION

Protocol No. 525

Formulation: Vitamins B_1, B_2, B_{12}
Classification: Miscellaneous **Dosage form:** Tablets/Injection
Standard preparation: Prepare solution of each vitamin in solvent separately to get 5–40 mg/ml. Apply 1 μl of each solution for linearity profile.
Solvent: Water–methanol (1 : 1 v/v).
Sample preparation: Powdered sample treated with solvent, sonicated, filtered and final solution contained 32 mg/ml (B_1), 32 mg/ml (B_6) and 0.32 mg/ml (B_{12}). Apply 1 μl of the solution for analysis. Injectable liquid can be used as such.
Chromatographic equipments:
Sample applicator: Hamilton syringe
Plate-coater: Camag hand-operated TLC plate coater
Development chamber: Camag flat bottom glass chamber, 20 × 20 cm
UV cabinet: Camag UV–cabinet
Densitometer scanner: Desaga CD 60 Scanner
Chromatographic conditions:

1. Stationary phase: Powdered bentonite (< 45 μm), washed with conc. HCl, dried at 120°C for 3 hrs. 8.8 g of treated bentonite mixed with fluorescent indicator, 0.5 g corn starch, suspended in 20 ml of water and slurry spread over glass plate with manual applicator to get 0.30 mm thick layer, dried at 105°C and used as stationary phase.
2. Mobile phase (MP): Isobutyl alcohol–methanol–chloroform–acetic acid–25% ammonia (7.5 : 1 : 3.5 : 0.4 : 0.5 v/v)
3. Standard/Sample application:
   Band length: 3 mm Volume applied: 2 μl Spacing: 5 mm
4. Chamber saturation: 20 min (MP)
5. RH (%): 55 ± 5 6. Temperature °C: 25 ± 1
7. Separation technique: Ascending
8. Quantity of mobile phase: 20 ml
8. Migration distance: 75 mm
9. Migration time: 20 min

Densitometric evaluation:
Wavelength: UV–275 nm Scanning mode: Reflectance/Absorbance
HRF: See densitogram
Linearity: 5–40 μg/band for all the three vitamins
Recovery (%): 95.6–101.4 for all the three vitamins
References: Abdul-Aziz Ramadan, Amer Bodakji and Ibrahem Mohamad, *Asian J. Chem.*, **22(4)**, 3283–3291, 2010.
Comments: The method validated for accuracy, precision, linearity, LOD, LOQ, specificity, robustness and ruggedness.

HPTLC : High Performance Thin Layer Chromatography
HPTLC Densitogram

No. 526

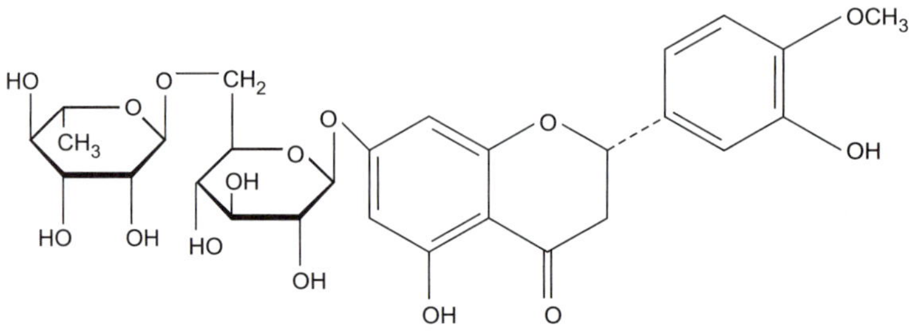

Hesperidin

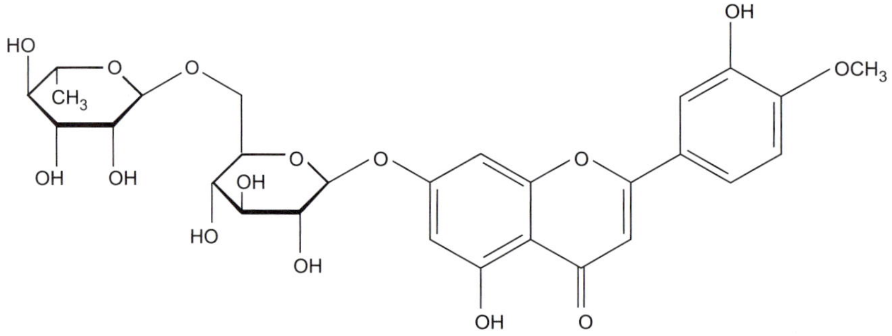

Diosmin

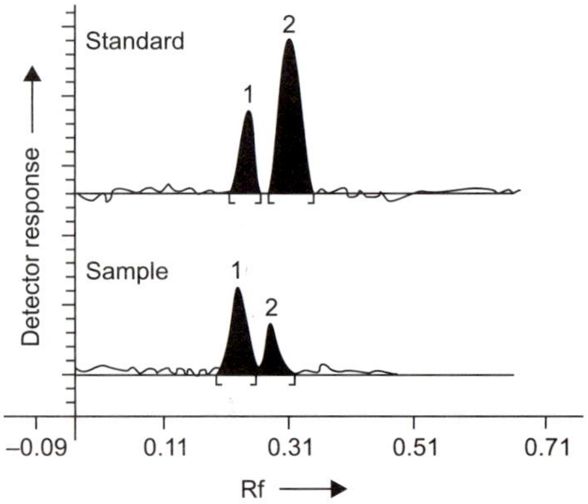

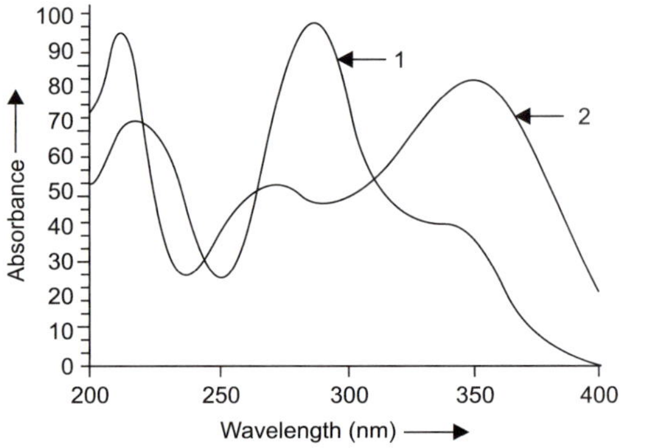

Overlaid UV-spectra of hesperidin (1) and diosmin (2) for selection of suitable wavelength for densitometric scanning

Typical densitogram of the standard and the sample containing hesperidin and diosmin. For detailed experimental and chromatographic conditions, refer to Protocol No. 526. Peaks identification: 1. Diosmin; 2. Hesperidin.

PROTOCOL FOR HPTLC ANALYSIS OF PHARMACEUTICAL FORMULATION

Protocol No. 526

Formulation: Hesperidin, Diosmin

Classification: Miscellaneous **Dosage form:** Tablets

Standard preparation: Prepare solution of both the compounds in solvent to get 200 μg/ml of diosmin and 500 μg/ml of hesperidin. Apply varying volumes (1–6 μl) of each solution for linearity profile.

Sample preparation: Powdered sample equivalent to 50 mg of hesperidin suspended in 90 ml of solvent, sonicated at 38°C for 30 min, diluted to 100 ml with solvent and filtered. Apply 4 μl for chromatographic separation, evaluation and assay.

Solvent: Methanol–DMSO (1 : 1 v/v)

Chromatographic equipments:

Sample applicator: Camag Linomat–IV

Development chamber: Camag twin-trough glass chamber, 20 × 20 cm

Densitometric scanner: Camag TLC Scanner–III

Chromatographic conditions:

1. Stationary phase: Silica gel $60F_{254}$ pre-coated TLC plates, 20 × 10 cm (250 μm) – Merck, pre-washed with methanol, dried at 60°C for 5 min prior to use
2. Mobile phase (MP): Ethyl acetate–methanol–water–acetic acid (25 : 2 : 2 : 1 v/v)
3. Standard/Sample application:
   Band length: 6 mm Volume applied: 1–6 μl Spacing: 4 mm
4. Chamber saturation: 30 min (MP)
5. RH (%): —
6. Temperature °C: Ambient
7. Separation technique: Ascending
8. Quantity of mobile phase: 30 ml
8. Migration distance: 70 mm
9. Migration time: 11 min

Densitometric evaluation:

Wavelength: UV–330 nm Scanning mode: Reflectance/Absorbance

HRF: Diosmin—23; Hesperidin—28

Linearity (ng/band): Hesperidin—25–750; Diosmin—100–3000

Recovery (%): Hesperidin—99.68–100.79; Diosmin—96.64–103.21

References: Eman Shawky, *J. Planar Chromatogr.*, **25(2)**, 138–144, 2012.

Comments: The method validated for accuracy, precision, linearity, LOD, LOQ and specificity.

HPTLC : High Performance Thin Layer Chromatography
HPTLC Densitogram

No. 527

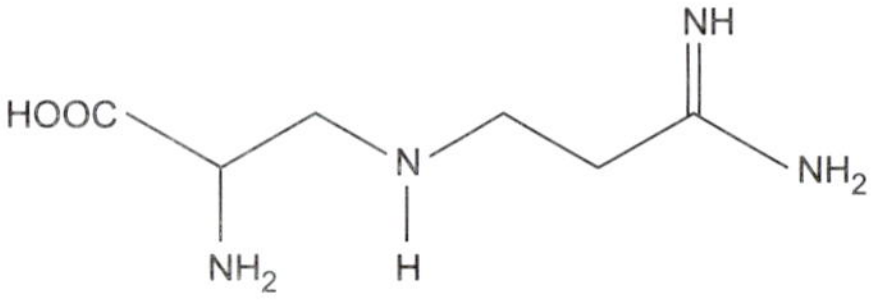

HOOC NH NH$_2$ N H NH$_2$

L. Arginine

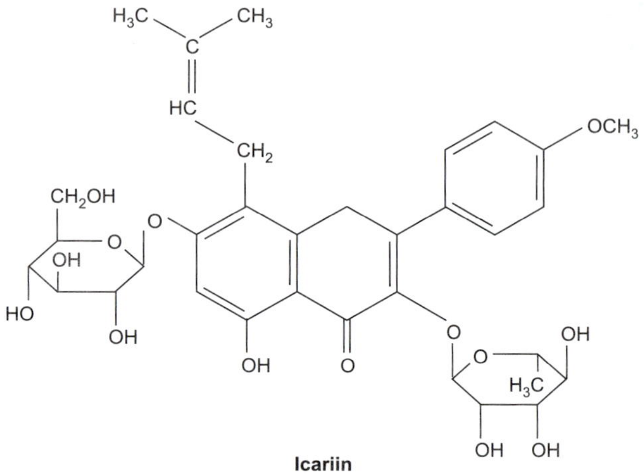

Icariin

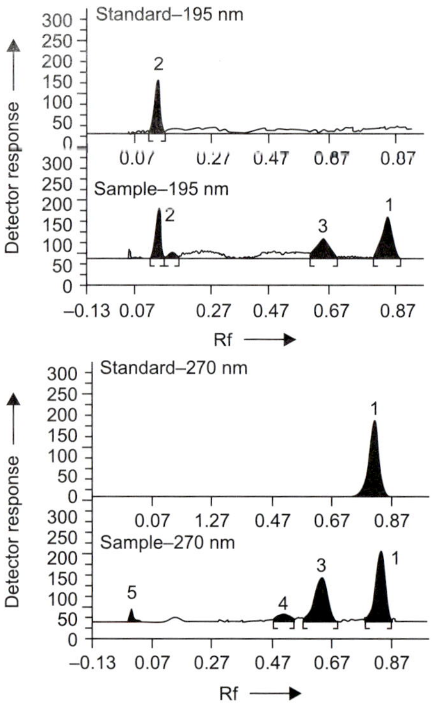

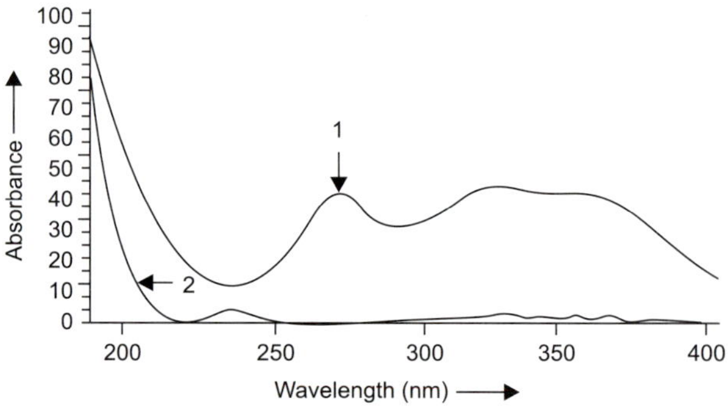

Overlaid UV-spectra of icariin (1) and L. Arginine (2) for selection of suitable wavelength for densitometric scanning

Typical densitogram of the standard and the sample containing L. Arginine and Icariin. For detailed experimental and chromatographic conditions, refer to Protocol No. 527. Peaks identification: 1. Icariin; 2. L. Arginine; 3, 4, 5. Unknown.

PROTOCOL FOR HPTLC ANALYSIS OF PHARMACEUTICAL FORMULATION

Protocol No. 527

Formulation: Icariin, L. Arginine

Classification: Miscellaneous **Dosage form:** Tablets

Standard preparation: Prepare solution of both the compounds in methanol to get 500 µg/ml (Icariin) and 1000 µg/ml (L. Arginine). Further dilute 5 ml of each solution to 25 ml with methanol and carry out linearity studies by applying varying volumes of each solution.

Sample preparation: Powdered sample equivalent to 20 mg of L. Arginine suspended in 15 ml of methanol, sonicated for 30 min, diluted to 20 ml with methanol, filtered and 2 ml of the filtrate diluted to 10 ml with methanol. Apply 5 µl of the resulting solution for chromatographic evaluation.

Chromatographic equipments:

Sample applicator: Camag Linomat–V

Development chamber: Camag twin-trough glass chamber, 20 × 10 cm

Densitometric scanner: Camag TLC Scanner–III

Chromatographic conditions:

1. Stationary phase: Silica gel $60F_{254}$ pre-coated HPTLC plates, 20 × 10 cm (200 µm) – Merck, pre-washed with methanol and dried at 60°C for 10 min, prior to use
2. Mobile phase (MP): Ethylacetate–acetone–glacial acetic acid–formic acid–water (12 : 2: 1 : 2 : 2 v/v)
3. Standard/Sample application:
   Band length: 6 mm Volume applied: 2.5–7.5 µl Spacing: 10 mm
4. Chamber saturation: 15 min (MP)
5. RH (%): 40 ± 5
6. Temperature °C: 25 ± 1
7. Separation technique: Ascending
8. Quantity of mobile phase: 19 ml
8. Migration distance: 80 mm
9. Migration time: —

Densitometric evaluation:

Wavelength: UV–195–nm (L. Arginine); UV–270 (Icariin)

Scanning mode: Reflectance/Absorbance

HRF: L. Arginine—11; Icariin—82

Linearity (ng/band): Icariin—250–750; L. Arginine—500–1500

Recovery (%): Icariin—98.26–98.77; L. Arginine—99.63–100.80

References: P.K. Gupta, V.V. Kuber, V.K. Ghosh, S.G. Bhope, V. Sharma and S. Purothi. *Acta Chromatographica*, **23(3)**, 447–458, 2011.

Comments: The method validated for accuracy, precision, linearity, LOD, LOQ, specificity and robustness.

HPTLC : High Performance Thin Layer Chromatography
HPTLC Densitogram

No. 528

Vitamin B_2

Vitamin B_{12}

Borate + **Diol** ⇌ **Complex (cyclic ester)**

Formation of cyclic ester from reaction of Vit. B_2 (1,2-diols) with borate.

PROTOCOL FOR HPTLC ANALYSIS OF PHARMACEUTICAL FORMULATION

Protocol No. 528

Formulation: Vitamins B_2, B_{12}

Classification: Miscellaneous **Dosage form:** Analyte mixture

Standard preparation: Prepare 100 μg/ml solution of each substance in methanol–water (1 : 3 v/v) and use for analysis. Store the solution in subdued light.

Sample preparation: —

Chromatographic equipments:

Sample applicator: Camag Linomat–IV

Development chamber: Camag twin-trough glass chamber, 10 × 10 cm

Densitometric scanner: Camag TLC Scanner–II

Chromatographic conditions:

1. Stationary phase: Silica gel $60F_{254}$ pre-coated TLC plates, 10 × 10 cm (Merck). The plate was washed with methanol–chloroform (1 : 1) to remove elutable components and then impregnating with 2% ethanolic boric acid, activated at 110°C for 1 h before use
2. Mobile phase (MP): Methanol–water–25% ammonia (7 : 3 : 1 v/v)
3. Standard/Sample application:
   Band length: 2 mm Volume applied: 5 μl Spacing: 5 mm
4. Chamber saturation: —
5. RH (%): 55 ± 5
6. Temperature °C: Ambient
7. Separation technique: Ascending
8. Quantity of mobile phase: 11 ml
8. Migration distance: 80 mm
9. Migration time: 15 min

Densitometric evaluation:

Wavelength: UV–254 nm

Scanning mode: Reflectance/Absorbance

HRF: B_2—71; B_{12}—97

Linearity: —

Recovery (%): —

References: Homayon Ahmad Panahi, Hossein Sid Kalal and Atyeh Rahini, *World Academy of Science, Engineering and Technology*, **42**, 193–195, 2008.

Comments:

- Boric acid forms complex with B_2 having diol group, thus leading to retardation in the movement of the vitamin; thus decrease in Rf value.
- The authors had tried several other solvent systems both on impregnated and non-impregnated plates, but described MP was most suitable.

Index

A

B

C

K

L

M

N

O

P

Q

R

S

T

V

Z